# Psychology Today

## HERE TO HELP

# taming
# BIPOLAR
# DISORDER

# Psychology Today

## HERE TO HELP

# taming
# BIPOLAR
# DISORDER

Lori Oliwenstein

ALPHA

A member of Penguin Group (USA) Inc.

ALPHA BOOKS

Published by the Penguin Group

Penguin Group (USA) Inc., 375 Hudson Street, New York, New York 10014, U.S.A.

Penguin Group (Canada), 10 Alcorn Avenue, Toronto, Ontario, Canada M4V 3B2 (a division of Pearson Penguin Canada Inc.)

Penguin Books Ltd, 80 Strand, London WC2R 0RL, England

Penguin Ireland, 25 St Stephen's Green, Dublin 2, Ireland (a division of Penguin Books Ltd)

Penguin Group (Australia), 250 Camberwell Road, Camberwell, Victoria 3124, Australia (a division of Pearson Australia Group Pty Ltd)

Penguin Books India Pvt Ltd, 11 Community Centre, Panchsheel Park, New Delhi—110 017, India

Penguin Group (NZ), Cnr Airborne and Rosedale Roads, Albany, Auckland, New Zealand (a division of Pearson New Zealand Ltd)

Penguin Books (South Africa) (Pty) Ltd, 24 Sturdee Avenue, Rosebank, Johannesburg 2196, South Africa

Penguin Books Ltd, Registered Offices: 80 Strand, London WC2R 0RL, England

International Standard Book Number: 1-59257-285-5
Library of Congress Catalog Card Number: 2004111435

06   05   04        8   7   6   5   4   3   2   1

Interpretation of the printing code: The rightmost number of the first series of numbers is the year of the book's printing; the rightmost number of the second series of numbers is the number of the book's printing. For example, a printing code of 04-1 shows that the first printing occurred in 2004.

*Printed in the United States of America*

**Note:** This publication contains the opinions and ideas of its author. It is intended to provide helpful and informative material on the subject matter covered. It is sold with the understanding that the author and publisher are not engaged in rendering professional services in the book. If the reader requires personal assistance or advice, a competent professional should be consulted.

The author and publisher specifically disclaim any responsibility for any liability, loss, or risk, personal or otherwise, which is incurred as a consequence, directly or indirectly, of the use and application of any of the contents of this book.

**Trademarks:** All terms mentioned in this book that are known to be or are suspected of being trademarks or service marks have been appropriately capitalized. Alpha Books and Penguin Group (USA) Inc. cannot attest to the accuracy of this information. Use of a term in this book should not be regarded as affecting the validity of any trademark or service mark.

*Psychology Today* is a registered trademark of Sussex Publishers, Inc., 115 East 23rd Street, 9th Floor, New York, NY 10010

Most Alpha books are available at special quantity discounts for bulk purchases for sales promotions, premiums, fund-raising, or educational use. Special books, or book excerpts, can also be created to fit specific needs.

For details, write: Special Markets, Alpha Books, 375 Hudson Street, New York, NY 10014.

**Publisher:** Marie Butler-Knight

**Product Manager:** Phil Kitchel

**Senior Managing Editor:** Jennifer Chisholm

**Acquisitions Editors:** Mikal E. Belicove and Paul Dinas

**Development Editor:** Christy Wagner

**Senior Production Editor:** Billy Fields

**Technical Editor:** Editors of *Psychology Today* magazine

**Copy Editor:** Jan Zoya

**Cover Designer:** Ann Marie Deets

**Book Designer:** Trina Wurst

**Creative Director:** Robin Lasek

**Indexer:** Angie Bess

**Layout:** Angela Calvert

*To my father, Jack Oliwenstein,*
*who escaped Nazi Germany only to face*
*his own emotional Holocaust.*

# Contents

# Foreword

It's hard to imagine a more puzzling condition than bipolar disorder. Not only do extremes of mood wax and wane on their own schedule, they create havoc in the lives—and minds—of those who have the disorder, not to mention the people around them. What is more, the manic phase of the disorder, at least in its early stages, can actually make people feel deceptively good with the energy and overconfidence it creates.

*Taming Bipolar Disorder* is designed to bring order out of the chaos of living with a condition that seems to be becoming more common, especially among the young. Although no one is sure what goes awry in bipolar disorder, it's now very clear that there is a great deal those who have it, and those who live with them, can do to curb its mysterious force and harness its creative energy.

However, there is so much information about what can be done to minimize the chance of manic or depressive episodes; to keep moods from spiraling out of control; to keep people from the self-destructive spending sprees, gambling sprees, talking jags, and personality clashes that leave so much wreckage in their wake. Never before have those with bipolar disorder had such a clear opportunity not just to normalize their lives but to actually thrive with this condition.

This book will do for you and your family what medications cannot. Necessary as they are, medications alone will not sustain a balanced quality of life. Only behavioral management can truly help achieve that goal. Author Lori Oliwenstein draws upon a broad array of expertise and personal experiences to help people understand the disorder, how to get good treatment, just what good treatment consists of, and how to both manage the condition day to day and plan for the long haul.

Lori Oliwenstein is uniquely qualified to describe the challenges of living with bipolar disorder. She is an experienced science writer who knows the condition from the inside out. Her father has it—and you will meet him in these pages. Of course she explains the cutting-edge research that has paved the way for this book, and she also describes the impact bipolar disorder can have on close relationships.

*Taming Bipolar Disorder* is the most comprehensive guide available on bipolar disorder. It discusses the challenge of diagnosis and the intricacies of treatment, including nutritional support. It offers coping skills and advice on work and relationships that can be both the cause and effect of episodes. This is the book that will get you, and those you love, all the way to the finish line.

Kaja Perina
Editor in chief
*Psychology Today*

# Introduction

When my father was diagnosed with bipolar disorder, it was actually a relief. Finally, a diagnosis that made sense. Finally, a foe we could name; one we could wrap our hands and minds around and do battle with.

He didn't feel that way right away, of course. He was scared and more than a little bit skeptical. Over the past few years, he's had to fight his own denial, resentment, and ingrained prejudice—that oft-spoken feeling that people who are mentally ill "just need to get over it"—in much the way he had to fight mania, anxiety, and debilitating depressions throughout most of his life.

How you're going to feel when someone speaks the words to you—or how you felt the first time they did—might be entirely different. But you and my father and the millions of others living with bipolar disorder have at least one thing in common: a drive to thrive. You're not going to take this lying down. You're going to fight this thing. And you're going to win.

Yes, it's hard having bipolar disorder. Yes, you're going to have to live with it for the rest of your life. Yes, it's going to affect the way you live that life. But yes, you can survive with your disorder. And yes, you can thrive with your disorder. It can even enrich your life and your experiences, if you're willing to accept it and work with it, rather than against it.

Know you are not alone. Scientists and clinicians are dedicating their lives to making yours more stable. The base of knowledge of bipolar disorder is growing daily. Some of these findings will have an immediate effect on how you grapple with this disorder on a day-to-day basis. Others simply add to the foundation of knowledge on which those larger findings are built. In *Taming Bipolar Disorder*, you'll hear about these people and what they're finding.

Then there are the people who love you and want to help you, people who might need some education or time to heal, to understand, but who will fight alongside you and grow with you. In *Taming Bipolar Disorder,* you'll learn how to help them along.

And then there are the people who know just what you're going through because they've been there themselves. In *Taming Bipolar Disorder,* you'll hear their stories. Maybe you'll even find one that's like your own. I hope you'll find ideas, inspiration, and hope.

**What You'll Find Inside** *Taming Bipolar Disorder* is organized into four parts:

In **Part 1, "Bipolar Basics,"** you'll find a primer on bipolar disorder: what its symptoms are (and what they feel like), the different types of bipolar disorder, what makes it different from other forms of mental illness, what's happening in your brain and in your DNA to get you here in the first place, and what you can expect from this disorder over time.

In **Part 2, "Gaining Control,"** you'll navigate the health-care system, peek inside the bipolar medicine chest, learn how to keep pace with your circadian and social rhythms, explore your other treatment options, and consider how best to put the brakes on bipolar disorder.

In **Part 3, "Taking Back Your Life,"** you'll learn how to resist the lure of danger, how to take responsibility and make amends, how to both get and give support in journeying from bipolar's poles back to life's more stable center, and what you can and can't expect in the workplace.

In the last part of the book, **Part 4, "Thriving With Bipolar Disorder,"** you'll consider the ways in which bipolar disorder affects your life at home as well as learn how you can approach its social challenges and come out a winner. You'll also look at bipolar disorder from some other points of view—from the point of view of a young child and from the points of view of the friends and family members whose own lives have been forever changed by your disorder.

**How to Use This Book**   In *Taming Bipolar Disorder,* you're going to hear from the experts themselves—both the scientific experts and the experts who've lived with and through this disorder—about what you can do to avoid the worst bipolar has to offer and how you can exploit the best of it.

This book is meant to help you on your journey to take back your life and make it even better. I talk to "you," the person living with bipolar disorder, throughout the book, but the information here is meant for anyone who wants to know more about the ways in which this underappreciated and misunderstood mental illness works, as well as the ways in which it can be tamed.

Read it cover to cover if you want, or dip into a relevant chapter for a quick coping tip. In addition to the main text, you'll notice a number of different sidebars, each meant to enrich your experience with the text: to expand on a point or consider one in more detail, to provide inspiration or explanation, or to let you know that you're not the only one dealing with what might feel like a very solitary burden.

As you read, dip, and flip through this book, you'll find these sidebars:

Q&A sidebars feature questions from people just like you and answers from the experts in that part of the field.

Web Talk sidebars encourage you to expand your explorations beyond this book by pointing out places on the web where you can go to get more information.

## GET PSYCHED

Get Psyched sidebars are filled with inspirational quotes and bits of advice from experts and people who have something to say that you should hear.

## PsychSpeak

PsychSpeak sidebars define, in plain English, a few of the more difficult or unfamiliar terms in the text. (For a more complete list of definitions, see the glossary in the back of the book.)

**you're not alone**

You're Not Alone sidebars tell the stories of people just like you; people who are working to find their way in a bipolar world and who might help you do the same.

In addition, at the end of each chapter, you'll find a section called "What You Can Do" that features a checklist summarizing some of the major points of the chapter and putting them into concrete form. These are meant to be some of your take-away points from the chapter; things you can do to have a better shot at stability and at thriving not just despite, but *with* your disorder.

**Welcome to *Taming Bipolar Disorder*** If there's one thing you'll hear again and again throughout this book, it's how important—even critical—educating yourself can be in your struggle to find your footing and regain your balance. You can't make good decisions about a disorder that you don't understand. As my father discovered, you can't really battle a foe you don't know.

But with information comes understanding. And with understanding comes the power to change, to get better, to reach your goals, and to fulfill your potential. This book is a first step. You can take it; you can do it. And we are here to help.

**Acknowledgments**  I talk a lot in this book about the importance of support. That's no less true for me than it is for anyone else. This book was made possible by the scientists and clinicians who work tirelessly and selflessly to understand, treat, and prevent bipolar disorder.

S. Nassir Ghaemi, M.D., director of the Bipolar Disorder Research Program at Cambridge Health Alliance and assistant professor of psychiatry at Harvard Medical School, was unfailingly generous and cheerful as he helped me better define the bipolar landscape and hone in on the most important and most relevant issues. His contributions truly made this book possible.

Terence Ketter, M.D., chief of the Bipolar Disorders Clinic at Stanford University Medical School, was equally generous with his time and wisdom as he helped me understand bipolar disorder's biological and psychological intricacies.

John Kelsoe, M.D., psychiatrist and medical director of the Mental Health Clinical Research Center at the VA Medical Center in San Diego, taught me everything I now know about the genetics of bipolar disorder and about the bipolar spectrum.

Ellen Frank, Ph.D., director of the Depression and Manic Depression Prevention Program at the Western Psychiatric Institute and Clinic, was invaluable in helping me see the issues involved in treating bipolar disorder with psychotherapy and was remarkably balanced in her assessment of treatment options—including the one she herself has developed.

There is no one better to explain the issues of bipolar disorder in childhood than Barbara Geller, M.D., professor of psychiatry,

Washington University School of Medicine in St. Louis, who literally wrote the book on the subject.

In addition, Hilary Blumberg, M.D., a psychiatrist from the Yale University School of Medicine, gave me firsthand insight into the bipolar brain.

And Cameron Quanbeck, M.D., from the University of California, Davis, helped me get a handle on bipolar disorder and the legal system.

I also got invaluable support from the folks at the Depression and Bipolar Support Alliance (DBSA). In particular, Lisa Goodale talked to me at great length about peer support and peer services. And Christy Hummel, from DBSA's external relations office, went above and beyond to help me find people who were willing to talk about their experiences with this disorder.

Similarly, thanks go to Jonathan Stanley from the Treatment Advocacy Center. Jon shared not only his expertise in the mental health field but also his own story of battling bipolar disorder.

Lynn Albizo deserves a similar note of gratitude, for sharing not only her experience as a mental health advocate and lawyer, but her personal experiences as well.

A hug and kiss go to my agent, Leslie Daniels, of the Joy Harris Literary Agency, who always, always watches my back.

Pure admiration belongs to the people of Alpha Books, especially Mikal Belicove and Christy Wagner, who kept me motivated and moving forward using humor and true empathy.

Hara Estroff Marano at *Psychology Today* was an incredible resource and collaborator. Thanks also to *Psychology Today*'s wonderful Lybi Ma, who made my participation in this project possible.

A huge debt of gratitude to Brenda Maceo and the gang at the University of Southern California's Health Sciences Public Relations Office, for giving me the time to take this on.

I wouldn't have made it through without the advice, free baby-sitting, and dinners provided by Ambre Ying, Debra Ritter, and Susanna Griffith, or without the indomitable Auggie Moms and their unflagging cybersupport.

My family has been amazing throughout. Thanks to my sister, Jill Vogelsberg, who lived the same story I tell in these pages; to my mother, Linda Hershfield, whose own life was affected by my father's bipolar disorder; and to my stepfather, Harry Hershfield, who has always been there.

Bruce and Jeffrey Kluger are my tireless champions and half the reason I was able to write this book. Steve Kluger is simply the greatest uncle and brother-in-law the world has known. I'm thrilled to call them all my family.

Heaps and heaps of love go to my amazing children, Emily and Noah Kluger, for whom the writing months must have seemed like a lifetime, and to my even more amazing husband, Garry Kluger, who did double-duty throughout yet still found the energy to be supportive and encouraging.

There aren't words to say how impressed I am with the people who thrive with this difficult disorder. To Alexis, Andy, Bobbi Jo, Christine, Jacqueline, Jon, Kay, Lynn, Mara, Natalie, Rachael, Shay, Stephanie, and especially to my father, whose struggles and triumphs I've witnessed firsthand: thank you for allowing me into your lives.

# Part 1

# Bipolar Basics

Before you got your diagnosis, you might not have even known what bipolar disorder was. Maybe you'd heard of manic-depression, but that's about all. Now you know what it is—and you're scared. Terrified, actually. Don't be. Knowledge is power, and in Part 1, you'll learn the bipolar basics—everything you need to know to become powerful.

# What Is Bipolar Disorder?

**B**ipolar disorder is about life at its extremes. It's about the deepest of depressions and, sometimes, the wildest of euphorias. It's about the struggle to get a grip on one's mind: to get diagnosed, find treatments, and forge a life out of chaos. And it's about surviving—even thriving—while riding this outrageous emotional roller coaster.

If you're bipolar, or if you live with and love someone who is, you know there's nothing easy about this condition—not its diagnosis, not its treatment, not even its definition. For every uncomplicated question you pose about bipolar disorder, you'll get an impossibly complex answer—if you get an answer at all.

Take something as simple and concrete as statistics. How many people are living with bipolar disorder today? The much-bandied-about number is 2.3 million Americans, or about 1 percent of the population—the same percentage of Americans who have schizophrenia. But almost anyone who deals with bipolar disorder— be it through personal experience or scientific research—believes that 1 percent is a low estimate. Almost everyone has a story to tell about bipolar disorder: a story about a friend, a relative, or even themselves.

The experts agree: 1 percent is too low. The real number is undoubtedly higher. But how much higher?

## PsychSpeak

**Unipolar depression** is a mood disorder in which a person experiences one or more episodes of persistent sadness and apathy, fatigue, and feelings of worthlessness, without any intervening episodes of mania or hypomania.

"The truth is probably somewhere between two and five percent, depending on your definition of bipolar," says S. Nassir Ghaemi, M.D., director of the Bipolar Disorder Research Program at Cambridge Health Alliance and assistant professor of psychiatry at Harvard Medical School. "That puts it at two to three times more cases of bipolar than schizophrenia, and about half as much as unipolar depression. I think that's probably right."

## Defining Bipolar

What *is* the definition of bipolar disorder? Simply, it's a mental illness in which you experience episodes of manias that range from mild to extreme, as well as episodes of depression. In reality, however, nothing is that simple. There are different types of bipolar disorder (see Chapter 2), and they all tend to look different in different people. Some people might experience the classic manic symptoms, while others might have upward mood swings that are so mild they're barely noticeable. Some might go through the classic manic symptoms of grandiosity and extreme elation, while others' manias might send them on shopping sprees and make them extremely irritable. Indeed, there are several different degrees of both mania and depression, each of which has its own variations on the general theme.

The importance of pinning down a definition goes well beyond semantics; the way bipolar disorder and its various parts are defined determines how you're diagnosed if you seek help from a clinician. The diagnosis you get determines the treatment you get, and the treatment you get might determine how well you are able to live with your disorder. And it all begins with a name.

# Manic-Depression vs. Bipolar Disorder

The first time bipolar disorder was described as a specific condition all its own, separate from the other forms of "hysteria" and "melancholia," was in 1851, when French psychiatrist Jean-Pierre Falret described what he called *folie circulaire,* or "circular madness," in which patients cycled through depression, mania, and a period free of disorder.

In 1899, German psychiatrist Emil Kraepelin—who is often referred to as the father of modern psychiatry—took this concept a step further. He differentiated between what he called "dementia praecox" (known today as schizophrenia) and "manic-depressive insanity," and gave psychiatrists the tools by which to differentiate between two conditions that can at times seem similar. At the same time, however, he took a step backward, as it were, by bringing together both the unipolar and bipolar forms of depression under the single manic-depressive umbrella.

Still, the moniker stuck. And thrived. In fact, a good number of the people who have the disorder today were likely diagnosed not with bipolar disorder, but with manic-depressive illness. Even now, if you talk about bipolar disorder, you might get a blank stare. But say, "You know, manic-depression," and the lightbulb will go off.

It wasn't until 1966 that not one, but two publications detailed the differences between bipolar and unipolar depressions in much the same way Falret had done. Falret's idea of bipolar disorder had been reborn, and the term "manic-depression" began to lose momentum. By 1980, when the American Psychiatric Association (APA) published the third edition of its *Diagnostic and Statistical Manual of Mental Disorders,* or *DSM,* the name change—and the shift in perspective—had become official. (The *DSM* is currently in its fourth edition, the *DSM-IV,* which was unveiled in 1994.)

*I spent most of my adult life thinking of myself as a manic-depressive; the name bipolar just doesn't seem to fit as well. Is there any chance the name will change back?*

"Probably not. There's force of habit to overcome, so unless there's a groundswell of support for a major change, coming from a majority of clinicians, things are likely to stay the same. Still, I do have to agree with you. Words have consequences, and what these words suggest is that people like you have poles. But because we now think the course of the illness is chronic depression with brief manic episodes, manic-depressive may be a better phrase.

"In addition, the bipolar/unipolar terminology is vague; it doesn't explain what the condition is very well. The distinction might work better if there was actually a clean distinction between the two, but the truth is the original impetus to distinguish between bipolar and unipolar depression is less powerful than it used to be." —*S. Nassir Ghaemi, M.D., director of the Bipolar Disorder Research Program at Cambridge Health Alliance*

## Mania

No matter what the disorder is called, mania is at its core. Mania is what makes bipolar disorder different from unipolar depression, different from schizophrenia, different from other forms of psychosis. And what makes mania is its energy. Sometimes it's a euphoric energy that propels you through life at breakneck speed, hurling thoughts and ideas at you with such force that you can hardly talk fast enough to keep up with them. And sleep? How can you possibly sleep when there's so much to do, so many profound insights to explore? It would all be too exhausting if it weren't for the psychic caffeine being pumped into your body day and night, sometimes for weeks on end. You feel as if you can accomplish just about anything. In fact, you know you will.

But not all mania is an exciting, if wild, ride. Sometimes manic energy is annoying, even irritating. It won't let you concentrate on one thing at a time. It won't let you sleep. It won't even let you sit down. You have to keep moving, you have to keep *doing,* no matter how much you want to stop. And so you seek out things that will help you slow down—drugs, alcohol, anything that will dissipate the energy, even just a little.

The classic concept of mania—of a person giddy beyond reason, full of energy and self-confidence and incredible delusions of grandeur—is true in maybe a quarter of the cases of mania, says Ghaemi. "Many people who are manic are angry or unhappy. They usually don't experience mania as a particularly pleasurable state."

**Symptoms** Mania really is the defining concept in bipolar disorder. After all, if you've never experienced mania or at least hypomania, mania's somewhat subdued sister (see the following "Hypomania" section), you can't be bipolar—at least not according to the guidelines put forth by the APA's *DSM-IV*. Depression, on the other hand, is not "required" for a bipolar diagnosis, which is somewhat ironic, considering that if you have bipolar disorder, you likely spend about a month depressed for every day you're manic. Of course, your mileage might vary.

Mania's symptoms are usually quite apparent—at least to the people around you. From the inside, it's more difficult to recognize. Mania often cloaks itself in denial and a lack of self-awareness, a sort of literal inability to see yourself clearly or recognize that you're exhibiting symptoms of mania. In fact, this so-called "impaired insight" (see Chapter 3) is itself one of the hallmarks of mania. Others include the following:

- Feeling euphoric, "high," speeded up, or irritable
- Having an inflated sense of yourself, of your importance and your power and your abilities (called grandiosity)

**GET PSYCHED**

"When I was manic, I owned the world. There were no consequences for any of my actions. It was normal to be out all night, waking up hours later next to someone I didn't know … I thought I knew what you were going to say before you said it. I was privy to flights of fancy that the rest of the world could scarcely contemplate." —*Patty Duke, actress, in "Through a Lens, Darkly," Psychology Today, August 2002*

- Needing little to no sleep, yet still being full of energy
- Talking more than usual, or so fast that it's almost impossible for others to follow you
- Jumping from thought to thought or idea to idea, and being easily distracted
- Being unable to slow down your thoughts or speech even if you wanted to
- Being physically agitated, unable to sit still, and hyperactive
- Behaving in a self-absorbed, self-destructive manner; drinking too much, taking drugs, having indiscriminate sex, or going on wild spending sprees

If you've experienced three or more of these symptoms at one time, you've likely had a manic episode. But the true test of mania is not so much the symptoms—after all, having a strong sense of self-esteem isn't necessarily a bad thing, and who among us hasn't experienced racing thoughts at one time or another in our lives? The true test of mania is that these symptoms have a real impact on your life, a negative impact such as damaging a relationship or putting you into severe debt or causing you to lose your job.

Another true test of mania is time. A day of euphoria after a promotion at work, a fleeting feeling of smugness after you pass a test most other people fail—that's not mania. In the medical world, you have to have these symptoms for at least a week to be diagnosed as manic (unless you've been hospitalized for manic symptoms, in which case the diagnosis is immediate).

In addition, true bipolar mania can't be explained away by some other medical condition, such as multiple sclerosis or Huntington's chorea, some symptoms of which can sometimes mimic mania. And you're not considered to have true bipolar mania if you've been using drugs associated with mania, such as amphetamines. In fact, although antidepressants can trigger mania in susceptible people, the *DSM* doesn't even consider manias caused by antidepressants to be bipolar manias. This can be problematic, of course, because so many people with bipolar disorder are initially misdiagnosed as depressed and put on anti-depressants.

**Hypomania** Although there's a fair amount of wiggle room in the guidelines for a manic diagnosis, it's not particularly difficult to recognize mania. *Hypomania,* on the other hand, can be much more elusive, if only because it's simply a subtler form of mania. Picking up hypomania—even just defining it—is, thus, significantly thornier.

To be considered hypomanic, you need to show the same three or more symptoms from the same list of clinical signs used to diagnose mania (given in the preceding "Symptoms" section). But in the case of hypomania, these symptoms need only persist for four days to qualify for a diagnosis. And although they should have a noticeable effect on your life   it's likely that your mood and your ability to function will be changed enough to be noticeable to others—they should not cause hospitalization or have a significant impact on your ability to work or hold together a relationship. If they do, you're manic—not hypomanic.

**Dysphoric Mania** As I'll discuss in Chapter 2, the psychiatric community is now beginning to recognize that mania is often more about negative feelings, even paranoid or destructive feelings, than it is about euphoria. Irritable manias are probably more common than the stereotypical grandiose, euphoric manias.

The next step up from irritability is dysphoric mania, in which the symptoms of mania are literally jumbled together with a few symptoms of depression. (On the other side of the coin is agitated depression, in which symptoms of depression are mixed with a few manic signs.)

The question that plagues researchers is what the mix of these symptoms does for the predictions we can normally make about the disorder's course or treatment or impact. True "mixed states," as discussed in the following section, meet the criteria for both mania and depression at the same time. But many clinicians and researchers in the field say this is just too high a bar to set. They say that even when only a few of depression's signs meet the full force of mania, the mania is changed somehow, in significant ways. And indeed, mixed states are more difficult to treat and get under control; in addition, people in mixed states have significantly higher rates of suicide than do people whose mania is straightforward.

How many symptoms of depression does it take to significantly change mania? At least one study has shown that the addition of a single sign of depression seems to make a difference in the way the mania plays out and how it responds to treatment. In addition, a study led by University of California, San Diego, psychiatrist Hagop Akiskal, M.D., found that it takes just two or three depressive symptoms to make mania look more like a mixed state in rates of suicide and ultimate outcome of the disorder.

**Manic Psychosis** What starts out as euphoria and degenerates into the dysphoria of depression can sometimes morph into the confusions and delusions that are the hallmarks of psychosis. One day you feel like a god; the next day God is talking to you. One day you're convinced that you're smarter than anyone around you; the next day you're convinced that you're being persecuted by everyone around you.

The symptoms of psychosis are as follows:

- Delusions
- Hallucinations
- Disorganized or incoherent speech
- Disorganized or *catatonic behavior*

If you show signs of two or more of these symptoms, you're likely to be diagnosed as psychotic; if you also or already meet the criteria for mania, then you'll be diagnosed as having a manic psychosis.

What turns elation into hallucination, grandiosity into paranoia? Lack of sleep, for one. The inability to slow down your thoughts, to concentrate, even to simply see what's happening to you, for another. But the truth is, no one really knows as yet just what makes one person susceptible to psychosis when he or she is manic as opposed to the next person. The only thing we know is that mania greatly increases your chance of having a psychotic episode; psychosis is much less common—indeed, almost unheard of—in hypomania.

**PsychSpeak**

Catatonic behavior, or catatonia, is a behavior disturbance during which you spend long periods of time in a virtual stupor. Physical symptoms characterizing catatonia include very stiff, rigid muscles, especially in the arms and legs.

## Depression

Mania might be at the core of bipolar disorder, but depression makes up the bulk of the disease's mass. After all, more than 90 percent of people living with bipolar disorder will suffer through at least one, and usually several, major depressions—and generally, they'll do it much more often and for longer periods of time than they will with mania. Depression is what makes most people seek a diagnosis in the first place and is what makes bipolar disorder most lethal, being the root of the disorder's 20 percent suicide rate.

Differentiating between bipolar depression and its unipolar cousin is a tricky business. There are real differences—bipolar depression is heavier, more physical, more deeply rooted in lethargy. And it's harder to treat. The usual antidepressants, which only work some of the time in unipolar depression, are even less able to turn the tide of a bipolar depression.

Still, debilitating as it is, depression does not bipolar make, says the APA—at least, not by itself. Without mania or hypomania, depression is its own debilitating disorder; without mania or hypomania, you don't have two "poles," and, thus, you don't have bipolar disorder.

"Static Turmoil"

Somehow, in sloping degree
I am impelled down, down, down
Not into some fearful hell
For in hell there is pain and pain can be fought
But into a saucer like a dried pea
Static and held in place by the gravity of being
So clearly I see over the bevelled rim to those who live
And I cannot join them
There is no joy in existence
Elation comes from living and knowing life
Existence in the saucer is merely breath
Had I the nerve I would scale this gentle slope
But it takes all of me just to be
There is no more of self
No reserve to start a climb
A static turmoil sheds the bark of the soul
To let my spirit weep away
You cannot see my hurts nor hear my muted cries
Yet these are the norms of my being
And they wear on me in constant fashion
Til I am eroded to a thin nothingness
That will not leave, will never leave
So I must leave
With desperate effort I conjure thoughts of force
To end the thudding aches
Borne into me breath by breath
—James H. Martindale, living with bipolar disorder (1990)

**Symptoms** The good news, as it were, is that when you're depressed, you're unlikely to lack insight the way you might during a manic episode. In fact, says Ghaemi, if you're depressed, you're probably hyperaware of how you're feeling. That makes depression particularly painful and difficult, but at least it increases the chances that when you start to pick up on depressive symptoms, you'll look for or ask for help.

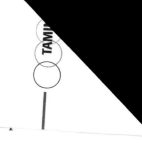

What are the symptoms of bipolar depression? T
cording to the *DSM*'s symptom lists (although not t
who experience them), identical to those of unipola
and include the following:

- Feeling sad, empty, or tearful for much of the day, every day
- Losing interest in people and activities you were formerly quite interested in
- Losing or gaining more than 5 percent of your body weight in a single month, even though you're not dieting
- Experiencing frequent bouts of insomnia or wakefulness
- Being either restless and agitated or noticeably slowed down
- Feeling tired and low on energy
- Constantly feeling guilty or worthless without any real reason to feel that way
- Having trouble thinking, concentrating, and making decisions
- Thinking about or planning death or suicide

If you're dealing with at least five of these symptoms (including both feelings of sadness and apathy), you're probably clinically depressed. But as is the case with mania, the true test of bipolar depression has less to do with symptoms than it does with the cause of those symptoms and the effect they're having on your life. Losing a job, the death of a loved one, the end of a relationship—all these can cause a major depression. Even relatively minor events in your life—not getting an award you were up for, getting reprimanded by your boss, a minor financial setback—can get you down for a while.

## GET PSYCHED

"You do get over depressions. More important, you are a better person for having had one. I seemed to wipe out many of my skeletons in a short period of time and discard many fears that had bugged me before. You become more sensitive and kind. In my case it was so."
—*Art Buchwald, political humorist, in "Celebrity Meltdown,"* Psychology Today, *November/December 1999*

The question is, can you pick yourself back up, or are the symptoms lingering, dragging you further down? Depressive symptoms that last a couple days are upsetting but common; it's when they cling to you for more than two weeks straight and when they start to have a big impact on your life and your relationships that they become a cause for concern—and a reason for a clinician to diagnose you as experiencing a major depressive episode.

Again, as in mania, a depressive episode isn't a depressive episode if you have a medical condition that can cause depression, such as a thyroid condition, or if you're using drugs associated with depression, such as barbiturates.

**Bipolar Depression vs. Depressive Disorders** Bipolar depression and depressive disorders share the same name and the same symptoms. But are unipolar depression and bipolar depression really one and the same disorder?

To some degree, it depends on your point of view. If you're looking at two people who are depressed—one with unipolar depression and the other with bipolar depression—they are likely to be indistinguishable from one another in terms of the symptoms of depression they're experiencing. It's only when you ask them about mania and about their family and medical histories that you might be able to tell one from the other. For that reason, some people insist that the two are indeed the same illness, only with slightly different courses. They believe that unipolar and bipolar depression are quite close to one another on the spectrum of mood disorders, and that they are more similar to one another than they are different.

Others, including Ghaemi, believe that the distinctions between the two forms of depression are significant enough to make them two different disorders—that although they are clearly on the same spectrum, they are on opposite ends of it and, at their core, are not the same disorder.

"In bipolar depression, you have increased sleep and increased appetite more commonly than in unipolar depression," says Ghaemi. "Psychotic episodes are more common in bipolar depression, as is postpartum depression, and there's an earlier age of onset in bipolar disorder. If you look at the symptoms, the course, the genetics, even the treatment response, on all of those features, bipolar and unipolar depression are different."

## Mixed States

Mixed states are exactly what they purport to be: a blend of manic and depressive symptoms, all hitting at the same time. Imagine a depression so deep you can barely get off the couch, while at the same time your thoughts are racing and you're unable to sleep. If there is anything worse than mania or depression, it's certainly having both at the same time.

The definition of a mixed state is undergoing a bit of a revolution. The *DSM* still insists that mixed states meet the "requirements" for both mania and depression in terms of numbers of symptoms, although they only need to last one week rather than the two normally used to diagnose depression. But others, including Akiskal—who is perhaps the most well-known proponent of rethinking the rigid definitions of all these states—say that it only takes a couple symptoms of depression to change mania into something more complex, and it only takes a couple symptoms of mania to similarly change depression.

Some clinicians see mixed states as a state of transition from mania to depression or vice versa; others believe they are as much a part of bipolar disorder as either of its parts alone. And still others claim that it can be a sort of transient, ever-changing state in each individual.

But almost all agree that, when mixed, mania and depression can become even more dangerous and even more explosive than they are when apart. As Frederick Goodwin and Kay Redfield Jamison point out in their classic textbook on the subject,

*Manic-Depressive Illness,* mixed states bring together a "critical combination" of depressive symptoms with the increase in energy and decrease in inhibition of mania. No wonder studies seem to show that if you're in a mixed state you're more likely to commit suicide than you are if you're either depressed or manic alone.

"You're highly agitated, sometimes even violent, and at the same time sad and hopeless," says Carol Ezzell Webb, whose mother committed suicide while in a mixed state. "It's a lethal combination."

## Diagnosing Bipolar Disorder

The reason so many people care so very much about the definitions and parameters of these bits of bipolarity is that diagnosing bipolar disorder has been—and continues to be—a major challenge. In fact, if you are an "average" person living with bipolar disorder, you had your first manic episode at the age of 19 and then went undiagnosed or misdiagnosed until you were about 40. That's a 20-year gap—two decades during which your symptoms could have been reined in and your disorder properly treated.

The problem is, misdiagnosis of bipolar disorder is positively rampant. Even if you exclude those people who experience a major depression as their first bipolar symptom—in other words, those who are rightly misdiagnosed, if there is such a thing—a full 40 percent of bipolar adults will be initially given the wrong label—and probably the wrong treatment as well. Children, too, are given diagnoses that don't quite fit—usually, behavior-based tags such as attention deficit disorder (ADD). In fact, bipolar children are even more likely to be misdiagnosed than are bipolar adults.

Why is proper diagnosis so critical? First of all, there are the obvious, true-for-any-illness reasons. Putting the right name to a set of symptoms points you and your physician toward specific treatments that you might not otherwise consider. And it enables you to steer clear of treatments that might only make your problems worse. Once you have the right name to put to your symptoms, you are finally empowered to make the choices that will enable you to have a good, full life. It will enable you to live, even thrive, with bipolar disorder.

Missing a bipolar diagnosis has more specific and destructive effects as well. Undiagnosed and, thus, untreated, bipolar disorder grows steadily worse over time, spawning more episodes that are more severe and that cycle more and more rapidly. In addition, a number of different research studies have shown that people whose bipolar disorder goes untreated through several episodes of mania and depression are more likely to find, when they finally are diagnosed, that the standard treatments for the disorder don't work for them. In other words, a misdiagnosis or lack of diagnosis doesn't only cost you years during which you could be free of mania and depression, but it might also cost you the ability to *ever* get the disease under control.

The costs of misdiagnosis are financial as well as psychological and medical. Studies assessing the monetary costs of bipolar disorder estimate that the disease costs somewhere between $10 billion and $45 billion annually. The question is, how much of that could be saved by getting better at diagnosing bipolar disorder?

Howard Birnbaum, Ph.D., and colleagues from the Analysis Group in Boston provided a glimpse at the potential savings in a 2003 article titled "Economic Consequences of Not Recognizing Bipolar Disorder Patients: A Cross-Sectional Descriptive Analysis," published in the *Journal of Clinical Psychiatry*. They looked at insurance claims data from 7 different large employers and found more than 9,000 people who had been treated for depression with antidepressants between 1998 and 2001. Of those, 623 were ultimately diagnosed as bipolar, with about half of them being correctly diagnosed during the period of time being analyzed and taking a mood stabilizer in addition to their antidepressant. The other half had been misdiagnosed as having unipolar depression and never received a mood-stabilizer during that time.

What Birnbaum and his colleagues found was that not only was bipolar disorder more expensive to treat than unipolar depression, but that the patients with unrecognized bipolar disorder cost their companies $1,179 per month—$378 a month more than the $801 spent on those who had been properly diagnosed. And those were only the so-called "direct" costs, for things such as prescriptions, doctors' visits, and hospitalizations. As it turned out, the undiagnosed bipolar patients were also more likely to incur higher indirect costs—absences from work, for example—than those already being properly treated for the disorder.

When all was said and done, the patients whose bipolar disorder was misdiagnosed as unipolar depression ended up costing their companies an extra $557 a month each as compared to those people with bipolar who were on a mood stabilizer.

*My sister's bipolar disorder was misdiagnosed as depression for several years, yet her mania seemed quite obvious to me. How could her doctor have missed it?*

"In the 1970s, bipolar depression was most often misdiagnosed as schizophrenia. In the 1990s, that problem was replaced by the misdiagnosis of bipolar disorder as unipolar depression. The nature of bipolar illness is such that depression is the predominant problem, and it's a much more noticeable problem. Most people with bipolar disorder spend the majority of their time in depression—and it's an especially onerous form of depression. Manic symptoms, on the other hand, are usually brief, and not always quite so severe. Because of that, they can be difficult to pick up. Add that to the fact that clinicians tend not to be very attuned to the symptoms of mania, and you wind up with a focus on depression and psychosis, both of which have received much more attention over the years." –*S. Nassir Ghaemi*

**Why Bipolar Is So Difficult to Diagnose** Most psychiatric disorders don't show up on an x-ray or an ultrasound or a blood panel. Bipolar disorder is no exception. Despite the fact that the search for the genes behind the disorder is going full-force, so far there's no test or measurement physicians can make to deter-mine the cause of the myriad psychiatric symptoms that go hand-in-hand with bipolar disorder. That alone makes diagnosis a challenge.

Of course, as is often the case with bipolar disorder, that's not the whole story. Diagnosing bipolar disorder is also particularly thorny because of the number of different masks the disease can wear.

More often than not, if you're seeking medical attention for bipolar-related symptoms, you're doing so as a result of a particu-larly ugly depressive episode. The depression, then, is what most physicians see and what most physicians treat. Without a family history of bipolar disorder or a voluntary admission of mania or hypomania—which is rare in the early days, when the manias still tend to be seen as positive experiences—the average clinician will tend to offer antidepressants to clear up the reported symptoms. The problem is that, in bipolar disorder, antidepressants can act like a match put to a powder keg, often propelling you into a mania that quickly spirals out of control and accelerating the rate of cycling between mood states—all while failing to help the depression that got you here in the first place.

Certainly, many mental health profes-sionals are woefully undereducated in the diagnosis of bipolar disorder—and even more general practitioners are outright ignorant about it. At the same time, those clinicians are dealing with patients grap-pling with the issue of "lack of insight," as described in Chapter 3, which leaves them literally incapable of recognizing or "seeing" their own manic symptoms, and thus incapable of reporting them accu-rately. There are also people who see mania simply as part of their personality, consid-ering themselves simply high-energy, or

**GET PSYCHED**

"There's no excuse in this day and age for seventeenth-century notions of mental illness. If you don't discuss it and you don't seek treat-ment, you can die, and ruin a lot of lives around you."
—Kay Redfield Jamison, psy-chologist and author living with bipolar disorder, in "Two Years Later: A Quieter Mind," Psychology Today, January/February 1998

excitable. Not to mention that during a major depressive episode most people are literally unable to recall a time when they were "up." Add into the mix a fear of the diagnosis and the significant stigma that can be attached to it, and you have a recipe for a diagnostic nightmare.

To better understand the extent of the problem, the National Depressive and Manic-Depressive Association (now the Depression and Bipolar Support Alliance, or DBSA) did a survey in 2000 of 600 people who had been diagnosed with bipolar disorder. They compared the results to a survey of 500 people they had conducted in 1992. The results were simultaneously encouraging and distressing:

- Although 36 percent of the 2002 survey respondents said they'd sought help within a year of first experiencing symptoms—compared to 30 percent in 1992—31 percent said that at least a decade had gone by before they had pursued help.

- Sixty-nine percent of the 2002 respondents had been misdiagnosed at least once; on average, they saw four physicians and received more than three different misdiagnoses before hearing the correct verdict.

- Although there was no difference in the prevalence of bipolar disorder by gender, women were significantly more likely to be misdiagnosed than men—72 percent versus 62 percent. When the women were misdiagnosed, they were given a diagnosis of unipolar depression much more often than the men. On the other hand, the men were much more likely to receive a misdiagnosis of schizophrenia than were the women.

- Overall, the 2002 survey respondents experienced a 10-plus-year delay between onset of symptoms and accurate bipolar diagnosis, with those who were misdiagnosed having a longer wait (an average of 12.5 years) than those who were diagnosed correctly upon seeking help (an average of 5.5 years).

# Man, Interrupted

"I knew my father was bipolar years before anyone uttered the words to him. "My father has always done everything big. He dreams big. He has a big temper, a big appetite. He makes big gestures of generosity, or hurt, or whatever he's feeling that day. And he spends big. He once told me, 'If I make a million dollars this year, I'll spend a million and one.' And then he proceeded to do just that.

"Today, my father will tell you he believes he may have been bipolar from childhood. But he knows for sure that the disorder had really begun to make itself at home when he was a young man climbing the corporate ladder. It's been with him through two marriages and a more-than-fair number of relationships; it's been with him while he's worked at a number of jobs in a number of different businesses.

"My sister and I have often talked about our father by describing his moods. 'Dad has his "voice of death," today,' she might warn me. Or when she asked me if I'd spoken to him and how he was, I might roll my eyes and say, 'Everything's f***ing amazing'—his phrase of choice during his manic phases.

"In the early 1990s, when he began having panic attacks—one after the other, for months on end—he finally broke down and saw a doctor, a psychopharmacologist recommended by a good friend. That doctor diagnosed him with an anxiety disorder and clinical depression and handed him a prescription for Prozac. Eventually, the doctor added a prescription for Klonopin, for those nights when my father said he wasn't able to sleep, 'because my mind was whirling.'

"My father made two real suicide attempts, once while living in Brazil, another time while in New York. He was hospitalized for both those attempts, as well as for an episode when he found himself wandering in Central Park in the wee hours of the morning. 'It was the one and only time I admitted to hearing voices,' he recalls. 'A police car stopped me, and the policeman asked what I was doing, asked if I was okay. And I said "no." I said the trees and bushes were talking to me, telling me to kill myself.'

"Yet it wasn't until he met a woman who had experience with bipolar family members that he began to question whether he was really suffering from anxiety and depression. And it wasn't until 1997—during yet another hospitalization—that a clear-eyed psychiatrist finally picked up on the mania, added bipolar to my father's diagnosis, and added Depakote to his growing pharmaceutical arsenal. The effect was almost immediate—and quite dramatic. My father had finally been properly diagnosed. He was 59 years old.

"'Before all this happened to me, if somebody came to me and said they were depressed or anxious or whatever, I'd tell them to snap out of it,' he says. 'I didn't believe in psychologists, psychiatrists. I was totally ignorant. And yet I always knew there was something wrong with me. I just didn't know what it was. For all those years, I didn't know what it was. Now, all of a sudden, my life had changed. I was in charge of my life again.'" *—Lori Oliwenstein, author of this book; her father, Jack Oliwenstein, currently resides in New York City*

**How the Diagnosis Is Made** In 1952, the APA published the first edition of its *Diagnostic and Statistical Manual of Mental Disorders*. By 1980, when the third edition of the *DSM* was published, what had begun as a categorization of mental illnesses had morphed into a comprehensive list of diagnostic criteria.

Today, there is a vast array of guidelines, checklists, and mania- or depression-rating scales used by an equally vast array of mental health professionals. But the current *DSM-IV*, published in 1994, really has the final word on the criteria that are used for diagnosis.

Of course, it's critical to keep in mind that lists of symptoms and criteria can only take you so far. Psychiatry, like football, is a game of inches—millimeters, even—rather than yards. One person's manic episode might be another's normally rapid speech pattern or naturally exuberant personality. One person's depression might be another's normal reaction to a stressful life event. That's why the APA points out that the *DSM-IV* is "meant to support the diagnostic process, providing clinicians with diagnostic guidelines, *not* a set of disorder 'check lists.'"

**WEB TALK:** Worried you might be manic? Fill out the screening questionnaire at: www.dbsalliance.org/questionnaire/screening_intro.asp

To that end, a good psychiatrist or psychologist will rely on more than a manual to figure out what's going on with you; he or she will also ask you about your medical history, family history, your own observations and feelings about your behavior, and the observations and feelings of those around you. In fact, because of the way bipolar disorder works on the brain, you might have a hard time recognizing your own symptoms or monitoring your own behavior. That's why it's a good idea to bring along a family member to your appointments, so the doctor can get another, more objective, point of view.

In addition, you might be asked to undergo some simple medical tests to rule out other conditions, and you might be asked to fill out any of a number of questionnaires that some professionals use as an indicator of mania, depression, or both.

Most good clinicians will also tell you that a diagnosis is a work in progress. Rarely will a patient fit neatly into a diagnostic shoebox; more often, adjustments need to be made over time. What a physician will see in you after a few meetings will be but a broad sketch; as time goes by, he or she can fill in that sketch with finer and finer levels of detail.

**The Bipolar Masquerade**  More often than not, if you've experienced at least one true manic episode—and especially if it was paired with a major depression—bipolar disorder is the culprit. But nothing is ever quite that simple when you're dealing with this wily mood disorder. There are, in fact, a number of medical and psychological conditions that can either cause or mimic mania or depression.

That's why one of the first things a good physician will do when evaluating someone for possible bipolar disorder—or really, for any significant mental health disorder—is to perform what is known as a *differential diagnosis,* which will rule out anything physiological in nature that might be behind the symptoms in question.

Medical conditions whose symptoms can mimic either mania or depression include the following:

- AIDS
- Stroke
- Hyperthyroidism
- Multiple sclerosis
- Lupus
- Hepatitis
- Influenza
- Head trauma

## PsychSpeak

**Differential diagnosis** is a systematic compare-and-contrast method physicians use to determine which condition a patient is suffering from when there are two or more possibilities that share a number of similar symptoms or signs.

A few others, such as Huntington's chorea and St. Louis encephalitis, can look a lot like mania, but not generally like depression. A larger number of diseases are depression-only impersonators. They include the following:

- Diabetes
- Hypothyroidism
- Coronary artery disease
- Tuberculosis
- Sleep apnea
- Viral pneumonia
- Mononucleosis
- Fibromyalgia

It's not just medical conditions that can look like, or kick off, mania and depression. A large number of drugs can have similar effects, which only serves to further muddy the diagnostic waters. Steroid use, for instance, can cause both mania (usually characterized by aggression) and depression. Mania can also be the result of amphetamine use, antidepressants, Ritalin, levodopa and bromocriptine (both used for treatment of Parkinson's disease), and drugs such as epinephrine and ephedrine.

Depression can be brought on by a variety of drugs almost too large to list. A few of them include indomethacin (a pain reliever for gout and arthritis), barbiturates, cimetidine (also known as Tagamet, a heartburn and stomach-acid medication), and certain chemotherapy drugs such as vincristine and vinblastine. The use of alcohol as well as withdrawal from amphetamines can also trigger depression.

And of course, a number of other mental illnesses or syndromes can look like bipolar disorder and need to be ruled out as well, including schizophrenia, psychosis, antisocial personality disorder, the early phases of dementia, and drug and alcohol abuse disorders.

# What You Can Do

Recognizing the signs and symptoms of bipolar disorder is the first step toward getting the right diagnosis, which is a huge step toward gaining control of your life. Here are some things to help you take that step:

☐ Know the symptoms of both mania and depression, and see a physician if you're experiencing more than one or two of them or if they linger for some time. The sooner bipolar disorder is diagnosed, the easier it is to treat.

☐ In the days or weeks before your appointment, keep an informal chart of your moods and symptoms and then offer the list to your physician.

☐ Be as truthful as possible when describing your symptoms. What you don't tell *can* hurt you.

☐ Consider letting friends or family members talk to your clinician. Better yet, bring them along to your appointment. They may well have insights into your behavior that you couldn't possibly provide.

☐ Take notes when talking to your doctor so you can better recall what you were told later on, when the memory is less fresh. You can also use the pad and pencil to jot down questions as they occur to you during your appointment.

☐ Never leave your doctor's office without having asked all the questions you came in with. Be sure you understand all the answers you receive.

# The Many Faces of Bipolar Disorder

**B**ipolar disorder is a 35-year-old Hispanic man who is struggling to hold down a job through his third depression in the past 12 months. It's a 72-year-old grandmother whose kids and grandkids are concerned because she seems agitated and depressed; they think she might have Alzheimer's. It's a 26-year-old mother of two who is suffering through a postpartum depression. And it's her six-year-old son, who is being evaluated for attention-deficit disorder at the urging of his first-grade teacher.

Bipolar disorder is you and me; it's our parents and grandparents and children. And like us, no two cases of bipolar disorder are exactly alike. Each will travel its own course and take its own twists and turns.

That's why trying to pigeonhole each individual case of bipolar disorder can be an exercise in frustration. Many clinicians are starting to believe that bipolar disorder is a *spectrum* of conditions that range from relatively mild to extremely severe and that you can slide from one diagnosis to another and sometimes even back again over a lifetime. They say that trying to pin names on each possible permutation of this incredibly complex disorder is unnecessary, possibly even harmful. Others disagree, saying the various forms of bipolar disorder are actually distinct diseases, each with its own slightly different set of biological causes, and it's important to differentiate one from the other.

No matter which of these viewpoints you adopt, what's important to remember is that manias, hypomanias, mixed episodes, and major depressions are just the ingredients for bipolar disorder. The disorder itself is the result of which of those symptoms make themselves apparent in what order and how severe they are when they do appear. Bipolar disorder, in other words, is quite often much greater than the sum of its parts.

Nonetheless, many—if not most—clinicians will still give your bipolar disorder a more specific name. They'll consider which symptoms you're experiencing and in which order. They'll look at how long it takes for you to go from one pole to the other and how much of a break you get between cycles.

That's why it's worth getting to know bipolar's most basic categories. There's bipolar I and bipolar II, the specifics of which almost everybody agrees upon. Some clinicians say there's a third form of bipolar disorder that is brought on by the use of

**Q&A**

*I know I'm bipolar, but I have no idea what "type" I am. Should I find out? Does it really matter?*

"Knowing your exact diagnosis does help to some extent to give you an appropriate understanding of the range of bipolar disorder. Some people just hear bipolar and think it's a whole lot worse than it is. Sometimes it's important for people to know they have a milder form of the illness; it removes some of the worry and stigma. Still, from a practical point of view, it can be a very difficult distinction for a clinician to make. And it doesn't really influence treatment decisions as much as you'd think. Ultimately, the distinction probably isn't as important as many people may feel." *—John Kelsoe, psychiatrist and medical director of the Mental Health Clinical Research Center at the VA Medical Center in San Diego*

antidepressants. Some include a bipolar variant called cyclo-thymia under the bipolar umbrella; others say cyclothymia, with its persistent low-grade hypomania, is only a precursor to true bipolar disorder. And then there's rapid-cycling bipolar disorder, a description that can apply to any and all of these categories.

To attempt to untangle this gnarled diagnostic thicket, here's a primer on the many masks bipolar disorder can wear.

## Bipolar I

Bipolar I is manic-depression at its dubious best. If you get a diag-nosis of bipolar I disorder, you've experienced at least one full-blown manic or mixed episode—and likely at least one major depression as well. Although it's true that in nearly three-quarters of bipolar I cases, mania and depression will switch off in a some-what orderly progression, there's really no rhyme or reason to the episodes: Depression might lead to mania, or mania to depression. They can be mixed in a single week or day, or they can be sepa-rated by months or even years.

Bipolar I is the most severe form of bipolar disorder. If you have bipolar I and you don't treat it, you're likely to experience as many as four mood episodes a year. Untreated manias might last for a month or more—an eternity spent in a world of frenzy. Untreated depressions can linger for months and months on end; some can even last for a year or more.

If your clinician diagnoses you with bipolar I, he or she will usually add a variety of modifiers—which are sort of like psycho-logical adjectives—to it. She might note whether or not you're experiencing psychotic features such as delusions and hallucina-tions. If you're a woman, your doctor might also consider whether your symptoms were kicked off or restarted by giving birth.

In addition, she'll note what sorts of symptoms brought you to her for diagnosis in the first place. There are six different subtypes that can be diagnosed in bipolar I, depending on your particular circumstances. They include the following:

- Bipolar I, single manic episode (This will be your diagnosis if you have never had a manic episode before.)
- Bipolar I, most recent episode hypomanic ("Most recent" in these subtypes refers to the episode you're seeking medical help for.)
  - Bipolar I, most recent episode manic
  - Bipolar I, most recent episode mixed
  - Bipolar I, most recent episode depressed
  - Bipolar I, most recent episode *unspecified*

## PsychSpeak

An **unspecified** bipolar episode is one in which your current symptoms of bipolar disorder do not meet the criteria (in terms of either time or severity) to be considered mania, hypomania, or depression, although one or most past episodes have met the criteria.

Bipolar I affects more than 2 million people in the United States, or about 1 percent of the population. Despite the fact that it is the best-known and most easily recognized form of the disorder, it is not the most common form. That particular dubious honor is reserved for bipolar II disorder.

## Bipolar II

If you're bipolar II, you've never been out-and-out manic, but instead you have gone through at least one or more hypomanias, as well as at least one major depression.

It's tempting to talk about bipolar II as "less severe" than bipolar I. Certainly, the symptoms of mania are less striking than they are in bipolar I, and if you're bipolar II, you're more likely to return to "normal" between hypomanic and depressive episodes. In fact, in a long-term study of bipolar II patients led by Lewis Judd, M.D., of the University of California, San Diego, the authors noted that although bipolar II patients spend a lot of their time with symptoms of depression, more often than not, those symptoms are relatively mild compared to those needed for a diagnosis of a major depressive episode.

## Dark Side of the Mood

For Christine, bipolar disorder is measured by depressions, not manias. In fact, Christine might not even know she's bipolar if it weren't for her mother, whose undiagnosed and untreated bipolar disorder eventually ended in suicide.

Christine's first depression hit at the age of 16, and lingered—unmedicated—for 4 or 5 months. Her second came barreling into her life midway through her senior year in college. "I never told my parents how depressed I was," she recalls. "I went to the psychiatric services counseling on campus but was never prescribed any drugs."

Then came the fall of 1987. As the days grew shorter, Christine's world grew darker. "I was so depressed I literally couldn't function," she recalls. "My brain felt as if it were filled with molasses. I couldn't remember things; I was disoriented to a really large degree.

"And then I began fixating on the idea of suicide. Although I hadn't really made any plans, I found myself thinking, every time I crossed a street, *Wouldn't it be great if a car hit me?* Then I started being careless when I crossed streets.

"At the time, I remember, I was working in a building with a center atrium that went up 14 floors, and it had glass elevators that you could look out of as you went up and down. I would look out at the crossbeams as the elevator rose, and picture my body seven flights down, draped over one of them. It was an utterly, utterly miserable time."

But it was a transformative time as well, because it prompted Christine to get help. At first, that help came in the form of antidepressants, but when they didn't quite do the trick, Christine's psychiatrist suggested giving lithium a try, especially considering her family history. It worked like a charm.

Still, Christine sometimes wonders about her diagnosis. After all, she's only suffered the mildest of hypomanias: "I'd get energetic, wouldn't sleep much, and would talk a lot. I had all this nervous energy, so I'd go running to burn it off. But I never did any of the injurious things."

In the end, though, Christine is just grateful to have gotten the help her mother never got. "Lithium could have saved her life," she says, "just like it saved mine."

But bipolar II has its own special brand of treachery. Those normal periods of time? They're shorter than in bipolar I. You're more likely to keep having episodes over time—bipolar II has a more chronic course than bipolar I. You're also more likely to experience rapid cycling (see the following "Rapid-Cycling Bipolar Disorder" section). And because of the amount of time you spend depressed, if you have a diagnosis of bipolar II, you're more likely to commit suicide than someone who is bipolar I. This is a particularly devastating issue, because bipolar II disorder is two to three times more common than is bipolar I.

"To paraphrase Kraepelin," wrote Judd and his colleagues in their 2003 *Archives of General Psychiatry* paper, "the nature of this deceptively 'milder' form of manic-depressive illness is so chronic as to seem to fill the entire life."

## Bipolar III

Bipolar III doesn't actually exist, at least not in strict medical parlance. But most people who work in the field say that there is definitely a third type of bipolar disorder—one in which you have a family history of bipolar disorder and you become hypomanic only after treatment with antidepressants for a major depressive episode. The problem is that although clinical experience demonstrates that treatment with antidepressants clearly stimulates mania in some people, the *DSM-IV* and other diagnostic tools all indicate that you don't have bipolar disorder if your mania or hypomania is brought on by drugs or medications.

Psychiatrist Hagop Akiskal, M.D., from the International Mood Center at the University of California, San Diego, is a widely renowned expert on the bipolar disorder spectrum and focuses especially on the disorder at the spectrum's fuzzier edges. In a 2003 paper on so-called "antidepressant associated hypomania," he and his colleagues examined whether what he calls bipolar III is actually caused by the antidepressants—in other words, as a side effect of the treatment—or is a pre-existing bipolar condition, indistinguishable from bipolar II, that is nudged to the surface by the medication.

The study, performed in France, involved 48 psychiatrists working in 15 different psychiatric centers with a total of nearly

500 patients with major depression. Of these patients, it turned out, nearly 40 percent had experienced one or more episodes of hypomania, and a quarter of those were the result of antidepressant treatment.

In general, the patients who were hypomanic because of antidepressants were very similar to those who were bipolar II. The main difference, the physicians noted, was that the people with antidepressant-induced hypomania were more severely depressed than the bipolar II patients. Nonetheless, Akiskal notes, they were just as likely to eventually be given lithium or another mood stabilizer as the bipolar II patients. The *DSM-IV*'s refusal to acknowledge these people as bipolar, Akiskal and his colleagues write, "flies against experienced clinicians who make the decision to treat them the way they treat other bipolar spectrum patients."

In the end, Akiskal believes, bipolar III disorder is actually "a depression-prone form of bipolar II." Figuring out what all this means in terms of the diagnosis and treatment of this form of the disorder is the next step.

## Cyclothymia

You get irritable a lot. You get depressed—but not *depressed* depressed, not clinically depressed. Still, you know something's wrong. It's been years since you really felt like yourself, like your old self, for more than a few days at a time.

Cyclothymia is the mildest of the bipolar disorders, but it's also the most persistent. If you're cyclothymic, you experience episodes of mild depression as well as episodes of hypomania that look a lot like depression—anger, irritability, sadness. And these feelings, these moods, hang around for years, never really quite letting go. In fact, cyclothymia is defined as two years of usually irritable hypomanias, with less than two months between each episode.

Mild or not, cyclothymia can have a real impact on your life. Constant cycles of irritability and mild depression can and often will take a toll on your career, your relationships, and your self-esteem.

And in as many as one in three cases, the mood swings will get wider and you'll wind up with a bipolar I or II diagnosis. In fact, some clinicians think of cyclothymia as a precursor to bipolar disorder rather than one of its forms. Others think it's basically indistinguishable from bipolar II. And still others wonder whether it's a disorder at all. When you snap at your kids or pick a fight with your spouse, are you just being cranky, or are you being cyclothymic? When you stay up until the wee hours of the morning sanding down some bookshelves, are you being industrious or cyclothymic? Isn't it possible that you're just a person with stormy, tempestuous relationships, possibly with a tendency to abuse alcohol, and maybe a creative or artistic bent? Is it really necessary to stick a label on you?

 *I've been moody my whole life. My wife says she's just learned to avoid me when I'm in "one of my moods." Is it possible that I'm bipolar or cyclothymic or something like that?*

"What distinguishes illness from temperament is impairment. When you're talking about cyclothymia, you're talking about people who have brief and milder fluctuations in mood on both the high and low side of things. If you're impaired in some way by these moods—your marriage breaks up, your job is in peril—then you're cyclothymic. But if not, if the same symptoms are just a touch milder, we wind up calling it temperament. If you're worried about your moods, talk to a physician. But if you're not experiencing any impairment in your life, if you're otherwise successful, you can just chalk it up to your personality." *—John Kelsoe, M.D., medical director of the Mental Health Clinical Research Center at the VA Medical Center in San Diego*

## Rapid-Cycling Bipolar Disorder

Rapid cycling isn't a "type" of bipolar disorder—if you have any of the diagnoses described earlier in this chapter, you can find yourself swinging from mania or hypomania to depression and back again. Rapid cycling, does, however, seem to pair itself most often with bipolar II.

Officially, rapid cycling bipolar disorder means you've had a minimum of 4 mood episodes in a 12-month period, interspersed with periods of normal or stable mood. It doesn't matter how severe those episodes are; it only matters that they're coming much too frequently.

It also seems that people who are rapidly cycling actually spend most of their time depressed. In Judd's *Archives of General Psychiatry* study, which followed 86 patients over a period of more than 13 years, he found that people with bipolar II spend 50.3 percent of their time battling symptoms of depression, both major and minor, but only 1.3 percent of their time dealing with the symptoms of hypomania.

What causes rapid cycling? No one's quite sure. It can come on quite precipitously and leave without as much as a fare thee well. You can cycle rapidly for years on end, or for just a short while; it can happen once in the course of your illness, or several times over. There really is no telling.

Still, there's some evidence to suggest that thyroid problems might contribute to cycling and its speed. In addition, a number of researchers think the rampant misdiagnosis of bipolar depression as unipolar depression—and the antidepressant use that results—is behind the problem. And it's a sort of self-fulfilling prophecy: you get misdiagnosed as unipolar, take a SSRI antidepressant, and start cycling rapidly. When you cycle rapidly, your predominant symptom is depression, which only reinforces the original unipolar diagnosis and antidepressant prescription.

Not everyone agrees with this assessment, however. A group of physicians and scientists from the National Institute of Mental Health's Collaborative Program on the Psychobiology of Depression studied 345 patients from that program who had been followed for anywhere from 12½ to 20 years. A quarter of those people had rapid cycling. The researchers found that although the rapid-cycling patients were more likely to have significant depressive episodes and to make serious suicide attempts, the rapid cycling tended to disappear within two years of starting and didn't seem connected to the use of antidepressants.

## The Bipolar Spectrum

You can juggle criteria, compare and contrast symptoms, scour the *DSM-IV*, and ultimately determine what form of bipolar disorder you might have. Or you can do what Hagop Akiskal has done and take a more panoramic view of the disorder, one that really gives you a chance to survey the landscape as a whole, to truly see the forest and not just the trees.

Akiskal sees the bipolar landscape as stretching from horizon to horizon—from psychotic mania to "strictly defined" unipolar depression, or what the *DSM-IV* calls major depressive disorder, and all the mood states in between. In other words, Akiskal simply doesn't see sharp delineations between different types of mood disorders. Instead, he looks at them all as shifting and changeable, without any real border over which you can step, where someone would be able to point and say, 'Ah. Yesterday she was suffering from unipolar depression, but today she's clearly in a bipolar depressed state.'

**WEB TALK:** To get a more personal view of bipolar disorder in its various guises, visit:

www.mcmanweb.com/index.html

"Akiskal would say that there is no unipolar disorder," laughs psychiatrist John Kelsoe, M.D., medical director of the Mental Health Clinical Research Center at the VA Medical Center in San Diego and one of Akiskal's close colleagues and collaborators. "But even he would say that's an extreme view. Still, his basic point is valid. He's basically saying that the core element of bipolar disorder is an instability of mood regulation. If you have a lot of instability, you have bipolar disorder. If you have just a little, you're unipolar."

Kelsoe not only treats patients, but dabbles in genetics as well (see Chapter 4), and he says Akiskal's spectrum meshes perfectly with his own pursuit of the genes behind the disorder. After all, it's been clear for some time now that bipolar disorder isn't caused by a single gene. It isn't caused by a pair of genes, or even a trio. There are likely dozens of genes that play a role in creating bipolar disorder. The idea is that you need to have a certain number of these genes, mutated in a certain way, to wind up with bipolar disorder. "It's a number rather than a yes or no," explains Kelsoe. "You get to a certain number of defective genes, and you pass a threshold and become what we call ill."

The bipolar spectrum is exactly the same thing. Every single person has mood swings, shifts, and cycles. In most of us, the amount of swinging and shifting plays a key role in making up our temperament. But at some point, a switch gets flipped or a line gets crossed, and what used to be a personality trait turns into a full-fledged medical condition.

"In the families we study, we see a lot of people who are never diagnosed as bipolar, but who are up and down and moody, or who are a little high all the time or a little depressed all the time," says Kelsoe. "One member of the family gets just the right balance of all those things and is unbelievably successful in life. Another gets too much of it, and they're ill. The spectrum is very obvious in interviewing these families."

Perhaps even more intriguing is the way the spectrum can play out in an individual. If you're bipolar, after all, your disorder shifts and changes; it's better one day, worse the next, better three months later, awful six months after that. Does your diagnosis change? Not under the traditional diagnostic criteria, and not according to the *DSM-IV*. But certainly, in a disorder characterized by change, it does seem somewhat rigid to insist on an unchanging diagnosis, a static medical picture of an ever-morphing disease.

> ## GET PSYCHED
>
> "You have just been told by a doctor that you are bipolar. It's an illness that affects your emotions, your thoughts, your mood, and your life in general. You will now be dealing with medication, therapy, and regular visits to the doctor's office. Is it a big problem? Yes. Can it be turned into a little problem? Yes. Will it destroy your life? Definitely not." —*Shay Villere, living with bipolar, author of* The Bipolar Disorder Manual, *www. bipolardisordermanual.com*

"I've seen individuals who at just the right point in their lives are extraordinarily successful," says Kelsoe. "And then the other two thirds of the time, they're totally incapacitated."

The call to consider bipolar disorder as a spectrum is not, however, a call to stop considering it a disorder in the first place. And it's not a call to stop treating it, either. In fact, says Akiskal, quite the opposite. Not recognizing the full spectrum of bipolar disorder, he wrote in a 1996 paper, "would deprive many patients with lifelong temperamental dysregulation and depressive episodes of the benefits of mood-regulating agents."

## The Changing Face of Bipolar Disorder

Once upon a time, bipolar disorder was a grown-up's disease. Today, it's an equal-opportunity employer who's ignoring child labor laws. It's also a disease of the elderly, whose symptoms were previously shrugged off as dementia. Today, bipolar disorder can look like almost anything—anyone—you can imagine.

Still, there are trends. If you look at the numbers, if you talk to the doctors, or if you visit with the people behind the diagnosis, you find that, like so many other things in our society, bipolar disorder seems to be marketing itself to a younger, edgier crowd.

**Younger Onset** Twenty-five years ago, the face of bipolar disorder was fully adult, with an average age of onset of 32. Today, with an average-onset age that hovers around 19, that face is more likely to be acne-prone.

What's behind the plummeting numbers? Certainly, a large part of the push over the precipice came from the recognition, over the past couple decades, that, yes, children can get depressed. That opened the door to the concept that, yes, children can be manic, too.

"In the early 1990s, our group was one of the first to begin looking seriously at bipolar in children," notes Barbara Geller, M.D., a professor of child psychiatry at Washington University

School of Medicine in St. Louis. "What we found was that children we had seen at the age of 10 for major depression, when they turned 20, almost half had become bipolar."

**Less Mania, More Irritability** With the recognition that bipolar disorder strikes indiscriminately came the recognition that, although grandiosity and euphoria are mania's calling card, they do not have to predominate. In children and adolescents, as well as in elderly people with bipolar disorder, euphoria tends to sour into irritability, anger, even violence.

And they're not alone. As our ability to pick up on bipolar disorder improves, we're able to focus more on mania's less-characteristic face. There are no longer any boundaries to mania: The sky—or the depths—is the limit.

**Bipolar in Children and Adolescents** The Juvenile Bipolar Research Foundation estimates that as many as 1 million children and adolescents in the United States are affected by bipolar disorder. And yet it's only in the past decade that anyone's really considered its implications for kids. In fact, notes Geller, in 1995 the National Institute of Mental Health awarded her group its first-ever grant to study the "natural history" of bipolar disorder in children—its prevalence, its course, what it looks like.

Research on childhood and adolescent bipolar disorder is sparse. But the good news is that it's rapidly growing denser as more and more researchers begin to take up the cause.

**WEB TALK:** Check out the Juvenile Bipolar Research Foundation at:

➤ www.bpchildresearch.org/

Still, there remains the dilemma of the slippery symptoms. Simply put, bipolar in kids doesn't really look all that much like the disorder in adults. For one thing, childhood bipolar disorder tends to be speeded up: Where an adult might cycle from mania to depression a few times a year, a child's cycles can often be measured in hours, morphing so rapidly into one another that they're often not even recognizable as one pole or the other. This is called ultra-rapid cycling.

In addition, mania is rarely seen in kids, at least not in the form with which we're most familiar. And when it does, it can be hard to recognize. After all, normal children are often excitable, full of themselves, and fearless. In bipolar children, however, these things are amplified. Oftentimes the mania manifests itself as outbursts of aggression and anger, followed by inappropriately silly, giddy, or rowdy behavior. This makes these children look a lot like children with *attention deficit/hyperactivity disorder* (*ADHD*) or one or another of the so-called conduct disorders. More often than not, that's precisely the diagnosis they will receive.

> **PsychSpeak**
>
> **Attention deficit/hyperactivity disorder (ADHD)** is a pattern of behaviors—difficulty paying attention, restlessness or constant motion, and lack of impulse control—that are out of synch with a child's level of development.

Those diagnoses are not necessarily wrong—just often incomplete. As many as 60 to 90 percent of bipolar children actually *do* have ADHD in addition to manic-depression. Indeed, the two are almost inextricably intertwined, sharing many of the same basic traits. Childhood bipolar disorder has a similar intimacy with conduct disorders, with an estimated 69 percent of bipolar children also fitting the criteria for a conduct disorder diagnosis.

As is the case with adults, the problems of diagnosis are further complicated by the fact that most pediatricians are not educated in the intricacies of bipolar disorder. A 2003 Consensus Statement on the Unmet Needs in Diagnosis and Treatment of Mood Disorders in Children and Adolescents—presided over by the Depression and Bipolar Support Alliance (DBSA)—noted that only child mental health specialists have adequate training in the field. General psychiatrists, pediatricians, and other primary-care physicians get little, if any, such training. Until that changes, the struggle to get a correct diagnosis in a reasonable amount of time will continue—for both children and adults.

**Bipolar in the Elderly**  With an average onset age of 19 and
the bulk of diagnoses made before the age of 40, it is perhaps not
surprising that the issues faced by people grappling with bipolar
disorder in their later years are woefully neglected. Indeed, as
the nearly 40 experts in the field who met in late 2001 to put
together the DBSA Consensus Statement on the Unmet Needs in
Diagnosis and Treatment of Mood Disorders in Late Life wrote,
"Late-life bipolar disorder is remarkably understudied."

What *is* known is that bipolar disorder in the elderly (which
for the purposes of most studies is defined as people older than
50) starts to look startlingly like bipolar disorder in adolescents—
with agitation and a sort of inward-turning form of depression
being the primary symptoms.

Researchers collecting data on the epidemiology of bipolar
disorder say that about 1 in 10 people who are bipolar are over
the age of 50. And they estimate that bipolar disorder is responsible for somewhere between 5 and 19 percent of mood disorders
among that age group. As diagnosis improves and baby boomers
continue to surge upward in age, those numbers are sure to only
increase.

Of course, improving diagnosis in the elderly is likely to be
an uphill battle. Along with all the other obstacles to a bipolar
diagnosis, older people who are agitated or depressed are often
assumed to have a medical condition such as Alzheimer's disease
or thyroid problems. And it gets even more complicated: Mary
Wylie and colleagues reported in a 1999 paper in the *American
Journal of Geriatric Psychiatry* that the older you are when bipolar
disorder kicks in, the more at risk you are for stroke and psychosis, both of which are likely to throw your physician off the
bipolar scent.

If you first develop bipolar later in life, you're likely to begin
with a depression that is followed, years later, by your first manic
episode. In other words, you won't know for years—15, on average, according to some reports—that the depression or (more

likely) depressions you've experienced are bipolar in nature. Your manias, when they finally come, will likely be more severe and less responsive to treatment, and you'll be more likely than younger adults to be kicked into an agitated mania or mixed state by antidepressant treatment. It's a recipe for potential disaster.

Actually, that potential was already there, it was just unmasked by inappropriate drug dosing. The issue of proper dosing of drugs in older people is one that's begun to plague the medical community in general. The problem is that most drugs are tested on younger adults, whose bodies process and react to drugs in a very different way than do the bodies of older adults. Take lithium, for instance. This first-line therapy for bipolar disorder has never been tested on older patients. What might be a good dose for a man in his mid-20s could be a significant overdose for that same man when he's in his mid-60s. In fact, some researchers have shown that elderly patients may need only 50 to 75 percent of the amount of lithium a younger adult would be prescribed.

The picture painted from what little research has been done on bipolar disorder in the elderly isn't particularly cheering. But with a push for increased interest from the medical and research communities, that picture should brighten considerably in the years to come.

## What You Can Do

Bipolar disorder can take on any number of hues. Its spectrum is a rainbow of moods and their manifestations. And it's changeable. Over the past few decades, the face of bipolar disorder has grown younger and its mood more irritable. At the same time, clinicians need to remember that all these young people will one day grow old and will be joined by others whose disorder has remained masked for decades at a time. No matter what your age, bipolar disorder requires attention and consideration. Here are some ways you can get—and keep—the upper hand:

☐ If you're interested, ask your doctor for your precise diagnosis. It might relieve some of your worries.

☐ Keep track of the length and frequency of your manic and depressive episodes, as well as of the symptom-free periods in between. Contact your doctor immediately if you notice your episode cycles are speeding up or growing more frequent.

☐ When you're trying to assess your behavior, focus not only on the symptoms of bipolar disorder, but also on the effect they're having—or not having—on your life. This might help you decide whether or not to seek help.

☐ Spread the word: Educate people about the bipolar spectrum and about the various forms bipolar disorder can take.

☐ If your child is showing signs of ADHD or conduct disorder, be sure he or she is also evaluated for bipolar disorder. These conditions share a lot of the same signs and symptoms but have radically different treatments.

☐ Don't assume you're "too old" to have bipolar disorder. The disorder is more likely to show its face when you're younger, but there is no bipolar cut-off age.

☐ If you're bipolar and over 50, be sure to discuss your medication regimen with your physician. The older you get, the harder it is for your body to metabolize the drugs you ingest. It might be time for your doctor to reconsider your dosages.

# The Bipolar Paradox

"**M**ania is fun," my father once confided to me." Being manic is fun. It may not be fun for the people who are watching, but it's fun for the person who's manic."

At first, his statement puzzled me. Mental illness is not supposed to be fun—not for anyone. It's supposed to be scary and off-putting. It's supposed to be an unmitigated Bad Thing.

But my father's words have since been echoed by almost every person I've spoken to who is living with bipolar disorder. Bipolar disorder, they say, is not at all black and white. It's full of gray. At times, it's full of vibrant hues, all the colors of the rainbow. It can even be full of energy and laughter and excitement.

Sure, there's depression. Bipolar depression is neither fun, nor vibrant, nor energetic. It's dangerous—even lethal. So lethal that if you're bipolar, you're 10 to 20 times more likely to commit suicide than someone who doesn't have the disorder.

But mania, the other side of the bipolar coin, has an undeniable upside. Even better is hypomania, which has all the fun of mania without its most serious consequences.

And therein lies the paradox of bipolar disorder. Some people insist that mania drives their creativity, is behind their determination to succeed in business, and is what enables them to love and live fully. And that's oftentimes true—to some extent. It's also true that mania, left unchecked, can lead to delusions, substance abuse, and impulsive, destructive choices that crush creativity, obliterate careers, and ruin relationships. Mania inches you closer and closer to the edge of a precipice, and the fall—into psychosis or full-blown depression—can be devastating. And it does so while keeping you blindfolded, unable to see what is happening to you.

Part of accepting bipolar disorder is accepting the fact that the negatives of the disease coexist with the positives. Pretending the positives don't exist won't help. One of the top reasons people with bipolar disorder give when they stop taking their medications—and each year almost one out of every two people with bipolar will do so—is that they feel that mood stabilization means deadening of thought, feeling, creativity, and energy. To some, it even feels like a sort of psychological suicide. As Stephanie, a 40-year-old writer who was diagnosed with bipolar disorder 3 years ago, says, "Hypo-mania is part of my personality; it's part of who I am. You can't medicate away my personality."

## The Allure of Mania

You're excited. You're interested in everything around you. Your mind is sharp as a tack. If there's a problem, you can solve it. You feel like you could squeeze beauty out of a stone. You feel like you could lead the world down the path to peace.

Mania. What's not to like?—aside from the irritability that starts to creep in and the voices you start hearing after your second week of no sleep, that is.

But no matter how bad mania can get, it still holds that shining promise of a near-perfect you in a near-perfect world. And all that is true. When you're in an early or mild mania, or when you're hypomanic, the world truly is your oyster. The energy feeding into you opens your mind just a little wider and gets you moving just a little faster. It lets you reach a little farther for what was previously just beyond your grasp.

The downsides are there, and if you've been there before, you know what they are. But that doesn't deny the beauty of the moment, the power that mania can hold over you.

"The couple of weeks before I was hospitalized for mania I was incredibly creative," says Rachael Bender, a 26-year-old graphic designer who runs her own business, Bender Consulting. "I did some of my best work then. I could work so much because I was sleeping less. I had such drive. My thoughts would speed up, so I could do things faster … until, of course, they were going so fast that I couldn't do anything because it was just too much.

"I know plenty of people who have gone off their meds because they want to be manic again. It's very alluring. On the one hand, you know it's bad, but on the other hand, you want it."

## The Gift of Creativity

The undeniable link between creativity and bipolar disorder has been considered from all angles. And one thing's certain: It's simply not possible to explain by chance alone the number of highly creative people, from almost every walk of life and every imaginable circumstance, who wind up being treated for bipolar disorder.

It seems that mania adds a spark of inspiration to the ideas already smoldering within you creative folk. What mania cannot do and will not do is provide the raw materials for creativity. Those either exist within you or they don't.

WEB TALK: Check out the list "People with Mental Illness Enrich Our Lives" at:

www.nami.org

Mania's spark seems to work in a number of ways. According to Kay Redfield Jamison, Ph.D., who wrote what is perhaps the most highly respected book on the topic, *Touched with Fire: Manic Depressive Illness and the Artistic Temperament,* people who are hypomanic actually have more advanced sorts of speech patterns. In addition to the rapidity of speech that is considered one of mania's symptoms, Jamison says people in hypomania's throes use both rhyming and alliterative words more frequently and

## GET PSYCHED

"In a sense, depression is a view of the world through a dark glass, and mania is that seen through a kaleidoscope—often brilliant but fractured." –Kay Redfield Jamison, "Manic-Depressive Illness and Creativity," in Scientific American, February 1995

tend to use a more advanced, quirky sort of vocabulary.

You might think that trying to use the ever-logical scientific method to pin down the essence of creativity in all its free-flowing, rule-bending glory is the ultimate exercise in futility. You might be right. And yet a number of studies done by some particularly creative scientists have yielded rather intriguing insights into the process of making art of almost any kind:

Nancy Andreasen, M.D., currently chair of psychiatry at the University of Iowa, did some of the very first work into the links between creativity and mental illnesses, particularly mood disorders, by studying 30 participants from the renowned Iowa Writer's Workshop and comparing them to 30 people who were not in "creative" fields. Overall, 80 percent of the writers had some kind of *affective disorder;* only 30 percent of the other group had similar diagnoses. And a full 43 percent of the writers were diagnosed bipolar, as compared to only 10 percent of the control group.

Kay Redfield Jamison, Ph.D., performed a study of both affective and bipolar disorder rates in a group of 47 highly celebrated British writers and artists. She found that 38 percent of the overall group had received some treatment for affective disorder. In addition, when she broke down the group into specialty, she found that the group most at risk was the poets, 33 percent of whom had needed to be medicated for depression. Even more striking, 17 percent of the poets had required lithium and a hospital stay, at a minimum, as a result of a manic episode. In addition, a full 89 percent of the participants in the study reported to Jamison that they had gone through at least one very intense period of creativity, which met many if not all of the criteria for hypomania or mania.

## PsychSpeak

Affective disorder is a disturbance of emotions, such as bipolar disorder, in which the disturbance is not caused by an unrelated medical problem.

Arnold Ludwig, a psychiatrist from the University of Kentucky, took a different approach: He read some 2,200 biographies of 1,004 prominent men and women and assessed them for signs of mental illness. Instead of publishing the results in a medical journal, however, Ludwig teamed up with the Guilford Press and published *The Price of Greatness: Resolving the Creativity and Madness Controversy* in 1995. He, like the others, found that artists, writers, and musicians were saddled with mental illness at rates significantly higher than other adults. He also found that these differences began during their teen years. For example, Ludwig showed that 34 percent of future musicians suffered from symptoms of mental illness, while it hit just 9 percent of the kids who were eventually to become scientists, athletes, and successful businesspeople.

Most recently, Terence Ketter, chief of the Bipolar Disorders Clinic at Stanford University Medical School, along with doctoral student Connie Strong, did a study comparing people with unipolar depression and bipolar disorder, healthy volunteers, and Stanford graduate students in fine art, product design, and writing who did not have bipolar disorder. Ketter and Strong had each of these subjects take the Baron-Welsch art scale, a test that measures creativity by looking at a subject's preference for simple or complex designs as well as symmetrical or asymmetrical designs. They found that the people with bipolar disorder scored 50 percent higher on the scale than did healthy volunteers and those with unipolar depression and scored similarly to graduate students pursuing creative vocations.

So many of mania's features, in fact, seem tailor-made for the creative mind that you might wind up wondering how it is that not every artist or writer or musician is diagnosed with bipolar disorder at one point or another. If you can function on little or no sleep, for instance, you might be able to get through that particularly knotty section in the middle of your novel without losing your train of thought simply by working through the night. If you're open to new ideas and to both painful and healing emotions, you'll be better able to transfer the vision in your mind onto a canvas.

**Q&A**

*How does mania lead to creativity?*

"In a study we did on creativity, we found correlations between scores on a test of creativity and having access to negative emotions. You can think of it as cyclothymia, dysthymia, irritability, or neuroticism. Or you can take a more positive perspective and call it noncomplacency. In any case, it turns out that dissatisfaction is the mother of invention; it creates creativity." *—Terence Ketter, chief of the Bipolar Disorders Clinic at Stanford University Medical School*

You can also look at the attraction between mania and creativity from the opposite viewpoint. As Ludwig points out in *The Price of Greatness,* the arts are compatible with the bipolar personality. So many of the arts are primarily solitary pursuits, with little pressure to conform and a great deal of acceptance of eccentricity. A manic personality is much more likely to thrive and succeed in a theater than in a cubicle at a large corporation.

Still, as much as mania giveth, it's capable of taking away so much more—and that is certainly part of the paradox. The very same artists whose manias are behind works of such breathtaking beauty and complexity that the rest of us can merely stare in awe are then driven by those same manias into psychosis or impelled by the depressions that follow to take their own lives. Virginia Woolf's decision to kill herself was based largely on her dread of the mania she felt approaching. As she wrote in her suicide note to her husband, Leonard, "I feel certain I am going mad again ... And I shan't recover this time."

The fascination with the effect bipolar disorder has had on so many great and creative minds has drawn in everyone from celebrity seekers and gossipmongers to scientists and clinicians. Psychiatrist John F. McDermott, M.D., from the University of Hawaii School of Medicine, inspired by speculation about Emily

Dickinson's mental health, did a full-scale analysis of all of Dickinson's poems and the dates on which they were created, considered that alongside her letters and other biographical materials, and concluded that the poet had experienced seasonal changes in her productivity, followed by a prolonged period of intense creative energy, which he speculates might have been the result of an undiagnosed bipolar condition.

Others—scientists, historians, physicians—have speculated on the mental disorders that might have plagued almost any creative individual you'd care to name. These posthumous postulations might never be fully settled, but they do serve a purpose. They bring to the forefront the names of people who led extremely successful, if sometimes equally tumultuous, lives despite—or perhaps because of—their experiences with bipolar disorder. For the general public, that can be an eye-opening and stereotype-shifting realization. According to the National Alliance for the Mentally Ill (NAMI), some of these people include the following:

- Ludwig von Beethoven, composer
- Robert Lowell, poet
- Virginia Woolf, author
- Gaetano Donizetti, opera singer
- Robert Schumann, composer
- Vincent van Gogh, artist
- Isaac Newton, scientist

**GET PSYCHED**

"For if Emily Dickinson was indeed the victim of the well-known Faustian bargain between affective illness and creative genius, it was her courage and imagination that enabled her to rise above the former and use the latter to transform powerful affects into metaphor." –*John F. McDermott, M.D., "Emily Dickinson Revisited: A Study of Periodicity in Her Work," in* American Journal of Psychiatry, *May 2001*

Other creative people have contributed to busting the stigma of bipolar disorder by openly discussing their relationship with their disorder. Some of them include the following:

- Maurice Benard, actor who works with NAMI as spokesperson for their bipolar disorder public service announcement campaign
- Patty Duke, actress and author
- Carrie Fisher, actress and author
- Connie Francis, singer and actress
- Mariette Hartley, actress; spokesperson for GlaxoSmithKline's bipolar disorder drug, Lamictal; and co-founder of the American Foundation for Suicide Prevention
- Margot Kidder, actress and advocate for natural and herbal treatments for psychiatric conditions
- Jimmy Piersall, baseball player and author
- Linda Hamilton, actress
- Jane Pauley, broadcast journalist, anchorwoman, author, and talk-show host

The core of the creativity paradox in bipolar disorder is not simply the tug-of-war between mania's creative benefits and its destructive tendencies; it is, rather, the lengths to which some people will go to maintain those benefits, even at the expense of their overall mental health. A full half of patients taking a mood stabilizer such as lithium will, at some point or another, go off their medication because of its real or perceived side effects, including a purported dulling of the senses. Indeed, many people complain that, like chemotherapy for the mind, lithium makes their creative hair fall out.

Jamison, who is bipolar and has a great deal of experience with lithium, points out that these sorts of medication issues wouldn't be issues at all if someone could develop treatments for bipolar disorder that stabilize moods without muting emotions. Then, you'd be able to stave off bipolar's most harmful effects without sacrificing a critical piece of your self.

**The Value of Overconfidence** In artists of all stripes, the relentless drive and energy of mania can be turned into creative expression that serves, at least for a while, as a form of release. Those same impulses—plus the natural grandiosity that can be part of being bipolar—can turn a shy, retiring type with a few interesting ideas into a true leader.

These are the sorts of people—men, at least in the earlier part of history—who seemed to possess a sort of cult of personality. They could draw people into their sphere and seemed to lead them almost effortlessly. They could inspire thousands with a single phrase. Indeed, a list of some of the most prominent of leaders with bipolar disorder (or at least suspected bipolar disorder) reads like a *Who's Who* of military and political history. Some of them include the following:

- Alexander the Great
- Napoleon Bonaparte
- Oliver Cromwell
- Lord Nelson
- Alexander Hamilton
- Abraham Lincoln (possibly)
- Theodore Roosevelt
- Winston Churchill
- Benito Mussolini

In more recent years, these driven and dynamic types have moved from the battlefield to the boardroom, where ambition of outrageous proportions is right at home. Take Ted Turner, for instance. The founder of Turner Broadcasting has talked openly about his diagnosis with bipolar disorder. How his disorder has affected his life and his career isn't clear, but certainly no one would argue his success, despite—or perhaps *to spite*—his condition.

Turner reportedly once quipped, "If I only had a little humility, I'd be perfect." Never before has there been such a concise, if unintentional, definition of manic grandiosity.

## The State of Denial

Although getting a correct diagnosis is, ultimately, a good thing, it can open a Pandora's box of issues and emotions. The truth is, nobody wants to hear that he or she has a chronic, lifelong mental disorder—especially one that carries a stigma, is difficult to treat, and is generally considered to be a lifelong condition. And nobody wants to hear that he or she is going to have to come down from the highs of mania.

These are some of the reasons why so many people with bipolar disorder wait so very long—a full decade, on average—to seek help in the first place. And they're some of the reasons why, when they do reach out, it's generally for the much more accepted condition of depression, rather than for mania or bipolar.

Still, once the box is open, it can't be closed again. Pretending nothing has changed won't make it so. Nor will pooh-poohing the seriousness of the condition or simply refusing to comply with your doctor's suggested therapy regimen.

This is more than an intellectual exercise: This is, in fact, serious stuff. A number of clinicians believe that those people who accept their bipolar diagnosis are more likely to comply with treatment—in particular, to keep up with the drug, therapy, and lifestyle regimens they're prescribed—and, therefore, have a better chance at a positive outcome.

## The Quandary of Impaired Insight

Denial is wanting not to hear what you're hearing; it's refusing to see what you're clearly seeing. Denial requires you to actively work against what you know to be true—to deny it access to your life or your plans or your consideration. Denial is something everyone goes through at one point or another—bipolar or not.

But in bipolar disorder, denial is just the tip of the iceberg. One of mania's most insidious side effects is called impaired insight. Impaired insight goes way beyond your desire not to see what's happening or being unable to recognize that mania is bad or destructive; it's not being *capable* of seeing it. It is, says Nassir Ghaemi, M.D., director of the Bipolar Disorder Research Program at Cambridge Health Alliance, an actual, biological phenomenon. In about half of all cases of mania, you literally can be physically incapable of knowing if and when you're manic. In fact, there's even a name for it: *anosognosia*.

> **PsychSpeak**
>
> **Anosognosia** is an inability to recognize, acknowledge, or act upon a set of symptoms, such as those of mania. Literally, it means "to not know a disease," and comes from the Greek words for "diseases" (*nosos*) and "knowledge" (*gnosis*).

There's precedence for this kind of bizarre lack of self-awareness, as anyone who's dealt with an elderly parent or friend with early stage Alzheimer's disease probably knows. In the beginning, when memories start to flee, many Alzheimer's patients will insist that there's nothing wrong with their memory. They'll become outright belligerent about it, in fact. And yet to the rest of us, the memory loss might be extremely obvious—so obvious, it seems almost ludicrous that they're denying its existence.

"That's lack of insight," Ghaemi says. "It's not that they know and are embarrassed; it's that they really don't know."

Physician and writer Oliver Sacks tells a truly astonishing tale about lack of insight in his book, *The Man Who Mistook His Wife for a Hat* (Summit Books, 1985). In the book, Sacks tells the story of one of his elderly patients whose stroke left her not only unable to move the entire left side of her body, but unable to even realize that she *had* a left side.

"She has totally lost the idea of 'left,' with regard to both the world and her own body," Sacks wrote. "Sometimes she complains that her portions are too small, but this is because she only eats from the right half of the plate—it does not occur to her that it has a left side as well."

The physical link between stroke, Alzheimer's disease, and bipolar disorder is that they may all involve some amount of impairment in the brain's frontal lobe, the seat of both thinking and emotions (see Chapter 4). Certain changes to that area of the brain might make it impossible for you to logically assess what's going on around you, yet you need just that sort of process when you're becoming manic so you might have a chance to pick up on the mania before it gets out of control. Instead, what you get is severely impaired insight—so impaired that when someone suggests to you that your behavior has turned somewhat manic, you begin to rant and rave, convinced that your friends are turning against you. You won't even consider the possibility that your friend might be right, that you might be becoming a bit manic, because you actually are unable to see what the friend is talking about, unable to recognize that anything is wrong or off.

When the mania disappears, however, so does your insight impairment. After the fact, you'll usually be able to recall most of what went on while you were manic. You'll be able to gain some insight into your disorder.

By then, however, it might be too late. A study done about 10 years ago by Ghaemi and his colleagues found that the lower the level of insight into the disease, the worse the person did over time. For instance, if you're unable to realize that you're manic, you'll be less likely to take your medications, and that makes you more likely to wind up being involuntarily hospitalized.

WEB TALK: The Treatment Advocacy Center has several fact sheets on impaired insight: www.psychlaws.org/

If you're having a hard time with insight issues right now, don't despair. Your level of insight is likely to shift over time without a discernible pattern. In addition, about a third of patients do better, insight-wise, once they've begun taking medication for an underlying affective disorder.

Interestingly—and in stark contrast to what we know about mania—bipolar depression is almost never marked by impaired insight. In fact, says Ghaemi, during depressive episodes, you're more likely to be even more in touch with your emotions than at any other time. "We call it depressive realism," he says. "They are more aware of themselves and their surroundings; they're more insightful."

## Differentiating Between "Normal" and "Disorder"

Yesterday, you were a mother or father, a lawyer or banker or school-bus driver. You were a person with a wry sense of humor, an avid skier, a weekend carpenter, a wanna-be novelist. Today, you received a diagnosis of bipolar disorder, and already you feel like it's taking over your identity.

Yesterday, you could be happy without being called manic or hypomanic. Yesterday, you could be sad without calling it a depression. Today, you wonder about every thought, every feeling, every action.

Any clinician will tell you that these are perfectly normal reactions to such a dramatic shift in your sense of self. Almost everyone with a chronic illness goes through it to some extent. You don't want to be labeled; you want to be normal, just like everybody else. You don't want to face a future in which you have to be bipolar for every single day of your life.

It's these sorts of feelings that drive people with diabetes to rage against the blood testing and insulin shots, even though they know that not complying with their treatment can mean blindness, kidney problems, even the loss of limbs. It causes people with heart problems to rebel against their low-fat diet, despite the possibility that the decision

> **GET PSYCHED**
>
> "Bipolar disorder is something that you have, but it is not who you are."
> —David J. Miklowitz, Ph.D., in The Bipolar Disorder Survival Guide (Guilford Press, 2002)

is a death sentence. And it's why, as for many people with bipolar disorder, taking your medication can be a daily struggle with yourself, even if you know all the dangers of going unmedicated.

For people with bipolar disorder, things can get even stickier than they do for those with diabetes or heart disease, mostly because it is exceedingly difficult to separate bipolar disorder from your natural personality or temperament. Trying to find the ever-shifting line in the sand between "moody" and "bipolar" can be frustrating.

Even more frustrating is the way bipolar disorder seems to take what you've always thought of as your personality and turn it into a disease, a disorder, something to be medicated and fought and conspired against. But as you'll see in Chapter 4, your personality didn't cause bipolar disorder, and it won't play a role in treating the disorder, either. When all is said and done, when you've had what will hopefully be a successful course of treatment, your personality will be exactly as it was before, except maybe better, because it will be able to shine through without fighting for space with your disorder. You'll still be you—you'll just be you minus the mania and the depression.

**you're not alone**

## Some of My Best Friends

For about three years now, Stephen has been one of my closest friends. He is a big guy with thick hair and a thick laugh. He is extremely smart and creative, both verbally and visually. He is also extremely funny. We share a sense of the absurd, and that is what first drew us into friendship.

And we are a lot alike. There isn't a facet of life in which we do not share an interest, from nanotubes to offbeat films. We both inhabit professionally the world of ideas and make our way by distinguishing good ones from bad ones in our respective spheres. We both have high standards and slog away at getting things right. We both are naturally inclined to stay up late and think nothing at all of having a midnight conversation, especially if one of us is stuck on a problem.

Does that make me manic-depressive? Because my friend Stephen is. And does that designation render his every action a signal of susceptibility?

"It's constantly an issue," Stephen told me, "questioning whether something is a normal problem of living or a subtle symptom of disorder. Just waking up tired on this rainy Monday: Am I depressed or just tired?

"Or is the new business venture I'm involved in sound? I think I'm thinking about it realistically. But the only flagrantly manic episode I ever had involved a business scheme for selling something on the Internet. It seems to me that there is an element of mania in every entrepreneurial venture. All new ideas involve a leap of faith. You get excited, and the energy feeds more excitement and that fuels planning. If you are manic the problem is whether the basic idea is warped; too much of it is a pipe dream. It's a very subtle difference. My psychiatrist said something wise to me: 'I'd hate for you to label as manic every entrepreneurial impulse you have.'"

The trouble is, Stephen says, a poorly trained mental health professional—and he knows, because he once had one—tends to label everything a manic-depressive does as mania or depression. "You cease being a person and become 'A Manic' or 'A Depressive.'

"Bipolar disorder does not affect just your emotionality. It involves the whole structure of your life. It's difficult to stay with things and to be a consistent personality. It's difficult to be in relationships, to stick to one time to get up in the morning, to one exercise program. You have a different way of approaching the habits of your life. I have to fight for every ounce of consistency in my life. 'Am I too tired, too happy, talking too much?' I'm constantly monitoring myself.

"I have a terrific psychiatrist who has taught me not to ascribe to illness what can be ascribed to the normal vicissitudes of life. My experience underscores the need to do medications and psychotherapy with someone who doesn't make you feel that you can't make your own decisions because you have manic-depression. Bipolarity is not the only mental apparatus that operates in bipolar people. There are other functions that are not amplified by the disorder."

*Hara Marano is* Psychology Today's *executive editor. She is also the editor and driving force behind a monthly newsletter called "Blues Buster," which focuses on depression and bipolar disorder.*

# What You Can Do

The paradox of bipolar disorder is that it can be beneficial—conferring a higher degree of creativity on many of those it touches, giving them ambition and focus and maybe a bit of grandiosity—while at the same time it can be destroying your life by destroying your family, spurring you on to shopping sprees, or making you contentious and argumentative. Trying to remain as clear-sighted as possible is your best bet for enjoying as many of the "benefits" of the disorder as possible without suffering too many of its burdens.

- [ ] Accept the gifts of creativity, and use them.
- [ ] Be proactive about getting enough sleep, staying on schedule, taking your medication, and going to therapy. Focus on all the things you can do to move forward, rather than on the things you used to be able to do.
- [ ] At the same time, try not to let the disorder take over your life. If you have people keeping an eye on you, and you're taking your medication and keeping to a schedule, it's okay to let yourself just be sad sometimes rather than assuming you're depressed. And it's okay to let yourself just be happy sometimes, instead of wondering if it's mania.
- [ ] Trust your instincts. If a mood or emotion seems somehow off to you, talk to your therapist or physician. If everything seems within normal boundaries—*and* you have a solid support system in place (see the next checkbox), you can let go of the worry that every fluctuation in emotion is a sign of impending doom.
- [ ] Listen to the people around you when they tell you something seems off. Give someone you really trust the permission to "go over your head" if it seems as if you're too insight-impaired to recognize a problem yourself.
- [ ] Remember, knowledge is truly power. Read up on bipolar disorder; dozens of additional resources are listed in Appendixes B and C. Join a support group or e-mail list, or become an advocate for others with bipolar disorder (see Chapter 12).

# Causes and Courses

I f you've received a diagnosis of bipolar disorder, your first two questions were probably "Why me?" and "What's next?" Why you? You drew the biological short straw. That's all there is to it. Bipolar disorder is a disease. It's a medical condition. It's not a punishment or a judgment on the way you've lived your life. It's not a weakness or a failure.

If you're living with bipolar disorder—actually, if you're living or dealing with any kind of mental illness—you've probably heard this all before. But as you probably know, hearing it is one thing; believing it is another.

The good news is that although bipolar disorder has been shamefully neglected in the past by scientists studying mental illness, those scientists are now amassing reams of data, all of which bolster the assertion that bipolar disorder is all about biology. Bipolar disorder is about changes in your genes that cause changes in your brain that cause changes in your behavior, your personality, and your emotions. You can no more control having bipolar disorder than you can control having blue eyes or a big nose or cystic fibrosis.

The good news is that although you can't control your biology and, therefore, can't control *having* bipolar disorder, you can control the course of the disorder itself through medication, psychotherapy, and being aware of environmental factors that play into your disorder. I'll discuss these more in Part 2.

What about the other question? What *is* next for you if you've received a diagnosis of bipolar disorder? What's going to happen to you?

The course of bipolar disorder—the road it travels, the trip it takes you on—is different for everyone. But clinicians can make generalizations, predictions that depend on which type of the disorder you have, whether you're having mixed episodes, and how fast you're cycling through your manias, hypomanias, or depressions.

There are no guarantees, but there are answers. There are scientists peering into the brain's inner workings and into the secret lives of genes. There are clinicians who've seen it all before and learned how to handle it. And there are other people who have been where you are. Talk to them. Harness the power that is knowledge.

## The Biology of Bipolar

Amassing scientific insight into the biology behind bipolar disorder is much more than an intellectual exercise. Pin down the genes that cause bipolar disorder, and you'll know what chemicals you need to keep an eye on—to test to make a diagnosis or to target with drugs and other therapies. Detail the changes in the structure of the brain, or in the quantities of *neurotransmitters* it produces, and you can begin to understand what causes the emotional symptoms that characterize the disorder.

### PsychSpeak

**Neurotransmitters** are a class of chemicals that travel from the end of one nerve cell to the beginning of another, giving that second cell the signal to fire—that is, to send its electrical message on down the line to the next nerve cell.

**The Genetic Link** Bipolar disorder has a genetic component; it can be inherited. If you have bipolar disorder, look around your family. Probably, at least one of your parents or grandparents or siblings are bipolar as well, or at least are battling unipolar depression or alcohol or drug abuse, all of which also seem to be linked at least to some degree to bipolar disorder. And if not your immediate family, it might be Uncle Joe or Cousin Sue, whose exploits have made your relatives' tongues wag for years now—or caused them to keep very, very silent. Bipolar disorder almost never simply appears out of thin air, even when it seems like it has.

It's worth mentioning up front, however, that genes are not destiny. Yes, people with a long family history of mental illness, and particularly of bipolar disorder, are likely to be at a much higher risk of developing the disorder. But if genes were the be-all and end-all of bipolar disorder, then they'd be more likely to kick in at birth. The way bipolar disorder works, most likely, is that a genetic predisposition reacts with environmental influences—the parenting you experience, the stresses you're under, the choices you make regarding the use and abuse of alcohol and other substances—to determine when and whether you ultimately develop the disorder at all.

Still, the genetic link to bipolar disorder is real, and it is based on a strong scientific foundation. Studies on twins have long been a great resource for answering these sorts of genetic inquiries. If a disease or disorder is indeed passed down through the genes, then identical twins, whose complement of genes is identical, will be more likely to both show signs of a particular disorder than will fraternal twins, who are no more genetically related than any other brother or sister pair.

Twin studies have made the case for a genetic link to bipolar disorder quite hard to ignore. As far back as the 1970s, researchers were able to show that, indeed, if one identical twin is bipolar, the other twin has around a 65 percent chance of being bipolar as well. On the other hand, a fraternal twin whose twin is bipolar has only about a 14 percent likelihood of being diagnosed as well. In fact, says Wade Berrettini, M.D., Ph.D., professor of psychiatry at the University of Pennsylvania, these twin studies tell us that as much as 75 percent of the risk of bipolar disorder is due to genetic, rather than environmental, factors.

If bipolar disorder followed the rules of simple Mendelian genetics (so named after Gregor Mendel, the Augustinian monk who essentially founded the field of genetics with his experiments with pea plants), there would be one gene for bipolar disorder, and it would either be a dominant gene (meaning you would only need to inherit one copy of it to get the disorder) or a recessive gene (meaning you would need to inherit a copy from each of your parents to get the disorder).

In the case of bipolar disorder, however, there are probably many, many genes that play a role in creating the condition, as well as many different changes and mutations to each of these genes that might increase your risk or susceptibility to the disorder. You might not have to have all those genes at the same time—in fact, it's most likely that you *don't* have to have them all—to develop bipolar disorder. This means that the handful of genes that caused your bipolar disorder probably aren't the same handful of genes that caused bipolar disorder in someone else.

How many bipolar genes are out there? "Certainly dozens," says psychiatrist John Kelsoe, M.D., whose research group at the University of California, San Diego, was the first ever to pinpoint a specific gene that causes susceptibility to bipolar disorder. "I'm just praying it's not hundreds."

*My father is bipolar I, and my uncle has been hospitalized for depression. What is my chance of developing bipolar disorder? What about my children?*

"On average, about 7 percent of the first-degree relatives—parents, siblings, children—of someone with bipolar disorder will have bipolar disorder. However, the risk for children if one parent is bipolar is about 10 to 15 percent; that doubles if both parents are bipolar. The risk in your question depends on whether the parent and uncle are on the same side of the family." *—John Kelsoe, M.D., psychiatrist and genetic researcher, University of California, San Diego*

Having multiple genes all involved in the same condition makes it much more difficult for scientists to track bipolar disorder back to its genetic roots, but it also makes it much more difficult for people to pass the disorder along to their children. A dominant Mendelian trait will be found in 50 percent of the children of someone who carries that trait. A recessive Mendelian trait will be found in 25 percent of that person's offspring—but only if the other parent carries the recessive gene as well. Bipolar disorder, on the other hand, is found in about 10 percent of children who have just one bipolar parent.

The gene Kelsoe and his colleagues found in mid-2003 was on chromosome 22. "We knew from previous studies that chromosome 22 had at least one susceptibility gene," Kelsoe explains. (A susceptibility gene is simply a gene that makes you more susceptible to a particular condition.) To figure out which gene or genes that might be, Kelsoe took DNA from animal cells exposed to amphetamines (to mimic mania) and put them on a *gene chip,* which enables scientists to look at the activity levels of hundreds of genes at the same time. "When we used the gene chips, we found that of the several hundred genes in the general area of the chromosome we were looking at, one underwent a 14-fold increase in its activity in response to amphetamine," Kelsoe says.

That gene, it turns out, is responsible for producing an enzyme with one of those impossibly dense names: G-protein receptor kinase 3, or GRK3. When the GRK3 gene is mutated, it fiddles with the brain's biochemistry and how it reacts to certain neurotransmitters. "We believe that a defect in GRK3 may make one super-sensitive to dopamine, somewhat like being born on cocaine," says Kelsoe.

When Thomas Barrett, M.D., Ph.D., an assistant professor at the University of

## PsychSpeak

A **gene chip** is a sliver of silicon that can grab and hold on to a very large number of DNA samples in a tiny grid pattern. Gene chips have enabled scientists to make genetic discoveries at a previously unimaginable pace, because they can now analyze the activity or function of hundreds of genes in the time it used to take to look at just one.

California, San Diego, who worked with Kelsoe on this project, looked into the human version of that same gene, he found a mistake in the part of the gene that determines whether the gene is turned on or off. He also found that same mistake in the genes of people who have bipolar disorder far more frequently than he found it in people who don't have bipolar disorder.

In the end, Kelsoe says, it looks as if GRK3 plays a role in about 1 in 10 cases of bipolar disorder. But it plays a big role in that small number of people. Kelsoe says it might be responsible for about 50 percent of the bipolar risk in those 10 percent of cases.

Right now, there are about half a dozen genes that seem to carry some of the responsibility for bipolar disorder in some percentage of people. And there are probably a dozen or more suspicious-looking patches of chromosomes that are being scoured in hopes of finding more of the genes.

This needle-in-a-haystack search for the DNA that drives bipolar disorder has also yielded new insight into the disease itself. When researchers from the University of Chicago tracked two overlapping genes on chromosome 13 and linked them to an increased susceptibility to bipolar disorder, they also noted that the same pair of genetic bandits had been previously indicted in the development of schizophrenia. Just a few months and several thousand miles later, researchers from the University of Cambridge in the United Kingdom provided another link between bipolar disorder and schizophrenia when they showed that both mental illnesses are the result of mutations to genes that put a protein coat called myelin around a neuron's axon. Without the myelin coat, the neuron short circuits, and the message being sent to or from the brain gets lost.

It's important to keep in mind, however, that as critical as the genetic influence is on bipolar disorder, genes are not the be-all and end-all of this condition. There are probably large numbers of people who carry the mutated genes for bipolar disorder yet never get the disease. In general, scientists assume that there need to be some outside or environmental influences—stress, drug use, antidepressants—that kick the mutated genes into destructive action.

# The Ties That Bind

Lynn Albizo has lived her life with a sword of Damocles hanging over her head, held aloft by a few strands of DNA.

Lynn was in first grade when her mother was hospitalized for the first time in Lynn's life. The initial diagnosis was depression. Eventually, after medications and electroconvulsive therapy and long stays in several different institutions, she was put on lithium. "Lithium was really a savior for her," says Lynn. "She finally became more stable, and learned to live her life."

It wasn't until college, however, that Lynn took a basic psychology course and realized what her mother's positive response to lithium meant for her diagnosis—and what that diagnosis might mean for Lynn herself. She began to have night-mares, echoes of the sleep terrors she'd suffered through during those long years without her mother. And then she found out about her grandfather.

"I knew my mother's father died when she was a baby, and I remembered that my parents used to say he had what my mom had," Lynn recalls. "But I never knew how he died, at least not until I was in college."

It turned out that Lynn's maternal grandfather had turned on the ignition of his car in a closed garage and killed himself when Lynn's mother was just an infant. She now knew where her mother's troubles had come from—and where her own might lie as well. "I felt so stupid not to have put two and two together before that," she says.

Although this new information might have increased Lynn's concerns about her genetic susceptibility to mental illness, the other shoe never did drop—or at least not in the way she was expecting.

Lynn might have dodged a biological bullet, but that doesn't mean bipolar disor-der has had no effect on her life. For one thing, she has to watch the disease wreak havoc on her younger brother. That experience, coupled with her mother's own struggles, undoubtedly led to Lynn's career as a lawyer who works with the mentally ill and advocates on mental health issues. And then there are Lynn's two children, the older of whom is now the age Lynn was when her mother was first hospitalized.

"I see my children, especially when they are acting temperamental, and I hope to God ... I don't even want to say it out loud," Lynn says. "But in the back of my mind ... I know that so often with mental illness it really comes out in the late teens and early 20s, and I look at my kids and I'm so scared that they could have to live with this. I just know I'm going to be so worried when my kids go away to college."

"There's the genetics, and there's the experiences you have in life," Lynn says. "For me, I really believe the things that have happened to me have affected the way I am. With my brother, he's had a lot of things in his life that are related to the fact that my mother was bipolar. And then he has the genetics on top of that. It's like a double whammy."

**Bipolar on the Brain** Bipolar disorder literally changes your brain—its shape, its chemistry, the way it handles the signals it is bombarded with on a second-by-second basis. In this sense, it is no different from any of the scores of neurological diseases—Alzheimer's disease, multiple sclerosis, Huntington's chorea. Bipolar disorder is a disease of the brain that primarily affects emotion and thought rather than memory or movement.

What differences are seen in the brain in bipolar disorder? For one thing, there may be enlargement of the ventricles, those spinal-fluid-filled cavities at the center of your brain. It also wreaks havoc with your amygdala, your brain's almond-shape "seat of emotion"—the place from which your feelings and impulses arise. (*Amygdala* comes from *amygdale,* Greek for "almond.")

Exactly what happens to the amygdala in bipolar disorder, however, is still being sorted out. A number of different researchers have done imaging studies that have shown that bipolar patients' left amygdala (you actually have an amygdala on each side, or hemisphere, of your brain) is larger than that of people without the disorder. Most recently, however, a Yale University School of Medicine team led by psychiatrist Hilary Blumberg, M.D., found a 15 percent reduction in amygdala size in both adults and teenagers with bipolar disorder as compared to adults and teenagers who do not have bipolar disorder.

WEB TALK: Find hundreds of links to scientific abstracts on bipolar disorder at:

www.neurotransmitter.net/bipolar.html

Similarly, researchers are still not sure whether these changes in size come before the disorder—and are, therefore, part of the cause of the illness—or come after, as a result of the disorder. Nor can they say just how a change in amygdala size is related to the increase in amygdala activity that others have found in bipolar disorder. Or how the "thought centers" of the brain, located in what is descriptively called the frontal cortex (because it's the gray matter, or cortex, found at the front of the brain), become less active.

"The amygdala is a more primitive structure found deep in the brain," says Blumberg, who uses a variety of imaging techniques to peer into the brain structures connected to bipolar disorder. "The frontal lobe is what makes humans human. It takes more complex information in from the senses and applies cognition and higher thought and then regulates amygdala functioning. That way it can help someone to have an emotional response that is just right for the situation they are in."

So if the frontal lobe falls down on the job, you wind up with emotions and impulses running amok, without a strong neurological voice of reason reining them back in.

"This is sort of a metaphor for what you see in cognitive behavioral therapy," notes Terence Ketter, M.D., chief of the Bipolar Disorders Clinic at Stanford University, who has also done a fair share of bipolar brain imaging and study. "The emotions are driving the thoughts. When patients recover from depression, however, that tends to correct itself."

Most of the studies on the structure and function of the amygdala were done in patients who were depressed at the time. Much less is known about mania, the fast-moving, often-underappreciated cousin in bipolar disorder. "What we'd all like to see is a kind of symmetry where the areas that are overactive during mania are underactive during depression, and vice versa," says Ketter. "But we're just not there yet."

Bipolar disorder also seems to mess with the circuitry in the brain—the connections between one *neuron* and the others surrounding it. These networks of neurons are at the bottom of every thought process or behavior you have, so it's not surprising that when these circuits are disrupted or otherwise rewired, your thoughts and behavior change as well.

## PsychSpeak

**Neurons** are the brain's signal-conducting cells. Neurons have a "body" surrounded by short, branching arms called dendrites, which pick up signals from nearby neurons. Those signals are then passed down the neuron's long, hairlike axon to get to the next neuron in the circuit.

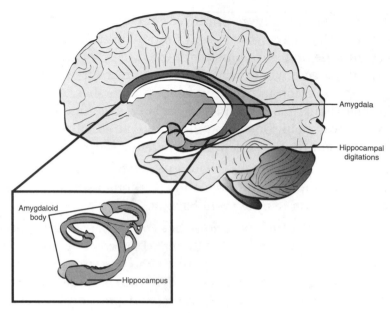

The brain's hippocampus is part of the limbic system, which is responsible for creating emotion and mood. The hippocampus is also where long-term memories are laid down and where some instinctual behaviors arise. The amygdala, which is particularly involved in generating emotions, appears to undergo physical changes in people who have bipolar disorder.

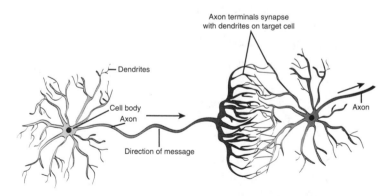

Neurons are the brain's impulse-conducting cells, receiving and sending electrical messages from all parts of the body. Neurons communicate with one another using groups of chemicals called neurotransmitters. It is when these neurotransmitters are either over- or underproduced that the nerve cell's message can become muddled.

Bipolar disorder does this rewiring job by taking advantage of your brain's Achilles' heel: the neurotransmitters, which send or transmit a message from one neuron to the next. These chemicals hang around in the spaces between the end of one nerve cell and the beginning of another. When the signal from one cell in a circuit finishes traveling down the neuron's axon, it gives a specific neurotransmitter a gentle shove over to the next neuron. Once there, the neurotransmitter slips into a receptor—a sort of cellular docking station—and prompts that cell to send a signal down its axon. And the entire process begins again.

Your brain's neurons are designed to be exquisitely sensitive to neurotransmitters so that even the slightest dip or surge in their levels can have enormous effects. Neurotransmitter levels can be affected by lots of things: too much or too little production; problems with the breakdown of the chemicals, leaving either too much or too little neurotransmitter floating around; or a change in the number of receptors on the surface of a neuron so the neuron receives too much or too little signal from its chemical messengers.

The effect these changes have on your brain also depends on which neurotransmitter you're talking about. In bipolar disorder, there are really five main neurotransmitters worth considering:

- Dopamine
- GABA (gamma-aminobutyric acid)
- Glutamate
- Norepinephrine
- Serotonin

Each of these chemicals has a critical role to play in the brain— and in bipolar disorder. Dopamine controls your movements and balance; too little could result in manic hyperactivity. GABA works to keep nerve cells somewhat calm, a clear barrier to mania. Glutamate is GABA's opposite; it excites neurons and prompts them to increase their signaling. Norepinephrine is one of the main neurotransmitters that respond to stress, which is certainly one of the guilty parties in the creation of episodes of mania and depression

71

in the first place. And serotonin plays a role in both memory and sleep; sleep, in turn, plays a role in bipolar disorder (see Chapter 7). In fact, if you've ever taken an antidepressant, it was probably of a type called an SSRI, a selective serotonin reuptake inhibitor, which works to keep serotonin levels on an even keel and lift you up out of your depression.

WEB TALK: For an easy-to-understand lesson about how neurotransmitters work, read:

bipolar.about.com/cs/neurotrans/l/aa0007_msngrs.htm

Using chemicals from a pharmacy to do battle with your body's own chemicals is a great way to right a biological wrong. And the fact that your body responds to them—or, at least, to the right one for the particular emotional symptoms you're going through—only underscores the disorder's biological roots. Lithium isn't going to calm you down if you just won the lottery—that's an excitement that comes from without and is appropriate to the situation. It will, however, help dampen the overexcitability that's characteristic of mania and that leads so many people with bipolar disorder down a devastating and destructive path.

**Stressing Out** When it comes to bipolar disorder, major life stresses—a death in the family, the loss of a job, a nasty breakup—can be the straw that breaks the camel's back—and a bipolar person's mood.

It's almost impossible to imagine a scenario in which stress alone puts you in a bipolar mania or depression. But it's not at all difficult to imagine how stress might interact with a genetic predisposition and an already-primed brain to tip the balance in favor of mental illness over mental health. Certainly, stress impacts a number of body functions: It raises and lowers the levels of certain hormones, reduces your ability to fight off germs and infection, and puts extra pressure on your organs. Stress messes with your body; it's no surprise that it also messes with your mind.

Severe stress can have long-lasting and devastating effects. Robert Post, M.D., chief of the Biological Psychiatry Branch of the National Institute of Mental Health, has pointed out that people with bipolar disorder who experience the stress of physical or sexual abuse as children or adolescents tend to wind up sicker than those people who did not have a traumatic childhood. They develop their disorder earlier, cycle more quickly, are more likely to be suicidal, and are more likely to abuse drugs and alcohol. Such stresses during development seem to permanently set the stress response system to a higher level of reactivity.

But stress has an even more frequent effect on all people with bipolar disorder, even those whose childhoods were perfectly normal or simply garden-variety stressful. Stress tends to be the spark that lights the bipolar fire, that acts as kindling to a brain blaze that's about to get out of control. In fact, as you'll see in the next section, this concept of kindling is a model that many believe helps explain the normal course of bipolar disorder.

> **GET PSYCHED**
>
> "Absolutely the best advice you can give to a bipolar patient about progressing with life is this—let go. That's it. Let go. Let go of your problems, let go of your preconceived notions about life … let go of stress. … It's a great world, but you've got to open your eyes to it. It's a little tougher when you're bipolar, but trust me, it *can* be done." —Shay Villere, living with bipolar, in The Bipolar Disorder Manual, *www.mental-health-matters.com/articles/ article.php?artID=550*

It does seem that stress has to shoulder at least some of the responsibility in the bipolar blame game. You might be born with a biological bias toward developing bipolar disorder, but it is stress that can push you over the edge. Stress determines the chemicals in your brain, and the chemicals in your brain determine not only how you respond to stress, but how you feel emotionally as well. Once these chemicals get agitated by stress, they can then push you into mania or depression.

But don't despair. The effects of stress can be reversed, or at least decreased. Once the stress has lifted, your brain chemicals may very well start to settle back down, and the stress-induced bipolar symptoms may lift.

## What Bipolar Looks and Feels Like Over Time

You've just been diagnosed with bipolar disorder. Maybe you're a little shell-shocked. Maybe you're a lot shell-shocked. You might be wondering what's going to happen next. You might be terrified about what's going to happen next. Will you need to be hospitalized? Will you ever be cured? Will your symptoms get worse or better over time?

"[T]here's no general rule that patients either stay the same or get worse or get better," says Harvard psychiatrist S. Nassir Ghaemi. "But there is definitely a subgroup that gets worse over time—about a third of bipolar patients are in that group. We don't really know why, or what characterizes these people, but we're looking for predictors."

In the nineteenth century, German psychiatrist Emil Kraepelin believed that the course of bipolar was such that it worsened over time, with patients experiencing more, ever-worsening episodes as the years went by. Of course, in his time, there were no mood stabilizers, no antipsychotic medications, no antidepressants; someone living with bipolar at that time would have had to battle his or her bipolar demons virtually unassisted.

Obviously that is no longer the case today. There is help available, and more seems to be coming every day. But still, there are ups and down and highs and lows with this disease. And there are trends—sketches of possible routes your disease might take rather than rules about how it will certainly go.

Between 5 and 15 percent of people with bipolar disorder will have a rapidly cycling course, with four or more mood-related episodes each year—either depressions, manias, hypomanias, or mixed episodes. If you have a rapid-cycling disorder, you do have a somewhat poorer prognosis; rapid cycling can be difficult to get under control, even with medications. But there are still options, and even if you are going to be prone to more swings each year, you can work to keep the number to a relative minimum.

## GET PSYCHED

"I was almost relieved when I got diagnosed. I was almost happy. I finally knew that there could be an answer and I wasn't 'just' crazy. I had a disorder that could be treated. I felt like, 'Now I'm going to get better. Now this doesn't have to keep happening.'" –Rachael Bender, graphic designer living with bipolar disorder

74

The relationship between the number of episodes and the course of the disorder is an intimate one. Data from a 2003 study presented at an international neuropsychopharmacology meeting by researchers from Case Western Reserve University in Cleveland showed that when bipolar I patients have four or more episodes of mania or depression in 12 months or less, they are no more likely to respond to mood-stabilizing treatment than to a placebo. It is indeed possible to predict the severity of bipolar disorder simply by looking at its frequency and how rapidly the moods cycle.

No matter how frequent your episodes, you're more likely than not to have periods between them when you're back to your "normal," fully functional self. According to the *DSM,* between 20 and 30 percent of people with bipolar disorder continue to have mild mood swings between major episodes. These moods might not be severe enough to qualify as official bipolar episodes, but they do tend to create problems with relationships and jobs.

There is no way to predict the course of an individual episode. A manic episode can turn psychotic seemingly without warning. Once you've had a manic psychosis, however, you are considered more likely to have another. There do seem to be individual patterns to how episodes follow one another—whether mania or hypomania, or depression comes first, how long your break between episodes is, and when and where those breaks come.

If you are bipolar II, you have a 5 to 15 percent chance over 5 years of experiencing the kind of full-out manic episode that's referred to as "frank" mania, according to the *DSM.* If that happens, your diagnosis changes to bipolar I. Cyclothymia, which generally begins in adolescence or when you're a young adult, is even more likely to ramp up. The *DSM-IV* refers to it as having "an insidious onset and chronic course." If you're cyclothymic, your risk of developing bipolar I or II is anywhere between 15 and 50 percent.

One of the ways the course of bipolar disorder can be viewed actually takes off from the biology of epilepsy. This isn't quite as bizarre as it sounds; as you'll see in Chapter 6, some anticonvulsant medications do seem to have a mood-regulating effect on some people with bipolar disorder.

*I recently heard a story about someone whose bipolar symptoms started disappearing as he got older. Can that really happen? Is there such a thing as bipolar burn-out?*

"If you listen to anecdotes from friends and family, you might come to the conclusion that it's common to be cured of bipolar disorder. Some people can get completely well, but they will always be at risk of having another episode. Once you've had a single manic episode, there's a high likelihood—over 90 or 95 percent—of future episodes. Still, in some cases, perhaps up to one third of cases, people will have either no more episodes or very few episodes if they respond well to a mood stabilizer—usually lithium." —*S. Nassir Ghaemi, M.D., director of the Bipolar Disorder Research Program at Cambridge Health Alliance*

The seizures that characterize epilepsy are thought to get underway by a process called kindling. The kindling model of epilepsy holds that the first seizure a person has increases their likelihood of having another—and that the more frequent the seizures, the more severe they are. It's almost as if it's much easier for a neuron to misfire again and again and again after it's learned how to become hyperexcited the first time. In addition, although the first seizures might have a real trigger of some sort, eventually the brain's circuitry is simply so messed up that future seizures will happen without any outside prompting at all.

Just as the name suggests, kindling in the brain is like kindling in a fireplace. To get the fire started, you have to add a little something that makes it easier for the fire to catch in the first place. Once that blaze is roaring, though, it does just fine on its own. It doesn't really need your help any more. In fact, unless you keep an eye on it, the fire can actually get out of control.

On the surface, that's just how things appear to work in bipolar disorder—and mania in particular. After all, more than 9 out of 10 people who experience a single manic episode will go on to have others. In addition, although the first episode might be triggered by a reaction to some life event or stress, future episodes are more likely to just happen, to be spontaneously generated. These episodes definitely tend to get worse and worse over time, particularly if you go untreated or if the usual treatments fail you.

But although the picture fits on the surface, nobody yet knows if the basic biology of bipolar mania fits the biology of epilepsy. That's why, to most bipolar researchers, kindling is more metaphor than model. "I don't think it's right to say that bipolar disorders are a form of epilepsy," says Terence Ketter, chief of the Bipolar Disorders Clinic at Stanford University Medical School and an associate professor of psychology and behavioral science. "But the idea that it may be a progressive disorder, that it may go from being reactive to spontaneous, with episodes becoming more frequent and severe, and ultimately resistant to treatment, seems to be realistic."

Ghaemi notes that making the link between the two is difficult: Studies that might do so are difficult to undertake, and a number of anticonvulsants are ineffective in treating bipolar disorder, despite the fact that some are quite effective. "We're also not sure that they are more effective in lithium-nonresponding patients," Ghaemi says. "That all makes it much less clear-cut."

**... When Treated** Treatment with a mood stabilizer has a huge effect on the course of your disorder. It smoothes out the moods, makes the episodes shorter and less severe, and elongates the time between episodes. In the best of cases, it even seems to banish them completely.

But bipolar disorder is a recurring illness, especially if you're bipolar I, where you run as high as a 90 percent risk of having future episodes of either mania or depression, even if treated.

Rachael Bender, a graphic designer from Florida who was diagnosed with bipolar I in 2002, says that the sense of impending doom is something she really had to get used to. "The truth about bipolar is, even when you're on medication, you're going to

## GET PSYCHED

"If you treat and get ahead of this thing, and you don't have episode after episode after episode, you in fact can do exceedingly well." *—Terence Ketter, chief of the Bipolar Disorders Clinic at Stanford University Medical School*

relapse eventually. According to my doctor, the medicine makes it longer between episodes, and it will make it less intense, but it's going to happen.

"In my last manic episode, I was really sick for about six weeks. I couldn't work. I had to be watched all the time," she adds. "To think that that could happen again is really a scary thing. No matter how well you plan, it's something you can't control."

**... When Left Untreated** When bipolar goes untreated, you can almost think of it as a degenerative disease. Everything starts to go downhill, and it picks up speed as it goes. Your episodes are likely to get longer and closer together. You might find that your depressions are deeper and your manias more manic. You're more likely to become psychotic or to attempt suicide.

What little research has been done on untreated bipolar disorder patients seems to suggest that without lithium or some other maintenance treatment, you'll go through about four episodes a year and that the interval between the episodes will diminish as you get older.

But the truth, Ghaemi adds, is that we're probably never going to have a really clear picture of what untreated bipolar disorder looks like. That's a good thing, actually, because it means that it's hard to find truly untreated people to study these days. If you've been diagnosed with bipolar disorder—even if that diagnosis took decades—you'll almost always be given some kind of medication. Same with people who are misdiagnosed: whether you're called depressed, schizophrenic, or psychotic, you were likely put on some form of pharmacotherapy. And although that might enable a scientist to test theories about how drugs for other illnesses work on bipolar disorder or how bipolar disorder responds to being undertreated or inappropriately treated, it still doesn't address the issue of going completely untreated. Today, a classical case-controlled study in which you look at patients who are being treated for bipolar disorder and compare them to people who never have been and never will be treated would be both impossible and unethical.

## Long-Term Effects of Bipolar on the Body and the Brain

Bipolar disorder wears you down. Not only do you have to deal with the day-to-day issues of your disorder and the especially nasty side effects some bipolar medications have, but bipolar disorder actually puts you at risk of developing certain other diseases and conditions.

First and foremost are the so-called comorbid psychological conditions—mental disorders that exist side by side with your bipolar disorder. If you're living with bipolar, you are also more likely to have attention-deficit disorder, anxiety, obsessive-compulsive disorder, and borderline personality disorder. You're also somewhat more likely to develop Huntington's disease and possibly Tourette's syndrome as well. Researchers have made connections between asthma and bipolar disorder, and intriguingly, it seems that lithium treatments can actually improve the symptoms of asthma. According to renowned bipolar experts Frederick Goodwin, M.D., and Kay Redfield Jamison, Ph.D., there have even been some nonscientific reports from people who swear they are less susceptible to colds and flu when they are on lithium.

Bipolar disorder has also been linked to an increased risk of developing diabetes. In a study performed by researchers from Dalhousie University in Nova Scotia, bipolar patients with diabetes were more likely than those without diabetes to begin rapid cycling and have a chronic course to their illness. They were also older and heavier and had a higher rate of high blood pressure than did diabetes-free bipolar patients.

## What You Can Do

You've accepted your diagnosis and the fact that your disorder comes from a place deep within you—your brain, your genes, your body's biochemical machinations. You know what's inevitable about the course of your disease and what you can change. Now you need to figure out what to do with that information. Here are some ideas to get you started:

- [ ] Know your family history. Did Cousin Sue spend time in a hospital after a suicide attempt? Was Grandpa depressed? Did Mom have wild mood swings? Bipolar disorder has a strong genetic link, and knowing your family history will help your doctor make your diagnosis.

- [ ] Keep your stress levels low, because stress can definitely set off both manic and depressive episodes. Sometimes stress can be avoided, but for the times when it can't, try meditation, yoga, a jog or brisk walk, or even a late-afternoon nap to take the edge off.

- [ ] Talk to your psychiatrist or psychologist about the prognosis for your disorder. Come up with a plan for how to handle possible relapses or recurrences of the disorder.

- [ ] Keep track of the ebb and flow of your disorder, which episodes come when, how long they tend to last, and what happens next. Once you've experienced your own personal bipolar biorhythm for a while, you can make an educated guess as to what's coming and try to prepare for it, if not prevent it.

- [ ] Stop blaming yourself for having bipolar disorder. It's not your fault. Nor is it your mother's or your father's. None of us gets to pick and choose our genes. Use the energy you're expending on guilt to get yourself better and get yourself to a better place in your life.

- [ ] On the other hand, don't take the biological basis of the disorder as permission to take no responsibility for yourself and your actions. You can't change your biology, but you can try to stop it from destroying your life and the lives of those around you. You are not responsible for your disease, but you are responsible for yourself.

# Part 2
## Gaining Control

Now that you know what you're up against, what can you do about it? Bipolar disorder can't be cured, but it can be controlled. From medication to psychotherapy, from food to sleep, here's everything you'll need to know to regain your stability—and start gaining control over your life again.

# Navigating the Health-Care System

S omething is wrong. Something is very, very wrong. Maybe you haven't slept in weeks. Maybe your thoughts are swirling so quickly through your head that you can't follow your own train of thought. Maybe you're so deeply sad that you can barely drag yourself out of bed each morning.

Whatever it is, you need help, and you know it. But getting that help ... well, that's an entirely different story. You don't have insurance or you can't remember whether your insurance covers mental health problems. You don't know whether you need to go to a hospital or a clinic. You don't know whether you need a referral. You don't know how to find a doctor. You don't know what kind of doctor to look for in the first place.

There's a reason why people call it "navigating the health-care system." When you're in the midst of it, you may very well feel lost, in need of a map or a compass. In this chapter, I'll provide that map and help you get your bearings. In fact, feel free to consider this chapter your own personal mental health care sherpa.

## Finding the Right Doctors

It's hard enough to admit to yourself you have a problem, much less admit it to a stranger—even if that stranger does have an M.D. beside his or her name. But to get help, that's exactly what you have to do. You have to admit you need help, and you have to seek it.

Unfortunately, admitting to a problem and seeking help is only the first step. In most places in the United States, finding a doctor is easy—you can't throw a metaphorical stick without hitting a physician. But finding one who specializes in bipolar disorder—and not only that, but one with whom you click, in whom you are willing to entrust your care, not to mention one who has openings for new patients and accepts your insurance or is willing to work with you to defray costs—well, that's a horse of an entirely different color.

It should come as no surprise that one of the biggest and highest barriers to getting the best possible care you can for your disorder is your insurance company. What you need—a highly trained specialist in bipolar disorder who you will see often and who will spend a lot of time with you and prescribe whatever the most effective medication may be for your situation—is usually at odds with what your insurance company is willing to pay for. It's difficult to push for what you need when you hardly have any strength left, but it's worth it. The right doctor and the right medications are worth their weight in gold.

## GET PSYCHED

"Many people worry about seeing a doctor to talk about mental health issues. Some think they will be labeled 'crazy' or that they will be judged. ... This is not true, and you are not 'crazy.' Seeking help is the best thing you can do for yourself, and the best way to start feeling better."
—"Finding a Mental Health Professional: A Personal Guide," from the Depression and Bipolar Support Alliance

When you do get to see a doctor, whatever her stripe, remember that you are no different than any other patient she sees. You are entitled to privacy and confidentiality. You are entitled to know—and understand—what your diagnosis is and what your options are for treatment. If you have special religious or cultural needs, those should be respected as well.

In a world of skyrocketing costs and managed care, it's sometimes easy to forget that you are the customer. Your doctors work for you—it is their job to help you to the best of their abilities, and it is your job to be sure your rights are protected and your needs are taken care of. You deserve nothing less.

Still, it can seem almost perverse that at a time when you're at your most vulnerable, you're supposed to find the strength and presence of mind to look up referrals and check credentials and listen to recommendations. But that's exactly what you need to do.

> **Of course, if you're having such a hard time that you're feeling suicidal, forget about referrals and credentials and recommendations. Call 911 or 1-800-SUICIDE (1-800-784-2433) so you can get the immediate help you need.**

The best way to figure out just whom you should be seeing, or what kind of help you need, is to consider what you're seeking help for. Do you think you might need to be hospitalized? Do you need medication? If so, you'll need an M.D.—either a psychiatrist or another physician who has experience in bipolar disorder—who has admitting privileges and the ability to write prescriptions. Do you need to work through some thorny problems in your relationship with your spouse or your parents? A psychologist or therapist or clinical social worker might fit the bill.

If you're really knowledgeable about the field of mental health, you might be able to take this one step further—to pinpoint what kind of specific psychotherapy you need and look for a clinician who specializes in it (see Chapter 8). Once you've done that, you can start to do your actual search.

You can also use physician-referral services, either by making a phone call or by accessing an online search engine that can pinpoint a psychiatrist or therapist by zip code or general area.

Some of these services, such as the following, are sponsored by professional societies and provide referrals to credentialed members of their organizations:

## GET PSYCHED

"The ability to deal with your doctor is a skill that is acquired over time. After being in the hospital five times and dealing with several doctors, I've realized that there is one key ingredient to establishing a wonderful relationship with him/her: the truth. Speak nothing but the truth to your doctor. Let him know absolutely everything. He's there to help, he's there to help you avoid having to come back, and he's there to improve your life in the long run." —Shay Villere, author of The Bipolar Disorder Manual, www.mental-health-matters.com/articles/article.php?artID=550

- The American Medical Association, where you can get referrals to physicians by name or specialty by calling 312-464-5000 or going to www.ama-assn.org/ama/pub/category/3158.html.

- The American Psychiatric Association, through which you can locate your state or district association by calling 1-888-357-7924 or going to www.psych.org.

- The American Psychological Association, where you can get a referral to a psychologist by calling 1-800-964-2000, or get the phone number for your state's chapter by going to www.apa.org/practice/refer.html.

- The American Association of Marriage and Family Therapists, where you can search for a local therapist by going to www.aamft.org/therapistlocator/index.htm or calling 703-838-9808.

- The American Mental Health Counselors Association, which has partnered with Provisions Consulting to put together a therapist referral service you can find at 67.100.221.186:8080/default.htm, or by clicking the links at www.amhca.org.

- The National Association of Social Workers, where you can find a clinical social worker in your area by calling 1-800-638-8799, going to search.socialworkers.org, or clicking on the links at www.naswdc.org.

Other organizations provide referral services as part of their outreach to the community:

- The Depression and Bipolar Support Alliance, at www.dbsalliance.org/Resources/Referral.html can provide physician referrals to bipolar specialists. You can also get patient-recommended doctors' names at www.dbsalliance.org/referral/search.asp.

- Harvard's Bipolar Research Program Referral Database includes physicians from all over the country and can be found at 64.95.78.5/partners-mgh/bipolar.

- www.psychologytoday.com provides a comprehensive find-a-therapist directory searchable by specialty, geographic location, and other features. Selection is aided by profiles enabling patient-therapist matching by multiple criteria.
- AtHealth.com/Consumer includes a therapist locator service.
- 1-800-THERAPIST is a psychotherapist locator service that also has a website at www.1-800-therapist.com.

This, of course, is not a comprehensive list. And you should be aware, when calling one of them, that not all therapists and physicians are covered by every insurance plan, nor are all always accepting new patients. Still, these lists should give you a head-start on what might otherwise be a completely disorienting experience.

## Who Should Make Your Diagnosis?

With no blood chemical to measure or gene to screen for, the diagnosis of bipolar disorder relies on the keen eye and ear of the mental health professional—preferably someone with experience in the diagnosis and treatment of mood disorders. In most cases, that means an M.D., specifically a psychiatrist.

That's not to say it's a bad idea to go to a general practitioner (GP) if you're feeling uneasy about symptoms you're experiencing. It's just important to be—and remain—aware of the limitations of a GP's training and the potential for misdiagnosis.

What a family physician or internist can do is point you in the right direction. Rather than go to your "regular" doctor with a list of symptoms, looking for a diagnosis, you might want to simply request a referral to a qualified psychiatrist—one who has been certified by the American Board of Psychiatry and Neurology.

If there's no one in your area who fits the bill, a psychologist should also be able to make a proper diagnosis. Psychologists can't prescribe medication, so they need to work with an M.D. to initiate the proper therapy.

**WEB TALK:** Find out if your physician is board-certified by checking with the American Board of Medical Specialties:

▲ www.abms.org

Another option for finding the right doctor is to seek advice from people who have been there. Organizations such as the Depression and Bipolar Support Alliance (DBSA), the National Alliance for the Mentally Ill (NAMI), and the Depression and Related Affective Disorders Association (DRADA) can often point you in the direction of a practitioner who has helped others in the organization. There are also literally dozens of online discussion groups that can give you the invaluable benefit of personal experience (see Chapter 12).

## When to Get a Second Opinion

Because the nature of the relationship between patient and doctor is especially important in mental health conditions, not every doctor is the one for you; not every therapist "fits." Among your rights as a patient is the right to pursue a second opinion if you're unsure about the care you're getting from your current doctor.

Deciding you want a second opinion is one thing; getting one is another entirely. The best way to find the right doctor for a second opinion is to get recommendations from people in the know. Some clinics actually specialize in providing a second look at mental disorders: the University of Chicago's Department of Psychiatry, for instance, has an Adult Consultation/Second Opinion Program that provides a review of your treatment; the development of a new, individualized plan; and a full psychiatric evaluation.

Terence Ketter, chief of the Bipolar Disorders Clinic at Stanford University Medical School, says he does a lot of second opinions, especially in cases where treatment isn't going well or the person in question has "atypical" symptoms. And then, of course, there are a fair number of people who simply have a hard time accepting the diagnosis and its stigma, connotations, and burdensome, side-effect-laden drug therapies.

If you're having trouble finding the right doctor for your second opinion, you can always ask your current doctor for a recommendation, as he or she is likely to know who his or her peers are. But this can be uncomfortable for many people, especially when you're talking about a second opinion for the treatment of a mental illness such as bipolar disorder, rather than for a more objective plan such as cancer treatment, for example.

*I like my doctor … a lot. I trust her. But I worry that I'm doing things wrong. Am I supposed to get a second opinion on my diagnosis or my treatment?*

"There's certainly nothing wrong with it, but if you've been properly diagnosed and you're responding to treatment easily, it really doesn't seem all that necessary. In fact, in some instances, seeking additional opinions may be counterproductive as it can delay appropriate treatment." —*Terence Ketter, chief of the Bipolar Disorders Clinic at Stanford University Medical School*

Once you decide to go for it, you'll also want to be sure your insurance will cover a second set of eyes and ears. Not all do, and they're not required to. That doesn't mean you can't get a second opinion anyway; it just means you might have to pay for it yourself.

## Getting—and Staying—Insured

For most people, having to pay out of pocket—be it for a second opinion, a first opinion, a hospitalization, or a drug prescription—would be ruinous. And thus mental health insurance was born to fill a void and meet a need. Today, well over half the people in the United States are covered to some degree by mental health insurance. But those numbers aren't nearly high enough.

NAMI—the National Alliance for the Mentally Ill—agrees. NAMI calls itself "the Nation's Voice on Mental Illness." In a recent survey of visits to its website in August 2003, NAMI noted that nearly 20 percent of its visitors were uninsured. More than half were covered by private health insurance paid (at least in part) by their employer. Another near-20 percent were paying for their own insurance out of pocket.

It was in talking specifically about mental health benefits that the survey results became truly disturbing. Just 17 percent of people with private health insurance were happy with the way it covered mental health treatment. A quarter of the people responding said they or someone they loved had trouble getting private health insurance because of a mental illness. And another quarter reported avoiding private insurance—staying unemployed, enrolling in Medicaid—because they knew they wouldn't be able to get adequate coverage for a mental illness. "Clearly discrimination in the field of private health insurance is a major problem within our nation's troubled mental health system," a NAMI report on the survey states.

Stephanie, a 40-year-old public relations writer who is living with bipolar disorder, agrees and adds that the discrimination isn't limited to health care. "When I list my medications on life-insurance forms or long-term disability forms, even though I was never hospitalized and I don't mention the suicide attempts, I am always turned down," she reports. "Because I am bipolar. Who knows what *she* might do?"

One solution to this problem, mental health advocates say, is *mental health insurance parity*, guaranteeing that mental illness is covered by insurance at the same level as other diseases. Do this, they say, and many of these issues melt away. Or at least they should.

Of course, this is not something you can do on your own. It's a political and legislative approach to ending discrimination against mental health care by insurers.

In reality, true mental health insurance parity isn't nearly as simple as it should be.

## PsychSpeak

People asking for **mental health insurance parity** are asking for mental health insurance that is equal in function to physical health insurance.

In 1996, the U.S. federal government enacted the Mental Health Parity Act, which made employers with more than 50 employees responsible for offering mental health insurance if they offer group health insurance, and that mental health insurance was to be capped no lower than the cap on physical illness. If your insurance put an overall lifetime cap of $1 million for physical illnesses such as diabetes and cancer and heart disease, for instance, it couldn't then put a cap of $50,000 on your mental health coverage, as was often the case.

It was, if nothing else, a start. But there were flaws. Big, gaping flaws. Flaws you could drive a truck through. For instance, although the caps had to be equal, the co-payments and deductibles and treatment limits didn't. And if the group health plan being used by a company didn't offer mental health coverage, the company wouldn't be forced to switch to one that did. And if your employer "believes" that adding mental health coverage to its insurance menu would drive up costs more than 1 percent, they could ask for an exemption from the law.

Today, NAMI and a large number of other organizations are fighting for newer, more extensive legislation—the Senator Paul Wellstone Mental Health Equitable Treatment Act has bipartisan support in both the House and Senate, as well as the stated support of President George W. Bush. "Our health insurance system must treat serious mental illness like any other disease," Bush stated in an April 2002 speech.

The pro-parity groups—which of course include essentially every mental health organization you can think of—point out that differentiating between mental and "physical" illnesses is based on nothing more substantial than ignorance, prejudice, and fear. "There is simply no scientific or medical justification for insurance coverage of mental-illness treatment to be on different terms and conditions than other diseases," notes a NAMI policy statement.

There is no real financial justification, either. A 1997 study from the National Institute of Mental Health and published in the *Journal of the American Medical Association* found that removing the cap on

## GET PSYCHED

"As the nation's largest organization representing individuals living with mental illness and their families, NAMI believes strongly that mental illnesses are real illnesses, that treatment works, and that there is no medical or economic justification for health plans to cover treatment on different terms and conditions." —*NAMI Policy Issue Spotlight, January 2004*

mental health benefits would cost employers offering a group managed-care insurance approximately $1 per enrollee. That's right: a single dollar bill per person on the plan.

"This research informs the debate over how much it would cost under the Mental Health Parity Act to provide insurance coverage for treatment of mental illnesses that is equal to that for other medical conditions," stated then–NIMH director Steven E. Hyman, M.D.

**Limits on Care and Services**  In 1999, David Satcher, M.D., then–Surgeon General of the United States, put together the first-ever Surgeon General's Report on Mental Health, a 500-page look at the issues in the diagnosis and treatment of mental illness.

"My message to Americans is this: If you, or a loved one, are experiencing what you believe might be the symptoms of a mental disorder, do not hesitate to seek effective treatment now," Satcher stated in a press release announcing the report's publication. "Insist on the kinds of services that this report makes clear can and should be available."

## PsychSpeak

An **employee assistance program (EAP)** is a program that offers professional support and education to employees who are trying to cope with emotional or behavioral problems that might have an effect on job performance. Oftentimes, an EAP allows you a certain number of visits, then, if further help is needed, provides you with a referral to an outside therapist covered by your insurance.

Limits, the report notes, can be both overt and covert. A health insurance plan that provides you with coverage to see the kind of psychiatric professional you need is a good thing, in concept. But if you're not comfortable talking about what your problems are to get the name of the right doctor for you, it's not going to do you much practical good. An employer who provides an *employee assistance program* (*EAP*) or an association that puts together an off-site, anonymous referral hotline are simple, relatively inexpensive ways to get past the stigma of mental illness and your fears of repercussions should you admit to having bipolar disorder.

Providing quality care is yet another area in which different insurance plans might have very different approaches. For example, one study has shown that although most managed-care insurance companies allow for a follow-up visit to a doctor after hospitalization for depression, some do a better job of communicating and even pushing that point than do others. In fact, the percentage of patients in that same study who took advantage of that follow-up visit varied from 30 percent in one plan to a whopping 92 percent in another. As with everything else, some insurance companies are better than others, even though they all operate in the same basic health-care climate.

**Getting Access to New Treatments**  Over the last couple years, there has been a veritable downpour of new, effective medications for the treatment of bipolar disorder. Others are in the pipeline, poised to hit the market as soon as the FDA gives them the nod (see Chapter 6).

But just because a new drug is available doesn't mean it's available to you—especially if you're looking to a private insurance company to buy the drug for you. The newest drugs are generally also the most expensive, priced to quickly reap a profit for the pharmaceutical firm that pumped millions and millions of dollars into its development and testing. Although you might have heard great things about lamotrigine or quietapine (see Chapter 6) and discussed them with your doctor, your insurance company is more likely to push Haldol or Thorazine your way, because they are significantly cheaper to buy.

Why is this a problem? If you've taken any of the older drugs, you'll know why—although oftentimes effective, they're burdened with a huge number of sometimes truly debilitating side effects. Burdensome side effects are among the very top causes of noncompliance with medication, and medication noncompliance almost always has some nasty results. On the other hand, when good treatments for mental illness are accessible and tolerable, NAMI says, their success rates beat those of the drugs fighting diabetes and heart disease.

The problem becomes even more complicated when you consider the fact that many of the drugs that are useful in treating bipolar disorder aren't approved for that specific use, but rather for other uses, such as treating epilepsy. It's perfectly fine and legal for your doctor to prescribe them to you "off label," as it's called, but oftentimes insurance companies will refuse to cover such prescriptions, claiming that the drugs are "experimental."

If you feel you're being denied the best treatment for your disorder, you do have options. Almost all insurance policies have an appeals or grievance procedure you can follow. Although you might find it difficult to get the information, the insurance company is supposed to provide you with the details on how to file a grievance or a complaint. If you're not satisfied with the response you get from that complaint, you're also well within your rights to take that complaint "outside"—to contact government agencies, your employer, your union, even the media. Whether those appeals will be successful is anybody's guess, but you do have the right to give it a shot.

If you've got the time and energy to really try to make a difference, you can channel your dissatisfaction into advocacy, joining groups such as NAMI and the National Mental Health Association in their attempts to get enacted legislation that protects your right to appeal the insurance companies' decisions, have access to adequate treatment and health-care providers, and more.

## Know Your Rights

In fact, the attempt to protect these rights—and addressing the many other specific needs of people who have to wade through the added layers of bureaucracy that often surround the mental health field—has led to an impressive show of strength from a large number of professional organizations involved in the mental health field. A group of nine professional associations—the American Psychiatric Association, the American Psychological Association, the American Association for Marriage and Family Therapy, the American Counseling Association, the American

Family Therapy Academy, the American Nurses Association, the American Psychiatric Nurses Association, the Clinical Social Work Federation, and the National Association of Social Workers—put together a document they call the "Mental Health Patient's Bill of Rights: Principles for the Provision of Mental Health and Substance Abuse Treatment Services." Six other prominent groups in the field have also lent their names in support of the principles.

The rights set out in this document are simple but empowering. If you are a mental health patient, you have the right to ...

- Know and understand the mental health benefits your insurance company or employer provides.
- Know any relevant information about the professionals from whom you're receiving treatment and to be informed of your treatment options and how effective they might or might not be.
- Be told of any contractual arrangements the insurance company has with your mental health provider, especially those that might play a role in treatment decisions, and to know just what information your clinician might provide to the insurance company to be paid.
- File a complaint or grievance against your health-care provider and to understand how to do so.
- Protection of your confidentiality to the full extent of the law and have any disclosures made only with your informed consent.
- Choose any licensed or certified professional to provide you with the mental health services you need.
- Have treatment recommendations made only by a licensed and certified professional and have treatment decisions made by you and your family, not by your insurance company.
- Have the same sorts of benefits for mental health and substance abuse treatment as you do for any other illness.

**WEB TALK:** Read the entire Bill of Rights online at:

www.apa.org/pubinfo/rights/rights.html

- Be protected from discrimination or penalties based on your disorder when you're looking for other health insurance or any other insurance benefits.
- Use the "full scope" of the benefits offered to address your needs.
- Receive the maximum level of protection and access to care.
- Have your treatment claims reviewed by professionals with adequate training and credentials, as well as someone without a financial interest in the outcome.
- Have your clinician held accountable in case of incompetence or negligence, have that clinician advocate on your behalf if payment is denied, and be able to hold your insurance company accountable for "any injury caused by gross incompetence or negligence or by their clinically unjustified decisions."

The idea of rights, of civil liberties, comes with a bit of baggage. After all, there are people who say that some people with extreme bipolar disorder are not in any condition to make certain choices or decisions on their own.

The possibility that impaired judgment might cloud decision-making has given rise to a not-for-profit organization called the Treatment Advocacy Center. It works "to eliminate barriers to timely treatment of severe mental illness" by getting legislation enacted that allows for involuntary outpatient treatment of people whose illness has all but run away with them. (The practice is called assisted outpatient treatment, or AOT.)

The Treatment Advocacy Center is considerably controversial. Critics say it is authoritarian and paternalistic, attempting to wrest the freedom of choice from legally empowered adults. But Jonathan Stanley, J.D., assistant director of the center, disagrees. "We can't take the freedom of choice away from people with severe mental illness. We don't *want* to do that," he says. "These laws only come into play once the person has lost that freedom already—to the illness."

He would know: Stanley has been living with bipolar disorder for 18 years—a bipolar disorder that got so severe he was hospitalized for almost 7 weeks at the age of 19 (see the following "You're Not Alone" sidebar).

Stanley says that the TAC's crowning achievement was the passage of New York's Kendra's Law in 1999. The law allows for family members to petition a court for AOT when a family member or loved one meets a number of requirements, including refusing to take medications, having been hospitalized at least twice in the past three years or having threatened, attempted, or perpetrated some violence in the past 4 years because of the symptoms of their mental illness, and being a potential risk to the safety of him- or herself and others. "Another key requirement," adds Stanley, "is that without AOT the person's condition will deteriorate to the point where there is 'a substantial risk of physical harm to the consumer or others.'"

Obviously, Kendra's Law and others like it are a last resort. The requirements for getting a legal petition to mandate outpatient treatment vary by state, Stanley notes, and require different levels of proof and requirements that must be met.

"What these laws generally do is require you to maintain your treatment in the community," Stanley explains. "You might be required to see your case manager a couple of times a week, or see a psychiatrist a couple of times a month. It's actually much less onerous to be on one of these outpatient laws than to be inside a hospital or a jail because of something your illness caused you to do."

**WEB TALK:** For more information on Kendra's Law and others like it, visit the Treatment Advocacy Center at:

▲ www.psychlaws.org

# Forcing the Issue

Jonathan Stanley joined the Treatment Advocacy Center in the early 1990s. But in reality, he says, his advocacy began a decade earlier, when he found himself standing, stark naked, on a plastic milk crate in the middle of a grocery store on the Lower East Side of Manhattan.

Jon was 19. He'd been experiencing the symptoms of bipolar illness for a couple years and even had a prescription for lithium but had chosen not to take medication. When his psychotic "break" occurred, he says, he'd been visiting a girlfriend in New York, as manic as he'd ever been. She had taken him to the airport to catch a plane to a wrestling match he was supposed to participate in, but once at the airport, Jon "realized" he was being followed by secret agents from the Navy. "The paranoia came sweeping in like a tidal wave," he recalls.

The girlfriend "freaked out," Jon says, and left the airport. Thus began a three-day journey in which Jon says he never slept and never ate but simply ran from the people he just knew were pursuing him. At the end of it all, he wound up in that grocery store, where he became convinced that the floor was "seething" with deadly radiation. He jumped up on the milk crate, he says, because it was plastic and would insulate him from the rays. He stripped naked, he says, because his clothes were wet and attracting the radiation to his body.

"The two Korean ladies in the deli were not overly thrilled with how this was coming down," Jon says with a characteristic wryness. "So soon after that, a couple of police officers came. I thank them, because they didn't take me to jail. I was so obviously mentally ill that they knew I needed a psychiatric hospital."

After that, Jon admits, his memory gets a little "sketchy." Jon was put on large doses of Haldol in an attempt to take him down from his psychosis. "And take me down they did," he says, recalling the dark days that followed.

The doctors at the emergency psychiatric unit told Jon's parents that, as sick as he was, he was not a threat to anyone but himself and they would only be able to hold him for 72 hours unless Jon were to voluntarily commit himself. Terrified of what might happen to their son, Jon's parents knew they had to get Jon to sign the admission forms.

"My dad told me that we went into a room and I signed a voluntary admission form." Jon laughs: "I'd love to see the signature on that form."

It was that signed form, and the parents who made sure it got signed, to which Jon says he owes his life—a life in which he went on to earn a law degree, got married, and is fighting to make a difference in the lives of other people like him. On medication, Jon Stanley hasn't had a single psychotic episode or experienced any of the major symptoms of his disease in almost 15 years.

"When we talk about laws requiring treatment, we're talking about the most chronically mentally ill people, people like me who lose themselves to the illness," Jon says. "When you're lost in your delusions, when you're psychotic, well, I think it's society's obligation to get you into treatment and make you better."

## Other Sources of Financial Help

It's a fact of life for millions of Americans: no health insurance, or insurance that's woefully inadequate to deal with an illness that requires expensive drugs, regular laboratory workups, and ongoing clinician oversight the way bipolar disorder can.

If you're one of these people, what are your options? First, keep in mind that you're not the only person in this situation, so don't be afraid to mention it to your doctor. Many will have sliding fee scales for people based on their income and level of insurance coverage.

You could also investigate the hospitals and clinics in your area. Many county or public hospitals offer free or low-cost care, for instance. If you're a veteran, contact your local Veteran's Administration office. Consider the possibility of using a clinic run by a charity or a religious organization, as they oftentimes provide free health care as well. And don't forget to check out your local medical school, if there is one. They are all affiliated with teaching hospitals, where care is often less expensive or scaled based on ability to pay. Many will also run clinics, including mental health clinics, that provide low-cost care.

If you're employed, you might be able to opt for a medical savings account, in which you'd put aside a set percentage of your salary—pre-tax—to be used for any medical bills not covered by insurance, including co-payments, prescriptions, and more.

## PsychSpeak

A **formulary** is a list of prescription drugs covered by a specific health plan. If a drug is not on a company's formulary, they generally won't cover its costs.

Of all the hurdles you have to get over, getting the drugs you need might be the highest, most difficult of them all. Even if you are insured, many insurance plans have limited *formularies* and don't cover new or experimental pharmaceuticals.

Once again, don't be embarrassed to ask for help. If money is a short-term problem, your doctor might simply give you samples pharmaceutical company representatives have left behind on sales visits. Over the longer term, there are programs that can help bring down the costs of medication for you. For instance, some companies will fill and mail-order your prescriptions for what might be a huge price reduction from your local pharmacy. You definitely want to be careful when dealing with these sorts of businesses, which can be found in places from A to Z: from Tucson, Arizona, to Zurich, Switzerland. Although some are quite legitimate, others can be less so. Still, if you do your research, you can probably save a very pretty penny.

For those who qualify in terms of income level and other parameters, prescription-drug assistance programs might also be available. These programs, sponsored by the pharmaceutical companies, offer either free or low-cost prescription drugs— usually in limited quantities—to people who are not insured or can't otherwise afford them.

WEB TALK: For more information and a copy of the PhRMA directory of companies with assistance programs, go to:

➔ www.helpingpatients.org

These companies, all members of Pharmaceutical Research and Manufacturers of America (PhRMA), have patient assistance programs that cover at least one drug you might be prescribed if you're living with bipolar disorder.

## Patient Assistance Programs

| Company | Product | Program Name | Contact |
|---|---|---|---|
| Abbott Laboratories | Depakote | Abbott Laboratories Patient Assistance Program | 1-800-222-6885 |
| GlaxoSmithKline | Lamictal, Paxil, Wellbutrin | Bridges to Access; Orange Card | 1-866-PATIENT (1-866-728-4368); 1-888-ORANGE6 (1-888-672-6436) |
| Janssen Pharmaceutica | Risperdal | The Risperdal Patient Assistance and Reimbursement Support Program; Senior Patient Assistance Program | 1-800-652-6227; 1-888-294-2400 |
| Eli Lilly and Company | Prozac, Zyprexa, Symbyax | Lilly Cares/Zyprexa PAP; LillyAnswers Card | 1-800-545-6962; 1-877-RX-LILLY |
| Novartis Pharmaceuticals | Clozaril, Tegretol, Trileptal | Novartis Pharmaceuticals Corporation Patient Assistance Program | 1-800-277-2254 |
| Ortho-McNeil Pharmaceutical | Haldol, Topamax | Ortho-McNeil Patient Assistance Program | 1-800-577-3788 |
| Pfizer | Geodon, Navane, Neurontin, Zoloft | Connection to Care Patient Assistance Program; Share Card | 1-800-707-8990; 1-800-717-6005 |
| Wyeth Pharmaceuticals | Effexor | Wyeth Patient Assistance Program | 1-800-568-9938 |
| Together RX (Abbott, AstraZeneca, Aventis, Bristol-Myers Squibb, GlaxoSmithKline, Johnson & Johnson, Novartis) | Many different products | Together RX | 1-800-865-7211 |

101

# What You Can Do

No one would deny that the health-care system has its downfalls, and those downfalls are only accentuated when you're talking about mental health. Still, you can and should do a number of things to help yourself—apply to programs, take advantage of services, accept help—that often go underutilized simply because not enough people know about them. Take advantage; take what's coming to you. Get the most out of what's available, and you're likely to get the best care possible.

- ☐ If possible, get a referral to a specialist—preferably a board-certified psychiatrist—and check on his or her credentials.

- ☐ Check out one of the myriad physician referral services available to find a doctor or clinician in your neighborhood or someone who specializes in providing the kind of help you need.

- ☐ Find out what your insurance plan covers with regard to mental health treatment—and what you need to do to be sure that coverage is and remains in effect.

- ☐ Investigate—and take advantage of—services provided by your city, county, and state to reduce health-care costs. Find out which local agencies serve your needs and what services they provide.

- ☐ Educate yourself on your legal rights in your state. What are the provisions for mental health insurance parity? Does your state have an assisted outpatient treatment law such as Kendra's Law?

- ☐ Support mental health insurance parity legislation by writing to your senators or congresspeople, getting involved in a local advocacy group, or simply spreading the word.

- ☐ Know how to file a grievance or complaint against your insurance company—and then follow through if necessary.

- ☐ Contact the manufacturers of your prescription drugs to see if they have a patient assistance program that can help you lower your out-of-pocket drug costs.

# The Bipolar Medicine Chest

The treatment of bipolar disorder usually begins with a pill. It doesn't end there, not by a long shot, but without the use of a *psychopharmaceutical*, a *psychotropic drug*, most of the rest of the therapies are virtually useless. Trying to provide you with cognitive behavioral techniques when you can't string together two coherent sentences is a waste of time. Trying to get a handle on the issues underlying your depression when you're so apathetic you can't even begin to verbalize them is a waste of breath.

But once you're on a drug—the right drug—the sky's the limit. A good, effective medication will work on the basic machinery in your brain's cells, helping bring any wayward responses back into line. Once your nervous system has been reset to a less sensitive state, your brain will be primed for techniques that can help you get the most out of your everyday life.

Of course, there's no magic bullet for bipolar disorder. Even if you get the disorder under control, you're likely to have to take medications for the rest of your life to prevent the disease from coming back. And yes, you're going to have to give up some of the highs that are so alluring. And yes, you're likely going to have to soldier through some unpleasant side effects—although you can and should work with your doctor to find the drug or drugs that give you the best results with the fewest side effects possible.

The good news? More and more options exist for you. Lithium is no longer the only game in town for stabilizing mood, although it is still a very effective, very useful therapy. New drugs are hitting the market all the time—and they are getting better and better at doing what they do. In fact, if you're willing to put up with a few potential ups and downs, or to consider taking more than one medication to treat your disorder, there's no reason not to look forward to the best "best results" imaginable.

## PsychSpeak

Psychopharmaceuticals or **psychotropic drugs** are chemical compounds that affect your mental state by acting on your mind.

**The information presented in this chapter is for educational purposes only. Please talk to your physician or health-care professional about which medications might be beneficial for you and follow his or her dosage recommendations. Work with your physician, and report any unusual side effects or concerns you have about any medications you are taking. Do not stop taking or change the dosage of any prescription drugs you are taking without first discussing it with your physician.**

# Why Pharmaceuticals Are So Important

Bipolar disorder has biological roots; it seems to come, at least in part, from an oversensitivity of the brain's nerve cells to the signals and chemicals that bombard them. Treating bipolar disorder, then, means somehow damping this sensitivity, recalibrating the way in which the nerve cells transmit messages to one another.

These biological roots go deep. You cannot will away bipolar disorder any more than you can will away cancer. And in most cases, you can no more get better without the use of some physical or biological treatment than a diabetic can control his or her blood sugar without the use of insulin.

Yet if you're bipolar, there's about a 50 percent chance you will, at some point, try to do just that. Even after struggling to be diagnosed and find just the right doctor to treat you, you're more likely than not to give up on your meds at one point or another.

Why? It could be because you're in denial that there's anything wrong with you. It could be because you're feeling so much better that you're pretty certain you're cured. It could be because you're starting to relapse into mania, and that lack of insight is once again rearing its ugly head.

It could be that you're just plain tired of popping pills every day, of having to stare your disorder in the face so wearyingly often, never getting to be "normal." As actress Carrie Fisher, who has made no secret of her battles with bipolar disorder, told *Psychiatry Today* in a November/December 2001 interview, "I'm on seven medications, and I take medication three times a day. This constantly puts me in touch with the illness I have. I'm never quite allowed to be free of that for a day."

Or it could simply be that the side effects are finally getting to you. There is, undeniably, an array of side effects with most of the drugs that work best against this disorder. It's not surprising that you might toy with the idea of just chucking it all.

You're not alone. One of the biggest problems in the treatment of almost every chronic disease is medication compliance, and bipolar disorder is no exception. It's also no exception when it comes to how dangerous that drug-halting decision can be. Discontinuing your medication is the number-one risk factor for having a relapse into mania or depression. And if you cease your medication abruptly, without going through a few weeks of weaning or tapering down, you're even more likely

## GET PSYCHED

"We encourage patients very strongly to expect a full remission of symptoms and not to be satisfied simply with a response, not to be satisfied simply with a change. We are looking to achieve full remission. We want them to be looking for that same kind of treatment effect." —*Ellen Frank, Ph.D., director of the Depression and Manic Depression Prevention Program at the Western Psychiatric Institute and Clinic*

to relapse—as well as to commit suicide—than those who go off their medications slowly.

It was this focus—the idea that only once your symptoms are under control can you really begin to work through the other issues brought forward by this disorder—that prompted the National Institute of Mental Health to fund the creation of the Systematic Treatment Enhancement Program for Bipolar Disorder, otherwise known as STEP-BD, in 2001.

Headed by Gary Sachs, M.D., from Massachusetts General Hospital, STEP-BD is an ongoing 5-year outpatient study aimed at looking at as many as 5,000 people with bipolar disorder to find out precisely which treatments, in which combinations, can stop depression and mania from coming back after they've been overcome.

Currently, nearly 20 sites across the United States are participating in the STEP-BD program. If you're interested in volunteering for one of these ongoing studies, or to find a site near you, call 1-866-240-3250 or e-mail stepbd@mailcity.com.

## Mood Stabilizers

There is no such thing as a mood stabilizer—at least not in strict pharmaceutical terms. In fact, the most recent revision of the American Psychiatric Association's guidelines for the treatment of bipolar disorder omits the term entirely because of "the absence of a consensus definition."

S. Nassir Ghaemi, M.D., director of the Bipolar Disorder Research Program at Cambridge Health Alliance, agrees: "The U.S. Food and Drug Administration does not approve anything as a mood stabilizer, which is a clinical term we psychiatrists, not the federal government, have invented."

Still, stabilizing your mood—no matter which pole you're currently at—is the true goal of any drug treatment you might take for bipolar disorder. If a mood stabilizer is truly effective, it will accomplish its balancing act without pushing you toward the opposite pole. In other words, a mood stabilizer needs to be able to bring you down from mania without causing depression, as well as bring you up from depression without making you manic. It would be even better if it could prevent you from developing future episodes of mania or depression as well—or at least reduce the number of episodes you have to swing through.

**Q&A**

*What is a mood stabilizer?*

A mood stabilizer, says S. Nassir Ghaemi, M.D., director of the Bipolar Disorder Research Program at Cambridge Health Alliance, is any treatment that works against two of the following three areas in bipolar disorder: acute mania, acute depression, or prevention of mania and depression. In other words, a drug that puts the brakes on mania and also works to prevent a new mood episode would be a mood stabilizer. So would a treatment that relieves depression and prevents further mood episodes. Finally, anything that can both bring you down from mania and up from depression would be considered a mood stabilizer as well.

**What Is a Mood-Stabilizing Drug?** Different clinicians seem to consider different drugs as falling into the mood stabilization category. Lamotrigine, one of the newest anticonvulsants to show significant muscle power against bipolar disorder, is a mood stabilizer according to many of these physicians; others would add the anticonvulsants valproate (Depakote) and carbamazepine (Tegretol) to that list as well.

But there is one mood stabilizer that rises above the rest; only one that's generally considered by at least some in the field to fit neatly into this category. And that, of course, is lithium.

### Lithium

*Brand names:* Lithobid, Lithonate, Lithotabs, Lithane, Cibalith-S, Eskalith, Eskalith CR

*Form:* Tablet, extended-release tablet, capsule, syrup

*Common dosages:* Between 300 and 600 milligrams 3 times daily

*Side effects include:* Weakness, dry mouth, increased thirst, drowsiness, dizziness, fever, tremor, confusion, diarrhea, unsteady walking, frequent urination, vomiting, slow and jerky movements, slurred speech, blurred vision, ringing in the ears, convulsions, a fast or irregular pulse, poor memory, upset stomach, loss of appetite, stomach bloating, stomach pain, headache, weight gain

*How long will it take to work?* 4 to 10 days, although some-times more

When you think *bipolar,* you think *lithium.* After all, as Paul Keck, M.D., chief of the Division of Clinical Neuroscience at the University of Cincinnati Medical Center, pointed out at a scientific meeting, "Lithium remains a first-line treatment for people with bipolar illness for a good reason."

For quite some time, lithium was the only drug on the market that could get its arms around the symptoms of mania. What makes it even more useful is that it also seems, in many people, to be able to make depression less frequent and severe and to stave off future episodes of both mania and depression. In fact, a study of lithium conducted by Keck and colleagues just a few years ago showed that once the initial manic episode was over, it was still important to keep lithium in the picture. "The odds of relapse, if you weren't on lithium, were four-fold higher than if you were on lithium for one year," Keck noted.

If you remember your high-school chemistry, you might re-member that lithium is one of the elements on the periodic table. It's a salt that's been in use in medicine since the mid-1800s, when it was used to treat gout. But it wasn't until almost a cen-tury later, in 1948, that Australian psychiatrist John Frederick Joseph Cade discovered, quite serendipitously, that lithium has a calming effect on people experiencing mania. (An intriguing side note: soon after Cade showed lithium's effects in humans, it was found to be responsible for the deaths of several heart patients in whom it was being used as a salt substitute. The Food and Drug

Administration [FDA] promptly banned the use of lithium in the United States, and it was shelved for two decades, until 1970.)

Today, lithium is still often one of the first drugs given to patients diagnosed with mania and bipolar disorder. It's effective in 50 to 80 percent of the people who take it, depending on the studies you look at. It can take a few weeks for its effects to show, however, and might even require a little fiddling with dosages.

You're more likely to respond well to lithium if you have "classic" euphoric mania and if you're not a rapid cycler. If you have a strong family history of bipolar disorder or depression, lithium is more likely to be the drug for you. If you have a lot of depressive symptoms or an ongoing substance-abuse problem, you're less likely to get lithium's full benefits, although that is by no means assured.

> ## GET PSYCHED
>
> "Lithium saved my life. After just a few weeks on the drug, death-based thoughts were no longer the first I had when I got up and the last when I went to bed … I'm not a Stepford wife; I still feel the exultation and sadness that any person feels, I'm just not required to feel them 10 times as long or as intensively as I used to."
> —*Patty Duke, actress, in Psychology Today, August 2002*

Lithium's main downside is its toxicity: few if any people taking the drug escape its side effects. Frequent blood tests are required to check lithium blood levels and other possible physical changes; they are annoying at best. Still, says Ghaemi, lithium's usefulness is far from over.

"My prediction is that people will be surprised at how much lithium will be used in the future," he says. "It really seems to affect the brain in beneficial ways so that some of the things wrong in the brain are improved by structural changes in the brain that come with long-term lithium treatment. On one level, it makes neurons live longer. It makes them branch, makes them have the right kinds of connections with other neurons. We can show in patients with bipolar disorder that when you get an increase in the number of episodes, you get a decrease in brain size. But bipolar patients on lithium are indistinguishable from patients who don't have bipolar disorder."

**you're not alone**

## Noncompliance

Natalie's mom has never liked taking her medication. "She's always hated the lithium," Natalie says. "Not so much because it muted anything—she was happy to feel like she finally had control in her life, I think. But it was her bladder. It just did terrible things to her bladder. When she has to go to the bathroom, she has to go *right now*. God forbid you're more than a few steps away from one. She's had accidents more times than I think she'll even admit."

Lately, however, Natalie's mom has been acting "different." Or rather, says Natalie, her mom's been acting the same way she did almost two decades ago, when she was first diagnosed bipolar when Natalie was 14.

"She had terrible mood swings," Natalie recalls. "I can't even remember more than one of my friends she liked—she thought they were all looking at her, that they all hated her. She was terribly paranoid, and she had these serious depressions, to where she was almost unable to function.

"Her manic episodes were to spend exorbitant amounts of money, run up her credit cards, spend all the cash she had. She'd buy clothes upon clothes upon clothes upon clothes … all for herself. She took up all the closets in the house with stuff she bought.

"All of that really went away with lithium, however. It was all really heavenly for my four years of high school. But lately … well, a couple of times she's said something about my husband and I've just had to say, 'You know, mom, we're not going there. We're not going to talk about Peter, ever.'"

Natalie didn't realize what was going on for a while, until her mother started refusing to let Natalie into her house. (They live just blocks from one another.) "I think she's gone off her lithium—I think she's been off it for a couple of years now—and her house is a telltale symptom of that. She's doing eBay, garage sales … Every popup that comes on her computer screen to tell her she needs to buy something, she buys it. I get the impression you can't even walk in her house; I know she hasn't let me inside the door in two years."

Knowing her mom is off her meds is one thing, says Natalie, who's an only child. Being able to do something about it is another. "I know nowadays there are times when she's up for 72 hours at a time, when she starts hallucinating," Natalie sighs. "I just don't know how to go in there and say to her, 'You need help again.' But she does. I know she does."

In addition, Ghaemi says, both lithium and Depakote seem to actually protect brain cells from further damage.

Finally, he notes, lithium seems to reduce the risk of suicide. A 2003 study led by Frederick Goodwin, M.D., one of the world's leading experts on the illness, found that fewer people committed or attempted suicide when on lithium than when they were being treated with Depakote.

"Lithium is the only drug that reduces the risk of death by suicide by an odds ratio of six to one," says Ghaemi. "I can say to a patient, 'If you take this drug, you'll live longer.' This is the kind of benefit that will keep this drug around for years to come."

# Anticonvulsants

The other two prongs in what is currently the bipolar treatment triumvirate are both anticonvulsants. Just how these drugs, normally used for the treatment of epilepsy, are able to calm manias—and sometimes even lift depressions—is still unknown. The assumption seems to be that the wayward electrical circuitry in the brains of people with bipolar disorder is, at least on some level, related to the kinds of electrical firestorms created during epileptic seizures (see Chapter 4). This means the drugs that block these impulses to stop seizures should also be able to block the rapid firing of neurons that creates many of the symptoms of mania.

So far, that assumption seems to be pretty accurate. Intriguingly, however, not every drug that's effective against epilepsy is equally effective against bipolar disorder. Some anticonvulsants pack a powerful antimanic punch, while others are much less aggressive in their mania-squashing attempts. And at least one— lamotrigine, the newest of the group—is actually much more useful in battling the depression in manic-depression than it is in the fight against mania.

## Divalproex/Valproate/Valproic Acid

*Brand names:* Depakote, Depacon, Depakene

*Form:* Injection, capsules, delayed-release capsules, delayed-release tablets, syrup

*Common dosages:* 750 milligrams a day to start, divided into 2 or 3 doses; dosage can be increased as needed

*Side effects include:* Serious damage to liver and life-threatening inflammation of pancreas, seizures, painful or upset stomach, loss of appetite, vomiting, dark urine, weakness, tiredness, lack of energy, facial swelling, yellowing of skin or eyes (jaundice), skin rash, easy bruising, bloody nose, unusual bleeding, fever, sore throat, drowsiness, headache, indigestion

*How long will it take to work?* May take up to 2 weeks

Valproate has become a real workhorse in the treatment of bipolar disorder since its FDA approval in 1995 for the treatment of mania. Its response rates are right up there with lithium's in that it stamps out *acute mania* somewhere between 50 and 80 percent of the time. Plus, according to Susan McElroy, M.D., professor of psychiatry at the University of Cincinnati College of Medicine, "Divalproex works better when you have depressive symptoms than does lithium." It also appears to beat out lithium in helping people who've had many past bipolar episodes. Valproate can also help prevent relapse, although perhaps not as quickly as some of the other drugs out there.

## PsychSpeak

Mania that comes on very suddenly, gets worse quickly, and lasts over a fairly short, defined period of time is called **acute mania.** In bipolar disorder, it usually refers to a single episode of mania.

Terence Ketter, M.D., chief of the bipolar disorders clinic at Stanford University School of Medicine, has a hypothesis regarding the way Depakote works in the brain. He has done extensive work looking at PET and MRI scans of people with bipolar disorder before and after they've taken Depakote. In these studies, they do what is called a "sustained sadness induction procedure," where they have the person recall some sad memories for 30 minutes while they take pictures of their brain and measure the levels of brain activity. In another study, they've looked at brain levels of a neurotransmitter called gamma-aminobutyric acid (GABA), which is thought to have some role in the symptoms and pathology of bipolar disorder.

"It looks like Depakote increases brain GABA," Ketter reports. "Something is going on here that is different from patients with unipolar depression, because in those patients, during depression, GABA levels are down. With bipolar disorder, during depression, GABA levels are near to normal."

## Carbamazepine

*Brand names:* Tegretol, Atretol, Carbatrol, Epitol

*Form:* Oral suspension, tablets, chewable tablets, extended-release tablets, extended-release capsules

*Common dosages:* As oral suspension, 100 milligrams up to 4 times a day to start; for tablets and chewable tablets, 200 milligrams taken 2 times a day to start; for extended release tablet, 100 or 200 milligrams taken 1 or 2 times a day to start; for extended-release capsule, 200 milligrams taken 1 or 2 times a day to start; all dosages can be increased as needed, but dose generally shouldn't exceed 1,200 milligrams a day

*Side effects include:* Blood disorders (unusual bleeding or bruising, fever, mouth sores, sore throat, fever), red or itchy skin rash, jaundice, irregular heartbeat, joint pain, faintness, swelling of feet or lower legs, seizures, drowsiness, upset stomach, hallucinations, insomnia, agitation, irritability, confusion, headache, difficulty coordinating movements, speech problems, dry mouth, impotence

*How long will it take to work?* A few weeks for full effect

Keck has noted that the jury is still out as to whether carbamazepine is an effective drug for maintaining a stable mood over long periods of time. Still, at least a couple of studies seem to provide some cautious optimism, declaring carbamazepine better than lithium at staving off relapse.

McElroy has stated that she, too, was concerned about carbamazepine's efficacy and was "so happy" to see the results of a recent study in which it was shown that "the drug really does work in acute mania."

## Lamotrigine

*Brand name:* Lamictal

*Form:* Tablet, chewable tablet

*Common dosages:* 200 milligrams per day as a target dosage

*Side effects include:* Serious—even fatal—rash, fever, swollen lymph nodes, redness of skin, swelling, changes in vision, clumsiness or unsteadiness, dizziness, drowsiness, headache, nausea, vomiting, diarrhea, loss of taste and appetite, irritability, insomnia

*How long will it take to work?* Several weeks to several months to achieve full and effective dosage levels

Lamotrigine is the new darling of the psychopharmaceutical world, garnering FDA approval in 2003. Unlike most of the other anticonvulsants, which work to put the brakes on mania, lamotrigine seems to be better at elevating a depressed mood. In addition, it's one of the very few treatments that seem to be able to even come close to helping people with rapid-cycling disorder.

Lamotrigine is not only effective at getting your mood up, but it's also effective at keeping it up—and not too far up. In a 2003 study led by Joseph Calabrese, M.D., of the Case Western Reserve University School of Medicine, one of the leading researchers in the development of this drug, lamotrigine was able to keep patients from sinking back into depression better than placebo could over an 18-month period. In the same study, lithium also was found to prevent mania better than a placebo. What needs to be done now, Calabrese noted, is to explore what might happen if clinicians started to use lamotrigine in combination with lithium over the long haul.

Unfortunately, lamotrigine's effects on mania are much less impressive. When put head-to-head with lithium, lamotrigine was no more able to prevent manic relapses than a placebo, while lithium showed a powerful anti-manic effect. All this, Keck said, suggests "lamotrigine's primary benefit for people with bipolar illness is in the depressed phase of the illness, an illness for which we clearly need treatment."

Still, Ghaemi predicts that lamotrigine is going to be a "good long-term alternative" to the drugs currently in favor. "Its main benefit is that it doesn't have the nuisance side effects that lithium and valproate have."

## Oxcarbazepine

*Brand name:* Trileptal

*Form:* Tablets

*Common dosages:* 300 milligrams 2 times a day to start; dosage can be increased as needed, but shouldn't exceed 2,400 milligrams per day

*Side effects include:* Red and itchy skin rash, seizures, shortness of breath, fever, swollen lymph nodes, joint pain, changes in vision, changes in walking or balance, depression, uncontrolled eye movements, dizziness, drowsiness, abdominal pain, heartburn, nausea or vomiting, runny or stuffy nose

*How long will it take to work?* A few weeks for full effect

Oxcarbazepine is not one of the more "popular" drugs for battling bipolar disorder, partly because researchers haven't done a whole lot with it in controlled clinical studies. Nonetheless, because it is an effective drug against epilepsy and because it has had some usefulness in treating anxiety, some scientists are beginning to look at it a little more carefully.

In a 2004 study published in the *Journal of Affective Disorders,* researchers from the University of Pisa in Italy looked at oxcarbazepine as an add-on treatment for 8 weeks in 18 patients whose bipolar disorder had not responded well to lithium. At the end of the admittedly short trial, 11 of the patients had shown a positive response to the oxcarbazepine, with 7 of them remaining stabilized in their moods throughout the trial period.

Still, before oxcarbazepine can be considered to be truly effective in the treatment of mania in bipolar disorder, it will have to be tested under placebo-controlled conditions in a much larger sample of patients.

## Topiramate

> *Brand name:* Topamax
>
> *Form:* Tablets, capsules
>
> *Common dosages:* 50 milligrams a day for the first week; increased as needed to a maximum of 400 milligrams a day
>
> *Side effects include:* Low blood sugar (shakiness, dizziness, rapid heartbeat, sweating, confusion, blurred vision, headache, weakness, fatigue, pale color, sudden hunger), tingling in fingers or toes, shaking hand, restlessness, crossed eyes, slow heart rate, breathing problems, problems with urination, unusual bruising or bleeding, slowing of mental or physical activity, increased eye pressure, problems with memory, speech or language problems, trouble concentrating, flulike symptoms, lessening of sensations or perceptions, loss of appetite, weight loss, blood in urine, decreased libido, swelling of tongue, increased saliva, dry mouth
>
> *How long will it take to work?* May take as long as 8 weeks to reach maximum effective dosage

Results of trials of topiramate on acute mania have been disappointing, although it's a useful drug in treating many of the other conditions that tend to go along with bipolar disorder such as alcoholism and impulsivity. "I thought this drug was going to work," McElroy admitted during a grand rounds presentation at UCLA. "It just shows how powerful bias can be."

Still, she noted, topiramate does still have a place in bipolar disorder therapy. It has been shown to be a good drug to induce weight loss and to treat bulimia, binge-eating, and alcohol dependence in people with bipolar disorder.

"I use this drug with bipolar disorder when I'm managing some of the schmutz that goes along with the disorder," McElroy said. "It's not a good acute mania drug, but it's a good after-the-acute-mania drug."

## Antipsychotics

Although antipsychotics were originally designed for the treatment of schizophrenia and its associated psychoses—hence the name *antipsychotic*—they've been found over time to be extremely useful in the treatment of mania. According to psychiatrist John Cookson of The Royal London Hospital, more than 80 percent of people with bipolar disorder manifesting as mania are treated with antipsychotics.

And we're not just talking about psychotic mania, either. In more than one study of people with bipolar mania who were treated with antipsychotics, the drugs were shown to have essentially the same positive effect whether or not the people being studied had psychotic features to their mania.

Antipsychotics are fairly rapid in their effects. "This is where the real value of antipsychotics in mania lies, in getting speedy improvement in mania," Cookson told an audience of clinicians at a 2003 conference sponsored by the American Psychiatric Association. "This improvement continues over the course of 14 days. By the end of that time, you can tell how much improvement the patient's going to get with an antipsychotic, and I think at that point you should decide whether to add a mood stabilizer if they're not improving enough."

There's evidence that you can get some amount of depression relief from the antipsychotics as well, especially if those symptoms

## PsychSpeak

Atypical antipsychotics are novel drugs that differ chemically from the older antipsychotics and are able to quell psychosis at doses that don't bring on the severe movement disorders common with the older drugs.

are tagging along with a manic episode. And among the *atypical antipsychotics*—the newcomers in this class of drugs—it seems that there's also a tendency to prevent mania from turning into depression during treatment.

The atypical drugs, Ghaemi adds, "have made a big dent in bipolar disorder." Still, there are some downsides. There are some concerns that these drugs predispose the people taking them to diabetes, for instance—a problem that recently has been noted especially with use of clozapine and olanzapine, both of which tend to cause significant weight gain. (Diabetes risk has long been linked to weight, and adult weight gain in particular.) Antipsychotics as a whole group also do tend to affect the way the body handles the sugar glucose. Still, Ghaemi believes that diabetes isn't going to be a class-wide phenomenon. "My hunch is that the other ones don't cause diabetes, or if they do, it's a very small risk."

Whether antipsychotics are good for maintenance—keeping mood stable and preventing people from relapsing into mania— is a subject of debate. The most recent studies seem to suggest that continuing to use antipsychotics after the manic symptoms are gone might not be the most useful strategy for preventing relapse—in fact, it might even increase the chance of depression. And because the antipsychotics carry a pretty heavy side effect burden in terms of things such as movement disorders and the like, some clinicians are beginning to recommend that treatment with antipsychotics remain limited to the acute phase of mania, rather than as a long-term prevention strategy.

### Risperidone

*Brand name:* Risperdal

*Form:* Tablets, oral solution

*Common dosages:* To begin with, 1 milligram per day total, given once or twice a day; dosage increased as needed to a maximum of about 16 milligrams per day

*Side effects include:* Cardiac arrhythmias (abnormal heart rhythms), seizures, difficult or rapid breathing, high fever, high or low blood pressure, increased sweating, confusion, severe muscle stiffness, loss of bladder control, pale skin, severe tiredness or weakness, difficulty speaking or swallowing, inability to move eyes, movement disorders, priapism (painful, prolonged erection of penis), shuffling walk, trouble sleeping, back pain, chest pain, extreme thirst, unusual bleeding or bruising

*How long will it take to work?* Several weeks

In early December 2003, the FDA approved Johnson and Johnson's antipsychotic Risperdal (risperidone) for the treatment of mania in bipolar disorder. It seems to work as well as lithium in treating acute mania and to be even more helpful as an add-on treatment, buoying the effects of lithium or any of the other effective mood stabilizers.

Since then, risperidone has continued to prove itself an effective treatment against mania. In a paper published in the June 2004 *American Journal of Psychiatry,* Robert Hirschfeld, M.D., professor and chair of the Department of Psychiatry at the University of Texas Medical Branch in Galveston, reported along with his colleagues on a placebo-controlled trial of risperdal on 259 patients with bipolar I disorder. Not only did the risperdal show a strong antimanic effect, they noted, but it did so quite rapidly, with differences between the experimental and placebo groups in terms of manic symptoms being seen just 3 days after the trial began.

"These findings, along with the established benefit of risperidone in combination with a mood stabilizer, suggest that risperidone has an important role in the treatment of patients with bipolar mania," they wrote.

Risperidone is now undergoing a large national, multicenter trial to see if it is equally effective in the treatment of bipolar mania in children.

## Olanzapine

*Brand names:* Zyprexa, Zydis

*Form:* Tablets

*Common dosages:* 5 to 10 milligrams once a day to begin; dosage then increased as needed

*Side effects include:* Seizures, uncontrolled jerking movements, fever, very stiff muscles, excess sweating, fast or irregular heartbeat, headache, agitation, drowsiness, constipation, dry mouth, upset stomach

*How long will it take to work?* A few weeks

Olanzapine's ability to squash mania has been proven in a number of different studies, which is probably why it was the first of the antipsychotics to be given the official FDA nod, in 2000, for use in treating bipolar disorder. Two fairly recent studies have provided evidence that olanzapine is just as—if not more—effective than divalproex (Depakote) is in fighting manic symptoms. A third set of data showed that over a 1-year maintenance period, olanzapine was better able to keep people from relapsing into mania and winding up in a hospital for treatment than lithium was. Those data have been echoed by other studies as well.

"Olanzapine is a good antimanic agent, not just a good antipsychotic," noted McElroy. "It works extremely well in non-psychotic manic patients."

## Quetiapine

*Brand name:* Seroquel

*Form:* Tablets

*Common dosages:* 25 milligrams twice a day to start; dosage usually increased to 300 or 400 milligrams a day divided into 2 or 3 doses, with a daily dose that usually doesn't exceed 800 milligrams

*Side effects include:* Tardive dyskinesia (a movement disorder), neuroleptic malignant syndrome (a drug reaction that includes muscle stiffness, stupor, unstable blood pressure, fever, sweating, and loss of bladder control), underactive thyroid, fainting, seizures, dizziness, dry mouth, constipation, upset stomach, stomach pain, headache, tiredness, excessive weight gain, blurred vision

*How long will it take to work?* May take several weeks

Clinical trials using quetiapine against the symptoms of acute mania have provided some early evidence that this atypical antipsychotic is both safe and effective. When it relieves mania, it does so fairly quickly; in two 12-week trials, quetiapine made a noticeable difference within 4 days in people taking it.

A study by Sachs and colleagues has also shown that quetiapine works well when added to lithium or divalproex, with both of those partnerships resulting in a higher rate of response in acute mania than either lithium or divalproex can get on their own.

And although some of the more typical antipsychotics are thought to have the ability to cause a switch into depression, quetiapine showed no such tendency.

Quetiapine was approved for use against acute mania in early 2004.

But that's not all it seems to be good for. At the May 2004 annual meeting of the American Psychiatric Association, Calabrese presented findings that indicate quetiapine can calm symptoms of anxiety associated with bipolar depression—making quetiapine the first antipsychotic to show efficacy against symptoms of depression rather than just against symptoms of mania.

### Aripriprazole

*Brand name:* Abilify

*Form:* Tablets

*Common dosages:* 10 to 15 milligrams once a day; no dose increases until after 2 weeks of therapy

*Side effects include:* Dizziness, fainting, blurred vision, irregular heartbeat, chest pain, swelling in extremities, seizures, difficulty swallowing, trouble breathing, unusual movements, confusion, sweating, high fever, urgent need to urinate, headache, nervousness, sleep disturbances, lightheadedness, upset stomach, weight gain, rash, dry eyes, ear pain

*How long will it take to work?* 2 weeks or more

Like quetiapine, aripriprazole is only now being looked at for its ability to counter the symptoms of bipolar mania. It's the latest of the atypical antipsychotics to be considered for treatment of bipolar disorder and seems to be generating a good buzz. In a recent study led by Paul Keck, aripriprazole proved to be better than a placebo in cutting down mania, with that difference showing up by the fourth day of treatment. Best of all, says Susan McElroy, it seems to be well tolerated, meaning that its side effects are somewhat less frequent and less debilitating than those of some of the other antipsychotics. It's currently under consideration by the FDA for approval as an anti-manic drug.

### Ziprasidone

*Brand name:* Geodon

*Form:* Capsules

*Common dosages:* 20 milligrams twice a day to start; may increase as needed to a maximum of 80 milligrams twice a day

*Side effects include:* Neuroleptic malignant syndrome (a drug reaction that includes muscle stiffness, stupor, unstable blood pressure, fever, sweating, and loss of bladder control), irregular heartbeat, muscle spasms, uncontrollable muscle movements, dizziness, fainting, priapism, seizures

*How long will it take to work?* Several weeks

According to McElroy, ziprasidone came onto the bipolar scene when scientists analyzing data from schizoaffective disorder studies noted that it seemed to have both antimanic and anti-depressant effects. There haven't been many clinical studies to back this up; however, one study did find that ziprasidone is better at treating bipolar disorder than placebo, and that the difference is noticeable quite quickly, as quickly as the second day of taking the drug. There are some concerns that ziprasidone might also have a tendency to induce mania, but further studies are needed to know for sure. The FDA is still considering the approval of ziprasidone for bipolar mania.

## Clozapine

*Brand name:* Clozaril

*Form:* Tablets

*Common dosages:* 12.5 milligrams once or twice a day, may increase as needed to a maximum of 900 milligrams per day

*Side effects include:* Agranulocytosis (a reduction in the number of certain white blood cells in the circulation), weight gain, increased diabetes risk, high cholesterol, seizures, sedation, low blood pressure, and increased production of saliva

*How long will it take to work?* A few weeks

Clozapine's usefulness in treating bipolar mania is not in doubt; however, with the addition of newer, less side-effect-laden antipsychotics, it seems to be beginning to fall out of favor with clinicians and patients alike. Clozapine has blood-related side effects that are so serious they require weekly blood tests. Clearly, this is not going to be your drug of choice—if you have a choice.

## Antidepressants

Treating bipolar depression has long seemed to take a backseat to treating mania. And yet it's the depression that leads to suicidal thoughts and actions; it's the depression that's longer-lasting and harder to bear.

"When you talk to patients, they will tell you that over time what ruins their life is actually the depression," said Lori Altshuler, M.D., director of the University of California, Los Angeles Mood Disorders Program and a professor of psychiatry at UCLA, during a bipolar disorder symposium held there. "As time goes on with the illness, the predominant reason people get hospitalized is for their depressions."

It could be argued that antidepressants were the wonder drugs of the 1990s; for the treatment of bipolar depression, prescriptions were written for a number of drugs, including the following:

- Tranylcypromine (brand names: Parnate, Nardil, Marplan, belonging to a class of antidepressants known as MAO inhibitors, in use since the 1960s)
- Moclobemide (brand name: Manerix)
- Fluoxetine (brand name: Prozac, the first of the SSRI anti-depressants)
- Paroxetine (brand name: Paxil)
- Citalopram (brand name: Celexa)
- Buproprion (brand names: Wellbutrin, Wellbutrin SR)
- Venlafaxine (brand names: Effexor, Effexor XR)

The development of the selective serotonin reuptake inhibitors (SSRIs) turned depression into a treatable condition—and one that could be taken care of for a relatively low side-effect cost. But the use of antidepressants in treating bipolar depression—as opposed to unipolar depression—remains quite controversial.

There is absolutely no question that antidepressants work—and work well. What is in question is whether they cause more harm than good in people with bipolar disorder by causing them to switch from depression into mania.

Because depression is the symptom seen most frequently and for the longest period of time, for most people with bipolar disorder, antidepressants are widely prescribed, notes S. Nassir Ghaemi. "That may be useful short term and give short-term benefit to people," Ghaemi says, "and that then translates into the assumption that 'if it ain't broke, don't fix it.'"

But Ghaemi believes that's not a good enough reason to keep treating people with a class of drugs he believes might actually be causing some number of them harm by switching them into mania. "In the case of new antidepressants, they're hardly studied at all, so we don't know if they're effective," he says. "Right now we're going on an extension of belief in the underlying assumption that if they work in unipolar depression, they'll work in bipolar depression."

According to Ghaemi, the data he's gathered actually suggests that antidepressants are safer and more effective in unipolar depression. "If we don't have data proving their effectiveness [in bipolar depression]," he says, "we shouldn't be using them.

"[A]t a very basic level, everything we do in medicine is Hippocratic: First, do no harm," he adds. "My experience is that most of the patients I see who are doing badly have been treated with many, many antidepressants and very few mood stabilizers. If we reverse the emphasis, I think we'll see real benefits."

"Antidepressants can precipitate mania, no question," Altshuler said. "Antidepressants can be like dynamite fueling the switch rates. But the rates may be overestimated. Some of what we might be attributing to a drug treatment may be part of the natural course of the illness."

In addition, Altshuler said, it's still not clear when switching occurs most frequently. Obviously, if you're taking an antidepressant and begin to exhibit signs of mania within the first few weeks of treatment, you should be taken off the drug and given something else to control your symptoms. But weeks or months later, once you've achieved remission and your depression is gone, how likely are you really to suddenly switch into mania? And does taking you off the antidepressant soon after your depression abates make you more likely to relapse into depression? Does it make you more likely to relapse than you are likely to switch into mania?

Altshuler and her colleagues have been studying these issues for some time now. In a 2001 study of 44 people with bipolar disorder who were being treated with antidepressants for an acute depressive episode, they found that cutting off antidepressants within the first year of treatment meant a much higher chance of relapsing into depression, despite the fact that these people were on a mood stabilizer throughout the study. Also, Altshuler said they found no increased risk of relapsing into mania.

The Stanley Foundation Bipolar Network did a similar study, of which Altshuler was a part, in which they looked at 84 patients who responded well to antidepressants and divided them into "continuers" versus "discontinuers." (The discontinuers had stopped before 6 months after remission.) The results of the year-long study, Altshuler pointed out, are quite striking. Of those people who stopped taking their antidepressants within 6 months, 71 percent relapsed into depression during the study period. Only 41 percent of those who continued taking the drugs relapsed, and that number itself could be divided into those who stopped taking the antidepressants between the sixth and twelfth months (57 percent of those who relapsed), and those who continued on for more than 12 months (just 29 percent relapsed).

How many of these people wound up manic because of the antidepressants? As many as 18 percent of the people in the study had manic symptoms during the follow-up period, which translated into 15 manic patients. Of those, six were on the antidepressants when they started experiencing mania and nine were not.

"So there didn't appear to be an association between being on antidepressants and relapse into mania," Altshuler noted. "The risk of relapse into mania after recovery from depression is much less than the risk of recurrence of depression."

That, however, is by no means the end of the debate. In early 2004, Ghaemi and his colleagues published a paper in the *American Journal of Psychiatry* that showed that people with bipolar disorder were 1.6 times less likely to respond to antidepressant treatment than are people with unipolar depression. More strikingly, they found a mania switch rate of 48.8 percent of the bipolar patients versus 0 percent of those with unipolar depression, with the propensity to become manic being much higher in those people who weren't also taking a mood stabilizer. And more than 25 percent of the bipolar patients began to cycle more rapidly after antidepressant treatment. (Again, none of the unipolar patients showed cycling, rapid or not.)

These results, says Ghaemi, weren't specific to any one form of antidepressant. In fact, they were found across the board in the drugs they tested, which included tricyclic antidepressants, monoamine oxidase inhibitors, and the newer selective serotonin reuptake inhibitors. These data do need to be replicated and evaluated by other researchers, Ghaemi says, but for him, at least, they underscore the importance of using antidepressants in bipolar disorder sparingly and judiciously, if at all.

## Other Pharmaceutical Agents

Aside from all the previously discussed psychopharmaceuticals, other medications are being looked at for the treatment of bipolar disorder as well. These drugs are generally used to treat entirely unrelated conditions but have been found to have a link to bipolar disorder. Research on all these types of drugs is generally preliminary at best, so none are currently being used as the main thrust of treatment in bipolar disorder. Still, they can be helpful adjuncts to treatment—and the insight they're giving researchers into the disorder might someday make the current treatments, with all their onerous side effects, obsolete.

### Calcium Channel Blockers

*Brand names:* Nimotop, Calan, Procardia, others

*Form:* Capsules, extended-release capsules, tablets, extended-release tablets, injection

How do calcium channel blockers work? The assumption is that because they can block the flow of electrical impulses in the brain, they might be able to make neurons a little less over-excitable and, therefore, calm manic symptoms. (In the heart, they work to relax blood vessels, increasing the blood supply to the body's tissues, including the heart tissues.)

Certainly, these are good, effective drugs in the treatment of various heart conditions, high blood pressure, and even migraines. Just how effective they can be in treating bipolar disorder, however, has yet to be fully explored.

So for now, these drugs are really only likely to be prescribed to you as a sort of add-on to other more established therapies, such as lithium or carbamazepine. Or if you don't respond or have severe reactions to the usual pharmaceutical suspects in bipolar disorder, your physician might try you on calcium channel blockers to see if they can give you some relief from your symptoms.

In a few small studies, calcium channel blockers (nimodipine, or Nimotop) typically used to treat angina and hypotension have been found effective for treating rapid cyclers. Calcium channel blockers stop the excess calcium buildup in cells, which might be some of the problem in bipolar disorder. They are usually used in conjunction with other drug therapies such as carbamazepine or lithium.

### Thyroid Hormones

*Brand names:* Levothroid, Levoxyl, Synthroid, others

*Form:* Tablets, injection

The connection between the thyroid—a gland located in your neck near your windpipe—and bipolar disorder has been the subject of increasing scrutiny. The thyroid, when prompted, secretes thyroid hormone, which is made up of amino acids (the most basic unit of a protein) with iodine attached.

Thyroid hormone is absolutely critical in your body's ability to function normally. It is the basis of your metabolism, telling your body's physiological engine how high to rev. If too much of it is pumped into the bloodstream, your body speeds up. High thyroid levels—called hyperthyroidism—can look a lot and feel a lot like mania. If you're producing too little thyroid hormone, everything slows down. Low thyroid levels—called hypothyroidism—often leads to the symptoms of depression.

It makes sense, then, that physicians and scientists have become interested in the link between thyroid function and bipolar disorder. When you first get your diagnosis, for instance, your clinician will undoubtedly run a blood test to look at your thyroid levels; if they're off in one direction or the other, you'll probably be treated to see if your problem is really all in your thyroid. In addition, lithium treatment seems to mess around with the functioning of the thyroid—sometimes bringing down hormone levels, other times raising them, oddly enough—so if you're taking lithium, your doctor will probably do regular thyroid checks and even give you thyroid hormones if necessary to reduce symptoms.

A change in thyroid function masquerading as bipolar disorder, or a change induced by lithium, is one thing. Thyroid problems as a potential cause of bipolar disorder—or perhaps being caused by it—is a much more complex situation. A 2002 study published in the journal *Biological Psychiatry* noted that autoimmune thyroid disorders (the kind in which your body essentially attacks itself) are found much more often in people with bipolar disorder—particularly women—than in people without mental illness or even people with other forms of mental illness. In fact, 28 percent of the people with bipolar disorder studied had antibodies against their own thyroid tissues, as compared to between 3 and 18 percent for the other groups studied. In 17 percent of the bipolar patients, those antibodies led to complete thyroid failure.

Other researchers have made a connection between rapid-cycling bipolar disorder and mixed bipolar symptoms and a greater chance of thyroid problems. And researchers from the University of Pittsburgh School of Medicine have shown that the lower your thyroid function is before you start treatment for bipolar depression, the less likely you are to respond to that treatment. Whether it's worth treating with thyroid hormones to bring up those levels before or while treating the depression, they said, "remains to be seen."

What does all this mean for treatment? Right now, you're only likely to get thyroid hormones added to your regimen if your numbers are low to start out with, or if they drop during lithium treatment. Some clinicians now also use it in addition to other drugs to treat rapid cycling. The jury is still deliberating over whether it has broader applications, but they're being given more evidence all the time. Stay tuned on this one.

## Why Combination Therapies Are the Way to Go

Clearly, there is no single drug that does everything you want it to do in controlling your bipolar disorder. Some drugs control symptoms of mania, and others control symptoms of depression. Some seem to prevent one type of episode or the other. Some work better in the short term, while others work better over time.

That is why most of the leading clinicians today will tell you that the way to treat bipolar disorder is with a sort of pharmaceutical partnership, pairing different types of drugs with one another to create the ultimate antibipolar cocktail.

There are studies to back them up. A 2002 paper published in the *Archives of General Psychiatry* found that olanzapine added to either lithium or valproate is a one-two punch that out-jabs either lithium or valproate on their own. In addition, Sachs and his colleagues have shown that people taking the antipsychotics risperidone or haloperidol (Haldol) in addition to lithium or valproate had more stable moods than those taking only the lithium or the valproate alone.

That point is underscored by the approval in late December 2003 of a new drug called Symbyax, which is the first-ever FDA-approved medication specifically aimed at bipolar depression. Symbyax, which was developed by Eli Lilly and Company, is actually nothing more than a combination of olanzapine (Lilly's version is Zyprexa) and fluoxetine, or Prozac.

In a Lilly-sponsored and -conducted trial published in the *Archives of General Psychiatry* in November 2003, researchers found significant improvement in symptoms of depression in bipolar I patients taking the combo without any increase in risk of mania. The only downside was that the study found higher rates of nausea and diarrhea in patients taking Symbyax as compared to those taking only olanzapine.

**Q&A**

*Is it okay to just take Prozac and Zyprexa separately to get the same effects as those found in Symbyax?*

"The approval of Symbyax is a very important development, as it's the first treatment ever approved for bipolar depression. But certainly, clinicians can prescribe Zyprexa and Prozac separately. What's crucial is that with the combination, the Zyprexa component provides robust antimanic protection that permits administration of Prozac—which allows robust antidepressant activity—without destabilizing mood." —*Terence Ketter, M.D., chief of the Bipolar Disorders Clinic at Stanford University Medical School*

Studies have backed the coupling of other drugs as well. For example, if you're on lithium or divalproate and you've got some lingering manic symptoms, olanzapine can boost their action as well. Risperidone and haloperidol have similar effects when added to lithium or divalproate.

Quetiapine also helps lithium and divalproate achieve a greater reduction in manic symptoms than they can get on their own. It ups the overall response rate to drug therapy as well.

When you first begin treatment for bipolar disorder, you and your doctor might decide to put you on just one drug at a time, so you can tell which drugs are actually effective. But if your bipolar disorder is at all refractory—psychspeak for stubborn or unresponsive to drugs—you might get better results from teaming up different types of drugs to give yourself the best and most diverse boost toward mental health possible.

Even once the worst of your symptoms have passed, you might want to hang on to a drug combination, especially if it's working for you. Paul Keck notes that most of the people with bipolar disorder he sees are being maintained on at least three different medications in an attempt to stave off any further episodes.

## The Next Generation

In 2003 alone, the FDA gave the nod to three different drugs for use in the treatment of bipolar disorder: lamotrigine (Lamictal), risperidone (Risperdal), and the olanzapine-fluoxetine combination found in Symbyax. In 2004, quetiapine became the first in what is expected to be an even longer list of new compounds given the thumbs-up for the treatment of bipolar disorder.

Clearly, notes Terence Ketter, M.D., chief of the Bipolar Disorders Clinic at Stanford University Medical School and the principle investigator for Stanford's arm of the STEP-BD program, there's been a real infusion of interest and energy into the pharmacologic treatment of bipolar disorder. But why bipolar? Why now?

"I think one of the things is the emergence of the atypical antipsychotics," Ketter says. "Once they were developed and launched in schizophrenia, their manufacturers started looking for other things to do with them."

Adds Ketter: "It's sort of natural that they went to bipolar disorder. The older antipsychotics had been used in the treatment of mania in the past, but they had unacceptable side effects. If you look at drug development, one pattern that can occur is to have a new treatment come out that will be better tolerated and then if you do have this treatment that's better tolerated, clinicians are more likely to use it. That's what seems to be happening here. It's a really exciting time in this field."

## What You Can Do

Psychotropic medications can be extremely effective—and extremely dangerous. The only way to avoid such issues as overdose and dangerous drug interactions is to know as much as you can about what it is you're taking.

But don't leave your physician out of the equation. Stopping or starting a psychopharmaceutical without being under a physician's watchful eye is simply foolish. You and your doctor need to be partners in this critical, personal endeavor, or it will most likely be doomed to failure.

☐ First and foremost, know the names and dosages of all your medications. Write them down on an index card if you need to, and carry it with you at all times. This is your protection against the mistakes that are made all too often in pharmacies and physicians' offices, and it's your passport to appropriate treatment in the event of an emergency.

☐ A complicated drug regimen can be made much simpler by getting a 7-day pill box and putting a week's worth of pills together at one time. Also consider making a list of your meds, doses, and timing and post it on your refrigerator, on your bathroom mirror, or in your date book.

☐ Ask your doctor if there's an extended-release or sustained-release form of your medication. This will mean fewer pills to take fewer times during the day and might make it easier for you to remember to take your medications.

☐ Don't just suffer through side effects in silence. Often you can try other treatment options that might reduce your suffering. Talk to your doctor.

☐ No matter how bad the side effects are, *do not just stop taking your medication abruptly.* In most cases, stopping these drugs cold turkey will make you sicker than any side effect possibly could. Call your doctor and ask how to wean yourself from the medication.

☐ Psychotropic medications can interact with any number of other medications, including those you can buy over the counter. They can also interact with some foods and with alcohol. The more medications you're taking, the greater the chance of a harmful interaction. Be sure both your doctor and your pharmacist know every medication you're taking, including any over-the-counter medications. Also, read the package inserts carefully and, if necessary, list and post the possible interactions somewhere you can easily find it.

☐ If you're having trouble finding the right medication for you, or if you're simply frustrated by the lack of options out there for certain forms of your disorder, consider joining an ongoing clinical trial. In addition to lowering your own medical costs, you'll be adding to the base of data from which future patients' treatment decisions will be culled.

# The Cycles of Sanity

The rhythms of our lives can be played *allegro,* as in the rapid *badum badum badum* of a beating heart, or *andante,* as in our more leisurely daily sleep-wake cycles, a woman's monthly menstrual cycle, or the even longer cycles of skin shedding, hair growth, and more.

In bipolar disorder, rhythm is almost everything. Cycles both define and plague this particular illness, with mood cycles and body cycles and external cycles all swirling around one another, intersecting here, conflicting there, and finding harmony another place. Understanding these rhythms and structures and cycles gives both insight into the disorder and opportunity to intervene.

The question is whether changes in cycles cause bipolar episodes or are the result of them. Or perhaps, as some researchers are convinced, rhythmic changes are both cause and effect. In other words, a misstep in your biological rhythm—such as putting off a night's sleep or missing one altogether—might very well cause you to become manic or depressed, which will then feed on that misstep, throwing off the rhythm even further, and worsening the bipolar episode. Eventually, you find yourself in a cycle of circadian arrhythmia, where your symptoms get worse and everything spirals out of control. In a sense, it's sort of the ultimate irony, the idea that changes in your biological cycles might set up a cycle of disease that is nearly impossible to put the brakes on. On the other hand, there's a real redemption here: taking control of your body's rhythms and getting inner and external cycles in synch is a simple but empowering way to help heal yourself, to take back control of a disease that is so often about being out of control.

## Circadian Rhythms

Deep in a part of the brain called the hypothalamus sits a cluster of neurons called the *suprachiasmatic nucleus* (SCN—you can just call it your biological clock). The SCN gets its name because it sits just above (*supra*) the so-called optic chiasm, where the optic nerves from both eyes cross at the base of the brain. This location is no coincidence: The SCN feeds off the signals sent by the optic nerves, relaying information to the pea-size pineal gland located behind the hypothalamus. The pineal gland's sole purpose is to produce melatonin, an amino-acid-based hormone. Melatonin is a sort of natural sleep aid.

It's a complicated system, but here's what you need to know about it: When it's light outside, the optic nerves signal the SCN, which signals the pineal gland to shut down melatonin production or, rather, to drastically cut back on it. Your body then quickly shakes off its nighttime stupor. When the sun goes down, or when its ultraviolet rays are no longer hitting the retina and sending signals down the optic nerves, the SCN sends the "all-clear" message to the pineal gland, melatonin production revs up, and your activity level naturally starts to wind down. Somewhere in our evolution the fundamental rhythms of night and day were etched into our brains, so that we would be organized in synchrony with our environment. We still operate most efficiently when inner and outer cycles are in harmony.

The SCN seems to have a memory as well. It becomes "trained" by the light it receives to send out its signals day after day in a manner choreographed by the light-dark cycle you experienced days earlier. That's why you get jet lagged when you travel across time zones: your SCN continues to keep time the way it was trained to until it has received a couple days' worth of new light signals. Eventually it resets itself, only to go through the same thing again when you return from your trip.

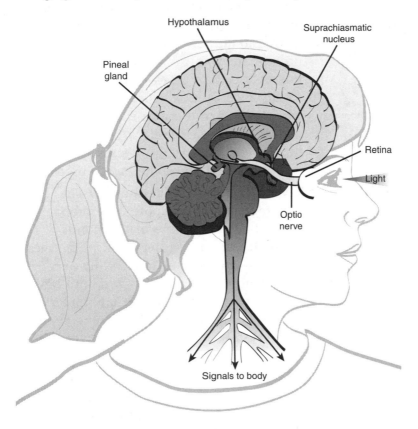

*Circadian signals are received in the form of ultraviolet light by the retina in the eye and then passed down the optic nerves. This signal is fed to the suprachiasmatic nucleus, or SCN, which sits right atop the optic chiasm, where the optic nerves cross at the base of the brain. The SCN relays the information to the pineal gland, which is located behind the hypothalamus, prompting the pineal gland to slow down its production of melatonin, which is a natural sleep aid. When the light signal ceases, melatonin production revs up again.*

For the record, the day night cycle—the so-called *circadian* rhythm—isn't only about sleeping and waking. It's also about hormone production, cell cycling, brain-wave activity, body temperature regulation, and more. Circadian rhythms are the rhythms of our days and our nights. They're what enable us to think on our feet when we're up on our feet, and to (usually) shut down our brains so we can fall asleep at night. They're what prompt our glands to pump out certain hormones at certain times—growth hormone, for instance, is usually produced in bursts while a child or teenager is asleep. Mess with the light-dark cycle your body is used to, and you're messing with some of your most basic and crucial biological processes.

## PsychSpeak

From the Latin *circa,* which means "about," and *dies,* meaning "day," **circadian** literally means "about a day." A circadian rhythm is a biological cycle that lasts for approximately 24 hours.

What does all this have to do with bipolar disorder? The short answer is: just about everything. If you're bipolar, you probably have an exquisitely sensitive body clock, one that responds quickly and almost violently to changes in the signals it receives. Disturb your clock in any way—stay up way too late, fly over a couple time zones, wake up before the sun rises—and both brain and body tend to rebel. (It's no wonder, actually, that bipolar disorder so frequently shows its face for the first time when you're in college, where disrupting your body clock with all-nighters is so common.)

And really, if you think about it, this isn't all that surprising. After all, bipolar disorder is all about cycles itself—cycles of mania, *euthymia,* and depression. In addition, sleep deprivation in and of itself is tied to many symptoms of bipolar disorder—irritability, sleep disturbances, trouble concentrating, changes in appetite, and more. People with jet lag, shift workers who have constantly changing hours, or new parents often "look" a lot like a person having a bipolar episode.

## PsychSpeak

**Euthymia** is a normal, tranquil mood. It's how you feel between episodes of mania and depression. It's the goal of treatment for bipolar disorder.

But if you're bipolar, the difference between you and the new mom next door is that your brain is wired a little differently, and you won't just bounce back simply by paying back your sleep debt. And although the new mom might stumble around a little, drop her keys, or forget where she put them, she's not likely to become frankly manic because the baby was up all night. You, on the other hand, might.

In other words, although a shift in your circadian rhythms might set off mania, it isn't the root cause. For circadian changes to make much of a difference, your brain needs to already be primed for liftoff by structural and chemical disturbances. But if you are primed, they can have a real impact.

Indeed, a disrupted circadian rhythm—a body clock gone awry—is a recipe for mania in bipolar disorder. Researchers have shown that less sleep does in fact cause mania, as opposed to mania simply resulting in less sleep (although it does that as well). In addition, says bipolar expert Ellen Leibenluft, M.D., from the National Institute of Mental Health, you can actually see this shift biochemically in people with rapid-cycling bipolar disorder. A study she conducted found that melatonin release begins about 90 minutes earlier during hypomania than during the depressive phase of the illness. "It is as if rapid-cycling patients might have an endogenous form of jet lag," she writes in a 1996 article in *Psychiatric Times,* "internally traveling back and forth over one or two time zones as they cycle between mania and depression."

Because it's become more and more obvious how influential sleep (or lack thereof) can be on the course of bipolar disorder and other mental illnesses, it's become a topic of interest for researchers, physicians, and mental health advocates as well. In 2004, the Depression and Bipolar Support Alliance (DBSA) announced results of a new survey on sleep and mental illness, and kicked off a campaign they're calling "Sleepless in America."

DBSA's survey of 1,464 volunteers found that as many as 75 percent of the respondents blamed racing thoughts as one of the main causes of lack of sleep. They also cited such common bipolar disorder symptoms as stress and restlessness.

According to a DBSA release on the survey, more than 93 percent of the respondents believed their sleeplessness had a direct impact on their mood, causing sadness, anxiousness, and irritability. Almost three quarters said it affected their relationships with friends and family. And yet less than half the people with sleep disturbances report them to their clinician.

That's why DBSA decided to launch its campaign. The Sleepless in America is aiming to create awareness about the links between lack of sleep and mental health, provide education about sleep disorders, offer tools to help you figure out if you have a sleep problem and if it's related to a mental illness, and provide tips on how to combat sleeplessness. For more on the Sleepless in America campaign, visit www.sleeplessinamerica.org or call DBSA at 1-800-826-3632.

Of course, there are other influences on your circadian clock besides light-dark cycles and sleep. Exercise, work, school, regular mealtimes, and even socializing can act as biological pacemakers or *zeitgebers,* a term used by circadian researchers that means "time-givers." (*Zeit,* in German, is "time"; *geber* means "giver.") And they all can have an effect on how your moods cycle, as well as how well you respond to treatment or how often you tend to relapse.

> ## GET PSYCHED
>
> "To stay healthy, I go to the gym and make sure I eat properly. I can get into a habit of not eating properly sometimes, and that really affects my mania. If I don't eat, I can start getting giddy and hyper. Also, I've cut out coffee and sugar, which also make me hyper. The good side of it is that my teeth are coming out cleaner!"
> —*Alexis Maislen, living with bipolar disorder*

# A Not-So-Good Night's Sleep

Sleep cycles are rightly called circadian—they are *about* 24 hours in length, but they aren't exactly 24 hours. Even under "normal" conditions, your body clock runs a little slow. Left to its own devices, your pineal gland, under SCN orders, would both wake you up and put you to sleep a little later each day. For most people, adjusting to this internal time conflict is a fairly simple matter: exposure to sunlight, especially in the morning, and even to some degree artificial light helps reset the biological clock. Plus, most people generally have a regular schedule they keep based on external cues such as alarm clocks, meowing cats, hungry children, or the timing of TV news programs.

But if you're bipolar, you're already at a disadvantage. According to research, you're much more likely to be significantly "phase-delayed," which is circadianspeak for a night owl. Left to your own devices, you'll go to sleep late and sleep in during the morning. And that's fine—if you can do it. However, what happens most often is you wind up going to sleep late and waking up at your regular time because of scheduling demands. And that, as you now know, can lead you right into the jaws of mania. Some studies show that a single night of sleep loss can be all your manic symptoms need to take over.

It's easy to see why keeping to a really strict schedule of both bedtimes and wake-up times is critical if you want to get a good, tight rein on your disorder. It's also why you should take even the very first signs of insomnia very seriously, especially if you're between episodes. It might be a clue that mania is on its way—and it might also be an opportunity to intervene while the intervening is good.

**Q&A**

*How am I supposed to convince myself to go to sleep when I'm really not at all tired?*

"We find that most patients with bipolar I disorders are night owls by nature or, in circadian system terms, are phase-delayed. They have a very strong preference for going to sleep late and rising late. The important thing, though, is to establish a regular wake-up time and to stick to it seven days a week. We encourage patients to avoid caffeine and stimulants, especially late in the day. If they're going to exercise, which does have certain stimulating properties, we encourage them to do it earlier rather than later in the day. We tell our patients to use their bed only for sleep and maybe one other thing (i.e., sex); not for reading, not for watching television. We want to establish a connection between their bed and going to sleep." *—Ellen Frank, Ph.D., director of the Depression and Manic Depression Prevention Program at Western Psychiatric Institute and Clinic in Pittsburgh*

The connection between wakefulness or sleep loss and mood can be seen on a daily basis. You're more likely to wake up depressed and have your mood improve as the day wears on than you are to wake up cheerful and slowly grow depressed.

There's a fair amount of data to back up these claims. For instance, a 1996 study from researchers at the University of Milan School of Medicine in Italy showed the connection between sleep loss and mania in a group of 34 manic bipolar inpatients at a local hospital. They noted that the relationship between the two was "bidirectional," with sleep reduction causing mania and mania causing sleep reduction. And they added that it was "self-reinforcing," leading to a mania that escalates out of control. "At the beginning of a manic episode, clinicians often observe a spontaneous sleep deprivation, due to the hyperactivity of the patient, resulting in an increase in manic symptomology and then in subsequent sleep loss," the researchers summed up in their paper, published in *Psychiatry Research*.

What they found was that the less these already-manic inpatients slept, the less cooperative and more manic in behavior they were the following day. Interestingly, however, the escalation of mania from sleep loss did not continue unabated. After about two weeks, the researchers could no longer predict how severe the manic symptoms would be based on the amount of sleep the bipolar patient got the night before.

Ironically, studying sleep itself—as opposed to lack of sleep—in manic patients is an extremely difficult task because if you're manic and unmedicated, you're probably not sleeping much, if at all. Still, there have been a couple studies that show that the basic disturbances in sleep in mania—interrupted sleep, less slow-wave or deep sleep, and a shorter rapid-eye movement or dream-sleep period—are similar to the disturbances seen in depressed patients, whether they are bipolar or unipolar. These similarities, some researchers say, only underscore the fact that mania and bipolar depression are simply different manifestations of a single disorder.

**"I** cannot even begin to tell you how important sleep is to a bipolar patient. The amount of sleep you get will make or break your life. Go to bed too late, get up too early, and suddenly the next day is *so much* harder than it normally would be. This is true for lots of people, even those who are not bipolar, but for those of us with the illness, the effect is tremendously magnified.

"Feelings kind of rule your world when you're bipolar. When your feelings are positive, life is a bowl of cherries, but when you feel tired, stressed out, or anxious ... man, life sure does get hard. So make sure to avoid undue problems—get your sleep. I'm not exaggerating when I say that it can mean the difference between life and death. The suicidal thoughts pop up with much more frequency and with higher intensity when sleep is escaping you. So if you're tired during the day, take a nap. If you have things to do early in the morning, go to bed when you should. Go through life as happy as possible. Get enough sleep." *—Shay Villere, living with bipolar disorder since age 16. Today, he is 27 years old, married, and working in the computer field. His free booklet,* The Bipolar Disorder Manual, *is available online at www.bipolardisordermanual.com.*

Conversely, when people who are experiencing bipolar depression are compared with those experiencing unipolar depression, it turns out that bipolar depression is significantly more disruptive to sleep cycles than is unipolar depression. Again, this shows the alliance of bipolar mood states—no matter what they are—as opposed to the alliance of depressive states.

The good news is that although bipolar depression is more destructive when it comes to sleep cycles, it's also much more responsive to a rather unique, and somewhat bizarre, treatment known as total sleep deprivation (TSD).

TSD is just what it sounds like—a night deliberately spent without sleep. And yes, it's a treatment for bipolar depression—part of the search for "benign" alternatives to medications and all their nasty side effects. In fact, it's an effective treatment, as far as it can go.

TSD has been studied on and off over the past 30 years as a treatment for depression and has shown effectiveness rates of as high as 60 percent. In a study published in 1998, Italian researchers led by Francesco Benedetti looked at the effects of TSD on people with both bipolar and unipolar depression. Fifty-one patients—17 of whom were bipolar—allowed themselves to be put through three consecutive cycles of TSD. Each cycle consisted of 36 hours without sleep, followed by a so-called "recovery" sleep of 12 hours. Benedetti and his team found that although the bipolar volunteers felt significantly better after the three cycles, those with unipolar depression were much less affected by the supposed anti-depressant effects of sleep deprivation.

"When patients are kept awake all night, they often show an improvement in mood that continues through the next day," note researchers Raymond Lam, Anthanosios Zis, and A. Dooley Goumkeniouk in *Bipolar Disorder: A Clinician's Guide to Biological Treatments* (Brunner-Routledge, 2002). "The mood changes can be dramatic, and many patients feel that their mood returns to baseline. Although it is difficult to design placebo-controlled studies, the fact that TSD is so counterintuitive to patients (most of whom think they will feel better if only they had *more* sleep) makes a placebo response less likely."

What makes the effects of TSD in people with bipolar depression different from the effects in people with unipolar depression? Well, there's the known tendency for people with bipolar disorder to respond to lack of sleep by developing symptoms of mania—that is, a "higher" mood. People with unipolar depression get a lift from TSD, as well, but they don't become pathologically elated—or rather manic—when sleep-deprived.

Of course, the tendency toward sleep-deprived elation in bipolar patients also raises some warning flags. After all, TSD isn't going to be a particularly useful therapy if it turns depressed people manic. Researchers are watching these risks carefully: The same group of researchers from the University of Milan have quantified the risk of someone with bipolar depression switching to a manic phase, and found that 4.85 percent of 206 bipolar patients in their study became manic after three cycles of sleep deprivation and that an additional 5.83 percent became hypomanic. That total rate, they noted in a 1999 paper, at 10.68 percent switchover to mania or hypomania, is equivalent to mania switch rates from antidepressant drug therapy.

Another potential roadblock to TSD is maintaining its mood-lifting properties. After all, you can't keep everyone with a bipolar depression awake for weeks or months at a time. Plus, once you've gotten a good "recovery sleep" under your belt, you have an extremely high chance of relapsing right back into depression—an 80 to 85 percent chance if you're not otherwise medicated.

The solution? Medicate. Or add light therapy into the mix. A series of different studies from Benedetti and his colleagues has shown that adding either lithium or light-box therapy (see the following "Seeing the Light: Light Therapy" section) to TSD maintains the benefits of TSD significantly longer. Intriguingly, all three in concert—TSD, lithium, and light—do *not* give any additional benefit. There is some concern that lithium might actually reduce light sensitivity in people with bipolar disorder, which would explain the lack of an additive effect, but that remains to be proven.

## Seasonal Affective Disorder

Seasonal Affective Disorder (SAD) is a real cause of depression, and it's a real issue for many people with bipolar disorder. SAD is a disorder tied to the shortened days and overcast weather that's characteristic of the winter months in most part of this country and, indeed, in distal temperate zones in other parts of the world that experience summers and winters of roughly equal length in time. It's aptly named: as less and less light stimulates the SCN, the pineal gland puts out more and more melatonin. All that extra melatonin brings with it decreased brain wave activity, lethargy, apathy ... in other words, depression. And it does so particularly

**WEB TALK:** For a list of trustworthy links on SAD, visit Medline Plus at:

www.nlm.nih.gov/medlineplus/ seasonalaffectivedisorder.html

well in a brain that is already vulnerable to the lowest of low moods.

Although SAD is more frequently associated with unipolar depression, estimates are that about 20 to 30 percent of people with SAD also have bipolar disorder.

Pinning down the numbers is hard, however, because SAD itself is a cycling disorder. When the winter "blues" begin to give way, the return of a simple good mood is hard to differentiate from the beginnings of a manic episode or—even harder perhaps—from hypomania. Still, clinicians estimate that about 20 percent of the people who escape the depression that grips them during the long months of long-nighted winter will slingshot well past "feeling good again" into feeling unbelieveably, hyperkinetically, pathologically great. And as you know, "great" can and often does turn sour very quickly.

**you're not alone**

Christine has known since her first depression that her disorder is inextricably tied to the changing of the seasons. Her depressions, she says, have almost always descended right around the time the first fall leaves begin skittering toward the ground. And her hypomanias—mild as they are—come swirling in with the first spring breezes.

And so, along with her lithium, her husband's watchful eye, and her psychiatrist's phone number, Christine keeps a light box by her side through the winter months. She spends just 30 or so minutes in front of its fluorescent rays each morning while reading the newspaper and having some breakfast. The difference it makes, she says, is real and quite obvious.

"When the daylight is at its shortest, I get a real diminution of energy," she confesses. "If I don't start up on the lights and continue using them through the winter, I could easily see myself falling back into a depression. And that's one of the last things I want to have to go through again."

Treating SAD means getting those rhythms back in synch—getting enough light to the SCN that it will hold off melatonin reduction for a while. Enter light therapy (which I'll discuss in greater detail in the next section). Light therapy—using exposure to bright light of very specific wavelengths—acts as an antidepressant for people who are suffering from SAD, no matter whether the depression is bipolar or unipolar in nature. The difference is that for people who are unipolar depressed without a seasonal influence, light therapy is not particularly useful; for those with bipolar depression, however, light therapy tends to lift mood no matter what the time of year.

## Can You Change Your Rhythm?

Yes. Absolutely. That's what makes the study of body rhythms so exciting and empowering. So much of bipolar disorder feels out of your control—your moods, your brain, your response to medication. But you can get a grip on your cycles. You can do something about them.

And best of all, righting your upside-down rhythms is something you can do for yourself, at least to some degree. You can set and keep a sleep schedule. You can be sure you get outside each sunny or even overcast day. You can be sure you're not overscheduled to the point of exhaustion and major stress. You can prepare yourself for the unexpected.

**Seeing the Light: Light Therapy** Light lifts moods. If you've ever dragged through a winter in the north or felt the almost adrenalinelike rush of spring fever, you know just how mood-lifting light can be. And if you suffer from SAD, you know light can have a dramatic and quick effect on you.

But if you really and truly want to appreciate the benefits of light, you have to do it with the eyes of someone with bipolar disorder, because bipolar depression is fantastically sensitive and responsive to light therapy, no matter what the time of year.

If you're looking for proof, look no further than a 2001 study in which Benedetti and his colleagues reviewed hospital charts and found that the side of the building a patient's room was on had a measurable effect on his or her length of stay. Those patients in rooms on the east side of the building, the researchers found, had more than 10 times the amount of light streaming in through their windows each morning than did patients whose rooms were on the west side of the building. The result? Out of 187 bipolar patients, those on the east side had significantly shorter hospital stays than those on the west—no matter what other treatments they were receiving. Perhaps just as telling, when the same review was done on the charts of 415 unipolar patients, there was no real difference in length of stay.

Because of data like this, a growing number of people with bipolar disorder are using light as an add-on to the more traditional medical therapies. Light's advantages are legion, although that's not to say there are no side effects from light therapy. There are, but they are minor and they don't involve chemicals that travel through your bloodstream or build up in your liver. Light therapy is so safe, in fact, that it's currently being investigated as a potential way of treating SAD and other forms of depression in pregnant women for whom continuing to take antidepressants and mood stabilizers might be dangerous.

## PsychSpeak

**Phototherapy** is a form of treatment for a disease or condition using light in carefully controlled doses.

A **lux** is a measure of illumination over a specified surface area. One lux is the uniform lighting of one square meter by one lumen of light. (A *lumen* is a measure of the energy of light in all directions.) Ten thousand lux is equivalent to 14.6 watts per square meter.

Enter *phototherapy* via a light box. The light box is a simple device with a fluorescent bulb that usually gives off 10,000 *lux* of light. For most people, a morning "dose" of phototherapy—anywhere from 10 minutes to an hour or more—is enough to lift or stave off depression. All you have to do is sit in front of the box, facing it with your eyes open. That's it. You don't have to look directly at the bulbs—in fact, you're encouraged not to—and you don't have to engage in any particular activity. You can read the morning paper, have breakfast, or even talk on the phone. Just so long as the light is reaching your eyes—and traveling from there down the optic nerves and to the SCN—you'll get the full benefits of the treatment.

But don't break out the tanning lotions just yet! Light therapy is indeed an attempt to simulate the beneficial effects of sunlight on hormone secretion and, thus, mood balance, but the treatment itself involves the use of fluorescent lighting, not the more dangerous ultraviolet rays that stimulate the melanin in your skin. The quality of the light used in a light box is critical to how well the therapy will work; the right light can work wonders, but light from the wrong part of the wavelength spectrum will ultimately do nothing for you. It's just another reason why you shouldn't try this at home. Not just any old light will do.

How does the light work? Well, in addition to resetting the body clock, there's evidence that a morning burst of light also boosts levels of the neurotransmitter serotonin throughout the entire day. Serotonin is a key player in the biology of depression; it's what the selective serotonin reuptake inhibitor (SSRI) antidepressants focus on. Anything that works to keep circulating levels of serotonin high will invariably lift mood.

But just how light turns into higher serotonin levels is still pretty much anybody's guess. It was thought for a while that perhaps serotonin—which is made from the amino acid tryptophan—might somehow be a byproduct of the production of melatonin. To date, however, that has not been shown to be the case. Researchers are still trying to pin down the precise connection between serotonin and light.

**WEB TALK:** For more about light therapy, visit the Society for Light Treatment and Biological Rhythms at: **www.sltbr.org**

One note of caution: Just because light therapy doesn't have chemically induced side effects does not mean that it's something to fool around with on your own. For one thing, the machines need to be carefully calibrated, and you need to be given an appropriate "dose" to take, which will depend on a number of factors involving your depression. For another, it's critically important that some sort of clinician keep an eye on you as you proceed through the therapy to evaluate if and when you cross the line from good mood into hypomania or mania. This professional also needs to be sure your various therapies aren't counteracting one another—for many people with bipolar disorder, for instance, an antidepressant plus light therapy might very well be a recipe for disaster. On the other hand, your doctor might want you to be on a mood stabilizer such as lithium during this treatment to augment and back up the light therapy (or vice versa), and to try to stretch out its benefits over a long period of time.

In other words, don't try this on your own.

**Avoiding Overstimulation** When you're in the grips of mania, or even hypomania, the idea of a nice, quiet life seems almost laughable. In fact, it probably seems downright undesirable. But the truth is, the quieter life you lead, the less burden you're putting on your twitchy, oversensitive, beleaguered brain.

*Quiet* doesn't have to mean *dull,* but it does mean cutting back and reducing the amount of stimulation you're bombarded with each day. It means learning how to relax, to slow down the pace of your life. It means cutting back on stress.

There's data to back this up. Susan Malkoff-Schwartz, Ph.D., and her colleagues from the University of Pittsburgh have shown that stressful life events quite often precede the onset of a manic episode. And stressful life events don't have to be bad things— they just have to be stressful. Moving, getting a new job, ending a relationship, beginning a new one—these are all well-known life stressors. But stress—and sleep disruption—can also come from simpler things, such as taking on too many projects at work or planning big dinner parties three weekends in a row, or having an activity scheduled almost every night of the week.

There are choices you can make—hanging out at a friend's home rather than going club-hopping, for instance—that can lower the level of stressful stimulation your body has to process each day.

"You have to find a balance between rest and activity, stimulation and boredom—something this population fears enormously," says Ellen Frank, Ph.D., director of the Depression and Manic

Depression Prevention Program at Western Psychiatric Institute and Clinic in Pittsburgh. "It can be hard adapting to these changes in routine."

These are not necessarily easy choices to make. Frank admits that many of the people she sees with bipolar disorder who make the choice to lower the social stresses and stimulations in their lives pay a price. "There are patients who, I think, rightly believe they need to markedly reduce the amount of stimulation they experience, [then] find themselves socially isolated, having lost many of their social contacts and many of the things that formed and shaped their social lives."

**Social Rhythms**  Knowing how critical all these rhythmic components seem to be in bipolar disorder, Frank and her colleagues developed a form of psychotherapy specifically for bipolar disorder that focuses on setting and maintaining a steady beat in your life as a way of staying emotionally steady.

Called Interpersonal and Social Rhythm Therapy (IPSRT), this treatment banks on the concept that if you're bipolar, routine is your best friend. Where stress and unpredictability create chaos, routine creates calm.

Basically, Frank says, this means looking at your daily schedule with a critical, circadian eye, and creating regular, reasonable routines you can stick to.

IPSRT goes beyond sleep schedules— although these are certainly a critical component. To do IPSRT right, you need to also schedule mealtimes, work, even recreation and leisure activities. In fact, says Frank, there are 17 different daily activities that an IPSRT therapist will discuss with you when you begin this therapy.

> **GET PSYCHED**
>
> "If I have to maintain a 9 to 5 schedule, then I have to go to sleep by 10, even if I'm not tired and have to lie in bed and meditate. If my thoughts are running fast, I take some deep breaths, think of peaceful situations ... I'll envision an ocean or a valley, I'll imagine myself running in the North Woods or the Grand Canyon, sometimes I'll just meditate on a scenic picture on my computer screen." *–Alexis Maislen, living with bipolar disorder*

The first phase of the therapy is identifying what these rhythms are; the second part is stabilizing the rhythms. This means finding a regular time to wake up, go to bed, take your meals, etc. "Initially, we tried to get those times in synch with the light-dark cycle," Frank says. "But many bipolar patients are phase delayed—their preferred good night time and their preferred good morning time are later than those of many other people. That's all right as long as it's regular and not completely out of synch with the light-dark cycle."

If you're doing IPSRT, you and your therapist will try to find your most unstable rhythms and start to work on those first, setting goals as well as "reasonable expectations" for change. "We recognize that trying to shift something by three, four hours in one week doesn't work at all," Frank says.

You then need to learn how to keep to that schedule, even when life starts throwing you some curve balls. In fact, you need to learn how to see those curve balls coming—to recognize situations that are likely to perturb your established rhythms and throw everything into chaos—and what you can do about them. (For more on IPSRT and other components of the therapy, see Chapter 8.)

*What are the main daily rhythms I should be looking at, and what is it about these rhythms that I'm supposed to be concerned about?*

"We ask patients to record at what time of day they carry out an activity and whether they do a particular activity alone or in company with others. These are things like getting out of bed, the first contact with another person, your morning beverage, breakfast, the first time you go outside, having lunch, watching a special TV program, going to bed. These are all activities we think might serve to set the circadian phase." —*Ellen Frank, Ph.D., director of the Depression and Manic Depression Prevention Program at Western Psychiatric Institute and Clinic in Pittsburgh*

# What You Can Do

Getting the rhythms of your life in synch with the rhythms of your body is one of the foundations of treating bipolar disorder—and one of the things you can actually control. Unlike the chemicals in your brain, you can reset your biological clock and retrain your body by using some simple behavioral tricks and adhering to a strict schedule. Here are some things you can do to get time on your side:

- ☐ Maintain a very strict sleep schedule, seven days a week. It's not as important to go to bed early as it is to go to bed at the same time each night. The same goes for waking up in the morning. To keep the lid on your bipolar symptoms, you likely have to forego sleeping in on the weekends.

- ☐ Try some of these tricks to help yourself get to sleep on time. Try carbo-loading in the later part of the day by having pasta for dinner rather than lunch. Try the time-worn "glass of warm milk" remedy. Avoid caffeine after noon, and preferably forego it altogether. Exercise in the morning rather than later in the day. Meditate. And if all else fails, just lie in bed with your eyes closed.

- ☐ Although total sleep deprivation (TSD) does seem to work to counteract bipolar depression, it's not something you should try to do on your own, especially because of its connection to the switch into mania. Talk to your psychiatrist or other mental health clinician if you think TSD might be something useful for you.

- ☐ Light therapy can be extremely useful for treating your bipolar depression, but doing phototherapy without a physician's oversight means risking a relapse into mania. Talk to your clinician if you think this is something that might benefit you.

- ☐ Eat three meals a day, at a minimum, and eat them at the same time each and every day.

☐ If you don't work a 9-to-5 job—something that's common among creative, impulsive people—you should still set a strict work schedule and stick to it, even if that means scheduling two hours in the late evening to work on your latest graphic design or write another section of your book. It's not the *when* that's important; it's the *regularity.*

# Other Weapons in the Arsenal

**M**edication is good. If you're bipolar and you've got your disorder under control, you know this. You know that when you take your meds as prescribed, you tend to feel better, and that when you don't, things go downhill quickly.

But the truth is, one cannot live by meds alone. Your pharmaceuticals are definitely, unquestionably, the foundation of your treatment plan. But bipolar disorder is a duplicitous foe. You might be able to force it into hiding, but you can't bury it. Bipolar disorder doesn't die. You need to have other tactics, other weapons, that you can employ to help yourself keep the stability you fought so hard to regain.

The best part? You play a major, active role in almost all these treatments. These are tactics that empower you and make you part of the solution, not just part of the problem. That alone should make them worth a closer look.

## Psychotherapy

Sometimes it seems as if people who talk about bipolar disorder are constantly contradicting themselves. Take psychotherapy, for instance. If bipolar disorder is a biological illness—a sickness just like cancer or diabetes, as everyone keeps telling you, then why do you need therapy? What good will it do you?

The answer to that, quite frankly, depends on what type of psychotherapy you're talking about. Traditional psychotherapy, during which you talk about your problems and issues and seek some sort of insight into them, hasn't been shown to be of much use in a biologically based disorder like bipolar—at least not in keeping the disorder from relapsing or in keeping you out of the hospital. But there are other forms of psychotherapy—more active forms, if you will, based on educating yourself and your family, or on relearning ways of thinking or acting with respect to your behavior and your disorder—that have been extremely successful in backing up medication to keep you stable and in remission.

*My brother is bipolar, and I keep trying to get him to go to talk therapy, but he refuses. He says that it wouldn't do him any good. Is he right?*

"I don't think there's any question that many patients who have bipolar disorder feel a profound need to engage in psychotherapy, but whether we can actually demonstrate that it makes a big difference in terms of outcome, that I'm not sure about. In fact, none of us who have been working for the last decade in psychotherapy for bipolar disorder thinks that traditional psychotherapy is in any way protective or curative in this disorder. We don't think that insight in the traditional sense of looking into what is motivating you unconsciously has anything to do with helping someone with bipolar disorder."—*Ellen Frank, Ph.D., director of the Depression and Manic Depression Prevention Program at Western Psychiatric Institute and Clinic in Pittsburgh*

What psychotherapies for bipolar disorder have in common—at least if they're going to be effective—is a focus on providing you with strategies. Some provide strategies to help you cope with the stresses that tend to bring on episode relapses, while others work on educating you about your disease so you can be a full and committed partner in your own treatment. And sometimes, of course, they will do both. "They're all very practical," says Ellen Frank, Ph.D., director of the Depression and Manic Depression Prevention Program at Western Psychiatric Institute and Clinic in Pittsburgh. "They're all very present and future oriented. They emphasize a big hunk of *psychoeducation,* and they all try to put some emphasis on regularizing the sleep-wake cycle and on self-monitoring of mood. And they almost all put some emphasis on trying to figure out what the particular patient's early signs of an oncoming episode are and developing some kind of plan for addressing those symptoms when they appear."

It might sound simple, but it's incredibly important, extremely effective, and unbearably understudied. As a 1996 report from the National Institute of Mental Health's Workshop on the Treatment of Bipolar Disorder noted, "Maintenance treatment with psychosocial therapies is progressing, although it still lags behind similar efforts for schizophrenia and major depressive disorder."

> ## PsychSpeak
>
> **Psychoeducation** is an intervention that teaches people with mental illness about their condition, what its effects and consequences may be, and concrete strategies that can be used to deal with those effects and consequences.

**Cognitive-Behavioral Therapy** Your credit card bills are piling up, your car payment is due, and you're two months behind on your mortgage. But you're not worried, because you know that somehow it's all going to work itself out. How? You don't know, and you don't care. It just will. And it will do so without your having to make any hard choices—or do much of anything at all.

Or maybe your credit card bills are piling up, your car payment is due, and you're two months behind on your mortgage—and you're beyond worried. In fact, you're overwhelmed. You can see only one way out: suicide.

Stress is an enormous danger to people with bipolar disorder. It can take a stable mood and knock it off-kilter with a single blow. And if you're not prepared, there's really nothing you'll be able to do about it.

Preparing you to deal with stress and life in general is the impetus behind cognitive-behavioral therapy, often shorthanded as cognitive therapy. Cognitive therapy has as its rationale the idea that people who become depressed or manic in response to life events are doing so at least to some degree because they are thinking about and processing those events in an inappropriate, or problematic, way. A cognitive therapist, then, seeks to get you to recognize these problematic thought processes and teaches you alternative ways to think about life stresses and other events.

The problem, such therapists will tell you, is that your biological predisposition to bipolar mood disorder doesn't work in a vacuum; things outside your brain and its chemistry can kick it into action. Things like stress, for instance. And the way you perceive stress is individual—it depends on your self-image, how you look at life events, and what you think your future is likely to hold. When your outlook is negative—or, to be more specific, when you engage in negative cognition or thought processes—you become more vulnerable to mood episodes. The same can be true for people whose outlook is inappropriately positive—a sure sign of mania or hypomania, or at least of their approach.

If you go to see a cognitive therapist, she will address your thought processes. She'll help you make an in-depth assessment of how you interpret things that happen in your life, and she'll teach you how to modify that interpretation to put you at less risk of a mood episode.

Most of the therapies for bipolar disorder are "team" approaches, and cognitive therapy is no exception. This is no passive experience. In addition to your active participation during therapy sessions, your therapist is likely to assign you "homework." Think of it as practicing the skills you've learned in each session, much the way you would if you were taking piano or tennis lessons once a week. Or think of it as a rehearsal for your future. In any case, these assignments might include keeping a mood journal or a behavioral journal, to help you and your therapist identify where your thought processes go "wrong." Or you might be asked to plan ahead for how you could respond to an upcoming event or stressor in your life.

Take, for instance, the bills-piling-up example given earlier. If you respond to legitimate issues by becoming manic or hypomanic, grandiosely assuming that the universe will provide for you without any effort on your part, a cognitive therapist might have you consider the scenario in which you do nothing to get out of your financial situation, and see what the consequences might be. He might ask you to try budgeting for a month to see if it actually does help you get a better handle on your finances. He might ask you to consult with your spouse or a financial adviser about your situation, to see if their take on it is any different than yours. He might play devil's advocate with you to get you to reassess your thought process.

If you respond to these issues by becoming depressed and suicidal, your therapist will likely try an entirely different tack, perhaps simply by helping you recognize and come up with workable solutions to your problem that stop well short of killing yourself.

**Q&A**

*How can I find the right therapist for me?*
"The sad thing is that most of these [new educational and psychotherapeutic] treatments are not available anywhere yet, because we're just beginning to see results from studies. It probably takes a decade from the time a new procedure is found to be efficacious for it to make its way into medical practice. Plus, we've got the problem of finding ways to train people to do these treatments. What you can do now, however, is go out and see if you can find someone who's espousing a present- and future-oriented treatment focused on the practical day-to-day problems of living with bipolar disorder. That's probably your best bet." *–Ellen Frank, Ph.D., Western Psychiatric Institute and Clinic in Pittsburgh*

He might also work with you to create a pro-and-con list regarding suicide and think about what it would or would not accomplish. He might ask you to force yourself to get involved in activities that were once pleasurable to you, so you again can begin to see the positive side of living. And he might ask you to sign a no-suicide contract that you and he negotiate together and that includes steps you can take to help yourself if you're feeling suicidal and steps the therapist will take to aid you in an emergency.

Cognitive therapists will tell you that their method helps keep your natural, bipolar disorder–derived impulsiveness in check, that it reduces your risk of suicide, that it helps you make important life decisions objectively, that it improves marital and family interactions, and that it reduces the stigma and shame that, all too often, come with a diagnosis of bipolar disorder.

And research does, indeed, back up at least some of these claims. In February 2003, Dominic Lam and colleagues from the Institute of Psychiatry in London, England, looked at 103 people with bipolar I disorder, half of whom received medication, regular psychiatric follow-up, and cognitive therapy, while the others received only medication and regular psychiatric follow-up. In the 12-month follow-up period, the group that got cognitive therapy had fewer relapses (44 percent in the therapy group versus 75 percent in the control group), and when they did have an episode, they spent less time in it (27 days versus 88 days). They had fewer mood symptoms and less fluctuation of the manic symptoms they did have. They were better able to cope with symptoms of an oncoming episode and to forestall that episode. And they had "significantly higher social functioning," meaning they were better able to maintain relationships and keep social commitments.

Adults aren't the only ones who can benefit from cognitive therapy. Researchers from the University of Illinois at Chicago reported in 2003 that a child-friendly version of cognitive-behavioral therapy had improved mania, depression, aggression, attention disorders, and sleep disorders in 34 children with bipolar disorder.

**Family-Focused Therapy** Mom's a perfectionist who's clearly disappointed with the way you turned out. Dad's an alcoholic who thinks you just need to toughen up and all your problems will be solved. Your brother treats you like you're an invalid. Your sister treats you like you're mentally retarded. It's enough to make you crazy.

When psychiatrist David Miklowitz, a professor of psychology and director of the clinical psychology program at the University of North Carolina at Chapel Hill, began working with bipolar patients, he was struck by just how often his patients' episodes coincided with periods of time when they were in intense conflict with one or more family members. Treating the people with bipolar disorder, he and his colleagues realized, would never quite solve the problems these people were experiencing. What they needed to do was to treat the whole family as well—or as much of it as possible.

"Communication breakdowns when families are coping with fluctuations of the disorder are common," Miklowitz said in 2000, while commenting on one of the first papers to be published on family-focused therapy (FFT). "Part of the treatment program involves coaching families to interact in a positive way and tackle problems systematically."

Thus family-focused therapy was born. Still in its testing phases, family-focused therapy is a 21-session program of education for both you and your family, given over 9 months immediately after you've achieved remission from a bipolar disorder episode. It focuses on educating you and the people around you about what bipolar disorder is and how it can be controlled. And it takes as its basis studies that have found that, in schizophrenia at least, negative attitudes in the people around the person with the mental illness can actually make the disordered person's outcome worse. On the other hand, these same studies showed, simply by teaching the family how to reduce stress, problem solve, and improve interpersonal communication, a person with schizophrenia can expect a significantly better course for his or her disease.

The question, of course, is whether the same holds true for bipolar disorder. And from the studies that have been done so far, the answer is a resounding yes.

"What Miklowitz and colleagues did was attempt to inculcate communication skills in families to deal with intrafamilial stress," noted Paul Keck, M.D., professor of psychiatry, pharmacology, and neuroscience and vice chairman for research at the University of Cincinnati College of Medicine, in a lecture at the American Psychiatric Association's 2003 annual meeting. "Specifically, they focused on expressing positive rather than negative feelings. In other words, putting something nicely and constructively instead of corrosively and critically, actively listening to the concerns and feelings of people with the illness, making positive requests for change instead of negative, and learning how to express negative feelings about specific behaviors; in other words, giving positive feedback as well as helping families with problem-solving skills."

In a 2003 study of family-focused psychoeducation in 101 volunteers with bipolar disorder, Miklowitz and his team found that, when used in addition to drug therapy, psychoeducation can make it easier for you to adjust to your disorder and can also make it more likely that you will adhere to your drug regimen. To be specific, Miklowitz and colleagues found that of the people given family-focused treatment along with medication, 52 percent went through the full 2-year follow-up without a relapse. The control group, which was given a less-intensive form of psycho-education dubbed crisis management, along with medication, had only a 17 percent relapse-free rate. This means, they noted, that family-focused therapy was threefold better at keeping relapses at bay than crisis management.

"Psychosocial interventions are by no means substitutes for psychotherapy, but they may augment mood stabilizers in pro-tecting patients from symptom deterioration as well as enhance compliance with maintenance treatments," the researchers wrote. The next and possibly most important step, they added, is to begin taking these sorts of approaches out of the laboratory and to the patients they're most likely to benefit.

**Interpersonal and Social Rhythm Therapy** Ellen Frank remembers the exact day when she came up with the idea for the newest form of psychotherapy for bipolar disorder. "It was July 14, my birthday," she says. "I had been invited to the annual meeting of what is now the Depression and Bipolar Support Alliance because of my work in unipolar disorder." Frank spent the day wandering from session to session, taking in all she could about bipolar disorder. "One experience after another during that day left me with the feeling that this was a disorder that had been abandoned by researchers, particularly in the psychosocial arena," she recalls. "I was stunned by how much difficulty navigating life these patients and their families were having, and I made up my mind then and there to dedicate the next decade of my life to working on this disorder."

And so she has. In fact, she started that evening, on the way home from the meeting, when she sketched out the basics of what would become interpersonal and *social rhythm* therapy, or IPSRT, on an airplane cocktail napkin.

## PsychSpeak

**Social rhythms** are daily routines that, when disrupted, might trigger the onset of a mood episode.

What she laid the foundation for that day is possibly the most practical of all these already-practical psychotherapies. And it was designed specifically—solely—for the treatment of bipolar disorder.

What IPSRT is mostly concerned with are your social rhythms—how often and when you eat, when and how long you sleep, whether you get out during the day, who you see. It looks at regulating 17 different activities each day in 3 phases. In the first phase, you get a bit of psychoeducation about your disorder and then you keep track of your daily activities—when you do them, how often you do them, whether you do them alone or in the company of another person. The second phase is when you work with your therapist to "stabilize" these rhythms, to get them to work in synch with both your natural circadian rhythms and the external rhythms with which they may conflict. (For more on circadian rhythms and their connections to IPSRT, see Chapter 7.)

Once the rhythms have been established, a therapist trained in IPSRT will move on to address the interpersonal part of your equation. "Many of our bipolar patients divide their lives into before the diagnosis and after the diagnosis," says Frank. "They see themselves as the person they were and the person they now have to be. Part of the work, we believe, is in helping the patient to grieve for the lost healthy self and come to terms with living with a chronic and, in a sense, life-threatening condition that sets certain limits on what they can do but does not preclude many of the accomplishments they hope to have."

Frank says that although it's great when psychotherapy can begin to lift a previously resistant depression or help calm an out-of-control mania, the ultimate goal is greater than that. "We encourage patients to expect a full remission of symptoms and not to be satisfied simply with a response, not to be satisfied simply with a change," she says. "We are looking to achieve full remission. We want them to be looking for that same kind of treatment effect."

## Electroconvulsive Therapy

Sometimes, nothing works. Sometimes, medication and psychotherapy and mood charting and support groups just aren't enough to pull you out of your bipolar quicksand. Sometimes, they're just not quick enough. What you just might need is to be jolted back to stability—literally.

You're probably shaking your head right now. "No way," you're thinking. "I saw *One Flew Over the Cuckoo's Nest*. Nobody's doing that to me." Electroconvulsive therapy (ECT)—shock therapy, in the vernacular—definitely does not have good PR. If you think mental illness carries a stigma, you ain't seen nothing yet.

But the truth is, modern electroconvulsive therapy is a pretty benign procedure. Here, briefly, is how it goes: You're given a muscle relaxant so your body doesn't move during the treatment and then you're anesthetized so you "sleep" through it. Only then is a small electrical current applied for about 2 seconds to electrodes attached to your skull, inducing a quick seizure. You don't feel a thing during the procedure.

**WEB TALK:** For a look at ECT by author Andy Behrman, someone who's been there, visit:

**www.electroboy.com/ electroshocktherapy.htm**

Scientists admit that they still don't completely understand how ECT works. But they know that it does. And they know that it seems to work best in the patients who are the sickest, which makes it a particularly useful tool.

ECT has long been known to be good at lifting an acute and deep depression—in fact, it's been shown to be as good as, if not better than, most antidepressant medications. And it appears to be just as good, or even better, at controlling mania. A number of scientifically controlled studies have shown that ECT can make you feel a lot better a lot more quickly when you're acutely manic than can lithium, or even a combination of lithium and the antipsychotic medication haloperidol (Haldol). Another study compared ECT to "sham" ECT—in which the patient was anesthetized, had electrodes attached, etc., but didn't actually have an electrical current applied—and found that ECT was significantly better at controlling mania.

ECT is also useful for pregnant women who find themselves in an episode that requires treatment but who can't take most of the mood stabilizers because their effect on a fetus is either unknown or known to be harmful (see Chapter 14).

There are those clinicians who say that ECT also has a place in the long-term maintenance treatment of bipolar disorder, and there is some evidence to back up that suggestion. For instance, one study of 22 medication-resistant or -intolerant people with unipolar or bipolar depression who had undergone 18 months of maintenance ECT treatment looked back at their response. Overall, they had had significantly fewer depressive episodes after the ECT maintenance than before, spent less time in the hospital, and had fewer episodes that required hospitalization. Other small studies have found similar results.

It's highly unlikely, however, that long-term ECT is ever going to become "popular," especially considering how resistant many people are to it in the short term. Still, for the relatively few people who simply don't respond to medication, no matter how many are trotted out and tried on them, or for those who simply can't tolerate their medications' side effects, ECT might very well be a good and effective choice.

Of course, like anything else, ECT has its own side effects. The main and most troublesome one is memory loss—a memory loss that isn't always recoverable. But the more modern versions of ECT carry much less risk than the ECT of *Cuckoo's Nest* fame.

**you're not alone**

## Hooked Up, Switched On, Blissed Out

"April 11, 1995. I'm in front of Barneys when it finally happens. My skin starts tingling, and I feel as if my insides are spilling onto the sidewalk. Everything moves in slow motion. I can't hear. I rush home and climb into the empty bathtub. I lie still for hours. As a last resort, I'm admitted to the hospital for ECT, electroconvulsive therapy, more commonly known as electroshock. The doctor explains the procedure to me. But most important, he tells me that I will get better.

"Seven A.M. The doctor and his team, as well as a group of residents, hover over me. Standing room only. I'm about to have my brains jolted with 200 volts of electricity while 10 note-taking spectators gawk. I'm joking incessantly to fend off the terror. Is it too late for the call from the governor? No call. The show must go on.

"I give the thumbs up. An IV of Brevital, an anesthetic, is stuck into my arm, silencing me. I struggle to stay awake—a losing battle. But I've been told what will happen. An IV of succinylcholine goes in next, relaxing my muscles to prevent broken bones and cracked vertebrae. The nurse sticks a rubber block in my mouth so I don't bite off my tongue, a mask over my mouth and nose so my brain is not deprived of oxygen, and electrodes on my temples. All clear. The doctor presses a button. Electric current shoots through my brain for an instant, causing a grand-mal seizure for 20 seconds. My toes curl. It's over. My brain has been 'reset' like a windup toy.

"I wake up 30 minutes later and think I'm in a hotel room in Acapulco. My head feels as if I've just downed a frozen margarita too quickly. My jaw and limbs ache. But I feel elated. 'Come, Electroboy,' says the nurse in a thick Jamaican accent. I take a sip of juice as she grabs my arm and escorts me downstairs, where my father is waiting with my best friend, a turkey sandwich, and a Diet Coke. I ask questions. Do I have a job? No. An apartment? Yes. A dog? No.

"When I get home, I reacquaint myself with my apartment. I'm not really sure it's mine. It feels as if I've been away for years. After a nap, I shower, get dressed, and hail a cab. By 8 P.M., I'm at a restaurant downtown, deliberating between the salmon and the veal.

"I have 19 treatments over the course of a year. I look forward to them. It's like receiving a blessing in a sanctuary. I become addicted to the rituals—fasting the night before, driving across Central Park to the hospital in the early morning, connecting to the machines that monitor my vital signs, closing my eyes, and counting backward.

"On the one-year anniversary of my first electroshock treatment, I'm clear-headed and even-keeled. I call my doctor to announce my 'new and improved' status and ask to be excused from ECT that week. He agrees to suspend treatment temporarily. Surprisingly, I'm disappointed. ECT reassures me. Soon I miss the hospital and my 'maintenance' regimen. But I never see the doctor again. Two and a half years later, I still miss ECT. But medication keeps my illness in check, and I'm more sane than I've ever been. If I could only remember the capital of Chile."
—Andy Behrman is the author of Electroboy: A Memoir of Mania (Random House, 2003). This essay was first published in The New York Times Magazine in 1999.

# Nutrition

It only makes sense, knowing as much as we do about the effects of food on our health, that what you eat—and what you don't eat—might have an effect on the biochemistry of your brain and on your moods in general. And it only makes sense that a lot of people who are interested in bipolar disorder would be attracted to research in this field.

The problem is that not all the people who are out there hawking supplements and formulations are looking out for your mental health. Many of them are instead simply looking out for their pocketbooks.

When it comes to assessing claims about the latest, greatest supplement on the block, there are three main points to keep in mind:

- It's almost always better to get your nutrition from foods rather than from a pill. Nobody really knows how various components of our diet interact, and when you take them out of their normal milieu and isolate them in a capsule, you might very well be stripping them of much of their power.

- Anecdotal evidence is not scientific evidence. You may have heard that your cousin's wife had an amazing response to some antioxidant cocktail, but that doesn't mean that cocktail is a cure for her illness or, more specifically, for yours. Until rigorous scientific studies have been done—in which people with the same basic disorder and similar characteristics are divided into two groups, one taking the cocktail and the other taking a placebo—you really can't extrapolate the experience one person—or even a dozen people—had to an entire population of people with that disease.

- The supplement industry is unmonitored and unregulated. What you see on the label might not be what you get in the pill. Be skeptical, and know not only what you're buying, but also who makes it and what their reputation is.

As with any other drug, some of these vitamins or other supplements can be dangerous for people with certain medical conditions, or people taking certain medications. Before adding any pill-based supplements into your diet,

## GET PSYCHED

"These [nutrients] are not going to work by themselves in most people, but they are adjuncts to medicines. You can get away with fewer medicines and maybe lower doses."
—Andrew Stoll, M.D., chief of the psychopharmacology research lab at Harvard's McLean Hospital, in Psychology Today's "Blues Buster" newsletter, November 2003

talk to your physician, and be sure he or she knows your medical and drug history. You don't have to be quite as concerned if you're simply modifying your diet, but if the changes are extreme or drastic, it would be a good idea to check in with your physician as well.

**Essential Fatty Acids** One of the biological theories of how bipolar disorder comes to be has to do with the way in which neurons signal one another. The thought is that bipolar disorder is rooted in overactivity in this signaling—in other words, there's too much talking back and forth between neurons. And so, the theory goes, if you could calm the brain's aimless, destructive chattering, you could calm mania, or maybe even lift depression.

Enter the *essential fatty acids,* or *EFAs.* EFAs have been all the rage for the past decade or two because of their importance in processes such as inflammation and their role in regulating blood pressure, heart function, digestion, and more. In studying them, it's become clear that some forms of these compounds can be taken up by the outer membranes of cells like neurons and that they might, thus, have an effect on how and when signaling between neurons occurs.

There are two types of essential fatty acids—the *linoleic fatty acids,* or omega-6 fatty acids, and the *linolenic fatty acids,* or omega-3 fatty acids. But when it comes to bipolar disorder, there seems to be only one that counts: the omega-3s.

Using omega-3 fatty acids as a treatment for bipolar disorder wasn't even on anyone's radar screen until the late 1990s, when Dr. Andrew Stoll and colleagues from Harvard's McLean Hospital began to really look at its utility.

> **PsychSpeak**
>
> Essential fatty acid (EFA) is a type of fat your body cannot synthesize and that, therefore, has to be included in your diet.

Their initial study was short—just 4 months long—and relatively small, including just 30 patients. But the results made a huge impact on the bipolar disorder community. What Stoll and colleagues found was that the patients taking omega-3 fatty acid supplements spent a longer time relapse-free and found their symptoms significantly reduced, as compared to those taking the olive-oil supplement placebo. "The striking difference in relapse rates and response appeared to be highly clinically significant," Stoll and colleagues wrote in their 1999 paper, published in *Archives of General Psychiatry*.

As soon as Stoll's study came out, experts—including Stoll himself—were practically tripping over themselves to be sure that all the caveats were heard and that people with bipolar disorder didn't start tossing their lithium and Depakote out the window in favor of fish-oil supplements. For one thing, the study itself had a number of flaws, not the least of which being the fact that the fish-oil supplements had a distinct aftertaste, so 86 percent of the participants in the trial were able to correctly guess whether they were in the fish-oil or placebo group.

Nevertheless, the results were both striking and exciting. So it's not surprising that since the publication of Stoll's initial paper, there have been a number of studies of the omega fatty acids and their relationship to bipolar disorder. Among them was an intriguing look by researchers from the New York State Psychiatric Institute at the connection between fish consumption and bipolar prevalence rates in a variety of countries. The researchers were able to show that countries in which fish consumption rates are high tend to have low rates of mood disorders. In fact, the connection between the two was so strong that they were able to use rates of fish consumption in a particular country to predict whether lifetime prevalence of bipolar disorder would be higher or lower than in other countries. The same could not be said for fish consumption and schizophrenia—which actually makes sense, considering that schizophrenia is not a mood disorder and the hypothesized connection is specifically between the fish oils and depression and/or mania.

But no study thus far has been able to get the same results Stoll and colleagues got. In fact, a 2003 report from the Stanley

Foundation Bipolar Network found no benefit to the oils in the treatment of acute depression or rapid-cycling bipolar disorder.

So should you start using fish oils? Unfortunately, you're going to have to go with your gut on this one, because science still isn't ready to give its verdict. Do some research and talk to your doctor. Maybe you'll want to start small and begin by incorporating more omega-3s into your diet instead of taking megadoses of supplements.

If you decide to give your brain a fish-oil boost through your diet, you'll want to get omega-3 fatty acids into your meals two or three times a day. But don't despair: it's not going to be as difficult as you might think. The omega-3s are found in a fairly wide range of foods, including the following:

- Fish such as salmon, trout, halibut, sardines, and tuna
- Nuts and seeds such as walnuts, mustard seeds, and pumpkin seeds
- Green leafy vegetables
- Canola or soybean oils
- Flax seed, or flax seed oil, which actually contains twice the omega-3 fatty acids as fish

In addition, a number of companies are now producing eggs that are especially rich in omega-3 fatty acids.

And even if it turns out that the omega-3 fatty acids aren't doing you much good mood-wise, your time and effort won't be completely wasted. Essential fatty acids have also been linked to better cardiovascular health and are believed to be able to reduce your risks of cancer, arthritis, and osteoporosis.

**Taurine** Taurine is an amino acid, one of the building blocks of proteins, and, thus, of pretty much every biological process you can think of. Taurine seems to work by inhibiting the production of neurotransmitters, working to keep the membranes of cells, including the brain's neurons, from becoming overexcited or

171

overexcitable. It's been used to help control epilepsy, and because of the increasing links between epilepsy and bipolar disorder—at least in terms of treatment with anticonvulsant drugs—taurine is now being looked at for bipolar disorder as well. In particular, because it does have mild sedative effects, it could possibly help to reduce manic symptoms. In fact, anecdotal reports have seemed to imply that it works best for people with rapid-cycling bipolar disorder, although whether that is actually the case remains to be scientifically seen.

Taurine can be dangerous if you take too much of it, so if you're going to give it a whirl, you'll want to keep it between 500 and 1,000 milligrams per day, and divide it into a couple doses.

**Other Dietary Modifications** Always keep in mind that dietary supplements are just that—foods or pills you add to your normal diet. And in bipolar disorder, they are also only supplementary to your drug regimen as well.

The B vitamins are well known for their role in keeping the nervous system functioning well. And they've been touted as a natural antidepressant—although a mild one—for quite a while. In particular, deficiencies in vitamins $B_6$ and $B_{12}$ have been linked to depression, so you'll want to be sure you're getting enough of both of them. But as with any antidepressant, be careful about overdoing the B vitamins, as there could well be a risk that they can also help switch you into mania. In particular, folic acid—which is crucial to your body's proper functioning at its normal dose—has been found to bring on mania when it's taken in unusually high doses.

If you're on Depakote or any other anticonvulsant, you'll want to add vitamin E into your diet because anticonvulsants tend to leach vitamin E out of your body. Minerals such as zinc and copper have also been mentioned in discussions of ways to nutritionally attack bipolar disorder.

Calcium and magnesium work hand in hand to regulate nervous system functioning and to help in the production of neurotransmitters in the brain. In moderate doses, they can be quite helpful in battling depression. In fact, they've been cited as particularly useful in calming or obliterating premenstrual dysphoria—depression that occurs in relation to a woman's menstrual cycle.

Another amino acid, tyrosine, has been considered for its potential to help in bipolar disorder. Tyrosine plays a role in forming neurotransmitters such as dopamine, norepinephrine, and epinephrine, all of which can lead to mood disorders when they're in short supply. And some nutritionists believe that it also keeps your thyroid gland functioning at its best. Hypothyroidism and hyperthyroidism can lead to depression or mania, respectively, so keeping the thyroid running smoothly could only be helpful in bipolar disorder.

The amino acid methionine—and its metabolite, SAMe (S-adenosyl-methionine)—have been touted for their antidepressant effects. And that touting has, to some extent, been backed up by research. But again, as with any antidepressant, it can cause mania in certain people with bipolar disorder; in fact, the risk of bringing on mania is so great that with SAMe in particular, it's not recommended for people with bipolar disorder.

Finally, a word about herbal supplements. You might be thinking that a "natural" approach is the way you want to go—no fuss, no muss, no nasty side effects. But the truth is, herbal supplements are medications. And as such, they carry all the risks of medications—side effects, contraindications, potentially dangerous interactions. Take, for instance, St. John's wort, widely acclaimed for its antidepressant qualities. More and more, clinicians are beginning to recognize that it can indeed lift depression—there are at least a few scientific studies that back up the claim. But they're also noticing that it has side effects—extreme sun sensitivity is one of them—and it can interact with prescription medications. Plus, like any antidepressant, it has the potential to switch you into mania.

But St. John's wort has one more problem that pharmaceuticals don't—it's not regulated. Nobody's making sure you're getting what the bottle says you're getting. Nobody's making sure you're getting the proper dosage, from the proper source. So if you're going to venture into the world of herbal supplements, be very, very wary. Be sure you know the company you're buying from, and be sure you know what the risks are. Otherwise, you might wind up doing yourself more harm than good.

## What You Can Do

When we talk about illness, we often fall back on military analogies. We talk about battling your disorder, fighting its symptoms, or treating disease with an arsenal of weapons, as I did in this chapter's title. For bipolar disorder, the big guns in the arsenal are the psycho-pharmaceuticals I discussed in Chapter 7. But what really keeps things stable after each individual battle has been won are the peacekeeping forces: education, psychotherapy, and nutrition. Here are some of the things you can do to give yourself the upper hand:

☐ Do some research on cognitive-behavioral therapy, family-focused therapy, and interpersonal and social rhythms therapy (IPSRT), and decide which approach is the right one for you. Then try to find a therapist whose approach fits the therapeutic model you've chosen for yourself.

☐ Even if you can't get the type of therapy you want (some are still in the experimental stage and not widely available), you can incorporate some of their concepts into your life. For instance, take a page out of the cognitive therapy book and keep a journal of what goes through your mind when you're faced with some kind of stress—a major decision, some type of rejection, an argument with someone close to you—and see if you can find ways to turn negative thoughts into useful energy.

☐ As you would in family-focused therapy, try to educate your family about bipolar disorder so they can begin to understand what you're dealing with as well as what they're up against. Then sit down as a team and try to brainstorm ways to make your interactions more positive.

☐ You can mimic at least some of the benefits of IPSRT by getting yourself on a strict schedule of eating, sleeping, and even socializing—and sticking to it as best you can.

☐ If you're having trouble finding the right medications to beat back your disorder, or if you're reacting badly to your medications, or you're pregnant, or you're simply so ill you don't have time to let the meds do their job, you need to seriously consider electroconvulsive therapy. Let go of your preconceived notions, and learn about it. Discuss it with your doctor. Then make your decision—and remember that it is yours to make.

☐ Consider whether or not you should add essential fatty acids to your diet, especially omega-3 fatty acids. If you decide to, you can do it simply by eating more fish or getting more flaxseed into your diet.

☐ Consider whether or not you should add taurine to your diet. You can do this simply by eating more meat and fish.

☐ Certain foods and food supplements may very well help you stabilize your moods or, more likely, keep them stable. But remember that, on their own, they are not and probably never will be enough to keep bipolar disorder in check. Do not stop taking your meds; no matter how good you're feeling, you most likely still need them.

# Stopping the Swing Before It Starts

I f only bipolar disorder were just a little less tenacious, a little less persistent—then it might not be nearly as devastating a diagnosis. But this mood disorder is tenacious, and it is persistent. It hangs on for ages and ages, and even once you think you've got it licked, all it's really doing is sitting right outside your perimeter, licking its wounds, waiting for another chance to strike.

That's why the truly visionary scientists working in the field of bipolar disorder have their sights set not only on getting you into a remission quickly and easily, but also on keeping you in that calm and quiet state. In other words, that's why the truly visionary scientists working the field are looking for ways to prevent bipolar disorder.

Prevention isn't just about keeping you away from the poles of your illness, however. It's also about getting you to a place where your life is good—where you're functioning well, you're working, and you're relating to people. And despite what you might think, that's a larger, more difficult goal to reach than simply not being manic or in a major depression. In fact, several studies over the past few years have found that one of the most debilitating things about being bipolar is that even when you're not in the midst of an "episode" per se, you're much more likely than other folks to be subsyndromally depressed—that is, living with symptoms of depression that are not quite severe enough to fit the criteria for a major depressive episode.

The harsh reality—*your* harsh reality—is that there is probably no way to completely prevent bipolar disorder from recurring. And there won't be until scientists figure out precisely what its biological cause is and how to fix the genetic or neurological errors at its base. But until that time—and it's undoubtedly coming, although not necessarily soon enough—there are things you can do to keep your disorder at bay and keep as much control as possible over your moods, your emotions, and your life.

## An Ounce of Prevention

Ask a couple clinicians if they can prevent bipolar disorder, and they'll immediately grow distant, even guarded. "Do you mean prevent it from starting in the first place?" they'll ask. "Or do you mean prevent it from coming back?"

The former, you see, is somewhat of a sore spot. Certainly, being able to stop people who are at risk for bipolar disorder from ever experiencing their first mania or major depression would be an immense, almost indescribable feat. But unfortunately, we're not even close to being there yet.

*I have bipolar disorder, and that means my son is at risk. Is there anything I can to do to intervene before he has to go through what I've gone through?*

"There's been very little work on this so far in bipolar disorder, though it is now becoming an issue of interest in schizophrenia. Unfortunately, the results so far have not been particularly encouraging. It's hard to know whether one can intervene in people you think are at high risk to prevent long-term illness. On the other hand, we do think that a number of the drugs we're already using might provide a prophylactic benefit, meaning fewer or less severe episodes over time in someone who's already developed the disorder." —*S. Nassir Ghaemi, M.D., director of the Bipolar Disorder Research Program at Cambridge Health Alliance*

But if you assure the clinicians you're only talking about preventing relapses, about keeping people stable for as long as possible after an initial episode, then they'll let their guard down. Because that they can do. They might not be able to do it perfectly, but they have tools, and research, and ideas.

Most tools and ideas and such center around the use of the very same drugs that are employed to get your moods stabilized in the first place. Take lithium, for instance. This well-studied drug has been shown to be pretty effective at keeping mania at bay. In fact, Paul Keck Jr., M.D., vice chairman for research in the Department of Psychiatry at the University of Cincinnati College of Medicine, told participants at a 2003 conference sponsored by the American Psychiatric Association that, "If you took all the relapse prevention studies with lithium and looked at relapse rates standardized at six months and one year, what those studies found was that the odds of relapse, if you weren't on lithium, were four-fold higher than if you were on lithium for one year." That means that if you go off lithium because you're feeling better and you're tired of dealing with its side effects, your chances of getting sick are four times higher than those of someone who sticks with the drug.

Another drug that seems to do fairly well at keeping symptoms hidden and preventing relapse is olanzapine (Zyprexa). Mauricio Tohen, M.D., of the Lilly Research Laboratories in Indianapolis and Harvard Medical School, and colleagues reported at the 2002 annual meeting of the American College of Neuropsychopharma- cology that they had studied olanzapine's effectiveness in keeping mania and depression at bay as compared to that of lithium and had found that olanzapine was actually better able to stave off mania than was lithium, while both were equally good at keeping levels of depression low.

Most recently, researchers from the University of British Colum- bia in Vancouver, Canada, have shown that lamotrigine (Lamictal) beats lithium in the prevention of depression relapse in patients who had recently been manic. Previous studies had indicated the same thing but had shown that lamotrigine is not particularly adept at preventing mania relapse as compared to lithium.

"It's a remarkably consistent story," Keck noted. "And it's also consistent with [Joseph] Calabrese and colleagues' study of lamotrigine in acute bipolar depression, suggesting that lamotrigine's primary benefit for people with bipolar illness is in the depressed phase of the illness—an illness for which we clearly need treatment."

As with the treatment of an acute episode, combination therapies seem, logically, to be a good choice for prevention of relapse into mania or depression. This is, however, one of those areas of research where clinicians don't yet have the numbers to back up their suppositions. The few studies that are out there, however, do seem to lean toward the idea that you get better relapse prevention from two or more drugs than you do from *monotherapy,* or just one drug working all on its own. For instance, a study led by Tohen quite recently found that people taking olanzapine plus either lithium or valproate (Depakote) enjoyed a much longer period of time without symptoms of either depression or mania than did people taking only lithium or divalproex.

"The results of this study suggest that, in patients who achieved remission from a manic or mixed episode after addition of an atypical antipsychotic agent such as olanzapine to previous treatment with lithium or valproate, the continuation of combination treatment reduced the rate of relapse of symptomatic bipolar episodes, compared with patients who stopped taking olanzapine and who continued on lithium or valproate monotherapy," the researchers wrote in their paper, which was published in the *British Journal of Psychiatry* in 2004. And the difference was significant: the addition of olanzapine kept people in the study symptomatically stable for almost five months. In comparison, those who were on only lithium or valproate stayed stable for an average of 42 days—less than 6 weeks.

## PsychSpeak

**Monotherapy** is a form of treatment that employs only one drug rather than a combination of pharmaceuticals.

An interesting side note to the study was that women were much more affected by the addition or subtraction of olanzapine to their regimen than were men, relapsing much more quickly without an olanzapine boost.

But there's a downside. As Keck has noted: "Additive drugs, additive side effects." Indeed, one study of combination therapy found that people with bipolar disorder taking two drugs had twice as many side effects as people with bipolar disorder taking just one drug. And Tohen's *British Journal of Psychiatry* study found that those people who continued on olanzapine gained almost 4.5 pounds over the 18 months of follow-up, compared to those people taking only lithium or only valproate, who actually lost almost 4 pounds.

Still, both clinicians and patients agree that when the drugs do actually work—and work well—it's a lot easier to pay the increased side-effect tariff than it is when they're not particularly effective. They also agree that as often as possible, you need to be using nondrug methods to control your moods and prevent relapses. After all, psychotherapy, mood charts, and patient education are pretty much side-effect free—and effective at what they're trying to accomplish.

## Mood Charting

Mood charting can give you a much-needed dose of control over your disorder. If you keep an honest record of your daily moods, how much of your medication you're taking (and whether you're taking it), how much sleep you're getting, and other factors that can change on a daily basis, you can take back the ability to "see" when things are starting to go awry—the very same ability that the disorder itself takes from you with its symptomatic lack of insights (see Chapter 3). It also can provide invaluable information to

**GET PSYCHED**

"People can have protective life events, like establishing or improving supportive interpersonal relationships or finding work they find meaningful or enjoyable. These sorts of things can be enormously beneficial." *—Terence Ketter, M.D., chief of the Bipolar Disorders Clinic at Stanford University Medical School*

your doctor, who might only see you weekly or monthly and who otherwise might miss the signs of an impending episode.

Just how you chart your moods isn't nearly as important as simply doing it. You can keep just a bare-bones notation of how you're feeling each day, or a detailed description of all the ups and downs you encounter. Positive experiences are just as important as negative experiences, too, so be sure to record those as well.

The Depression and Bipolar Support Alliance has a free six-month diary that includes entries for medications and dosages, hours of sleep each night, a rating of your overall mood each day (on a scale of 0 to 100), the number of mood changes per day, the severity of individual episodes, records of significant daily events (including medication side effects and other medical or psychological issues you might be having), and, for women, a way to keep track of where you are in your menstrual cycle and how that might be affecting your moods.

You don't even have to keep a formal chart if that seems somehow restrictive to you. A personal journal will do the trick as well, although it can be harder to pick up on trends and changes without also keeping some sort of graphic or numeric picture of your moods. You can talk into a tape recorder if you'd like and then transcribe the information once a month or so. You can create a chart on your computer and fill it out each evening when you check e-mail. Whatever works.

WEB TALK: Get your diary/ personal calendar at:
**www.dbsalliance.org**

You don't even have to do a daily mood chart, although you're most likely to have the best results with one. If you have a slowly cycling version of the disorder and you can't face daily mood charting, keep a weekly chart. The idea is simply to do it often enough that you'll be able to see the patterns that emerge and hopefully figure out the warning signs or triggers of an oncoming mania or depression. And if you do see one or more of those warning signs, call your doctor immediately. The sooner you grab a mood swing, the easier it is to wrestle it to the ground.

There are many mood charts available to you. To give you options beyond the DBA's more-than-adequate offering, here are just a few of the other ones you can get for free online. Check them all out, try them all out, and then decide which one works best for you:

- Download a free, printable mood chart at www. psycheducation.org.
- Get a blank mood chart or see an example of a completed mood chart at Harvard Bipolar Research Program's website, www.manicdepressive.org/moodchart.html.
- Another set of blank and completed mood charts are available at www.psychiatry24x7.com. Search for "mood diary."

If you have a child who is bipolar, there are child-friendly charts (with symbols to show mood, for instance) you can find and download from places like the Child and Adolescent Bipolar Foundation at www.bpkids.org. And if you want to get even deeper into mood charting, books such as *The Mood Tree* are available that teach you not only how to put together a chart, but also how to analyze the charts you produce.

**WEB TALK:** You can purchase *The Mood Tree* at:

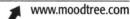 www.moodtree.com

## Heeding Warning Signs of Mania

You've been here before, to this place of energy and excitement and agitation. This isn't the first time you've felt this sense of incredible power and irritation at people who don't seem to understand what you understand. Your parents have been here before as well, as have your partner and possibly your friends. That's why all of you—as a team of sorts—are in the best position to notice when things start to go awry.

Once you or someone close to you notices the start of a shift, you need to take the next step—to tell people, to get help, to follow through. And of course, while you're in the best position to pick up on the earliest harbingers of mania—grandiosity sending up its first green shoot, euphoria warming itself in the sun, paranoia building a nest in a nearby tree—you're not necessarily in the best position to do much about them. Between the denial, the impaired insight, and the sheer enjoyment of the early stages of mania, you're more likely to ignore the signs, deliberately or not, than you are to speak up about them. That's why having a strong support system is so essential to carrying out a prevention plan for mania. And it's why your best bet is to put together an emergency plan with your clinician at a time when you're perfectly healthy. Think of it the way you do the writing of a will. You don't particularly want to ponder these issues when you're healthy and happy, but it's the only way you'll be able to have a say in what goes on when or if things start to go wrong.

## PsychSpeak

**Rescue medication** is a drug that brings quick relief from an acute episode or attack of an illness.

Generally, a prevention plan is fairly simple. It includes lists of symptoms that characterize your first steps toward mania, a means for contacting your doctor or an on-call emergency physician, and instructions or prescriptions for small supplies of some sort of *rescue medication*.

Some of the signs of oncoming mania are pretty broad—that is, they occur in a large percentage of people with bipolar disorder. But there may also be certain symptoms that you'll notice are rather unique to you and you alone. For instance, in a 1999 study of early manic symptoms, one person noted that wanting to take more than one bath in a day almost always preceded his or her mania. Another was able to point to a specific food for which he or she would develop a craving as a signal that something was about to go awry. If you have symptoms like these, don't ignore them as too quirky to be useful or worth mentioning. They are, rather, likely to be one of the most important symptoms for you to monitor and may help you avoid a number of the consequences of undetected mania.

Other studies have looked at how often the various symptoms pop up in both mania and depression and how much time you have to do something about them. In one review study of a number of different sets of research data, the amount of time between when the disorder fired its first symptomatic warning shot and when the mania hit its peak was anywhere between one day and four months. On average, however, the people in the studies under review got between 21 and 29 days to pick up on the psychological hints being left by their bipolar disorder and get their mood under control.

What can you do to help yourself in just a couple weeks? Plenty. For one thing, you can put into place some predefined coping strategies to help you discharge some of your energy, or at least exert a little control over yourself. And for another, you can begin to take a new drug or up your dosages of your old ones to try to nip things in the bud. (Of course, don't try this at home. You should never play with medication levels or types without the supervision of a medical doctor of some kind.) These drugs, which often take weeks and weeks to kick in fully, can make a big difference in a short amount of time if you start them before things really begin to get out of control.

> **GET PSYCHED**
>
> "I take things day by day. When I feel my mood shift, I limit my self-indulgence and I talk about it, joke about it. The two most valuable things someone with bipolar disorder can have are a sense of humor and a good support system." *—Tina, living with bipolar disorder*

"We have found that a small amount of rescue medication in the hands of responsible, well-educated patients can be absolutely lifesaving," says Ellen Frank, Ph.D., director of the Depression and Manic Depression Prevention Program at the Western Psychiatric Institute and Clinic. "We try to educate patients about their early warning signs and then give them a small supply, usually of an antipsychotic medication, that they can use any time."

In addition, Frank says, they encourage their patients to call, day or night, and they back that up by offering a 24-hour answering service that can hook you up with a clinician at any time of the day or night.

"We've found that it can be very helpful in de-escalating a crisis simply to talk to a professional clinician, and that, especially for mania, intervention in the first hours or the first 24 hours can be critical," says Frank.

**Q&A**

*What are the early symptoms I should be looking out for so I'll know if I'm about to relapse into mania?*

The symptoms of mania are pretty individual. But there are some that seem to occur more frequently than others. In a review of the literature, British researchers noted the following symptoms popping up again and again:

- Sleep disturbance (77 percent)
- Symptoms of psychosis such as delusions or hallucinations (47 percent)
- Mood changes of any magnitude (43 percent)
- Speeded up movements as a consequence of mood change (34 percent)
- Loss or increase in appetite (20 percent)
- Increased anxiety (16 percent)

*(From "A Systematic Review of Manic and Depressive Prodromes,"* Journal of Affective Disorders, *May 2003)*

**Lack of Sleep** You've noticed that lately you're having trouble falling asleep. In fact, the other night you sat up for a few hours— well after your wife had gone to bed—and caught up on a little extra work. Your mind was sharp, and today you don't feel par- ticularly tired, even though you didn't really sleep in much this morning. Somewhere in the back of your mind this rings a warn- ing bell, but you're so pleased with all the work you got done, you don't really want to listen to it.

Sleep—or lack thereof—can be one of the most sensitive mood barometers, letting you know when there are rough winds ahead or when there's likely to be smooth sailing over your emotional seas. In fact, in 1999, psychologists Grace Wong and Dominic Lam from the United Kingdom reported on the "development and validation" of the Coping Inventory for Prodromes of Mania, and noted that sleep was an early warning sign of mania in more than 50 percent of the people in the study. And in a 2003 review of studies on the earliest symptoms of mania, that number went even higher. Overall, 77 percent of people with bipolar mania had sleep disturbance on their list of early symptoms of relapse.

**Lack of Inhibition** Normally, you're a pretty private person. But just the other day, you found yourself telling your whole life's story to the grocery checker. It was kind of funny, actually. But definitely out of character.

Or maybe you were at a party recently and found yourself the center of attention. You were telling jokes, people were laughing, and you just fed off all that positive energy. You were a little surprised when your husband took you by the arm and said, quietly, "That's enough now, honey." What a party pooper.

Or maybe you're talking just a tad faster than usual; after all, you're feeling sharp these days, and you've got a few great ideas that you want to pursue. Nothing too far-fetched, just some creative thoughts. In fact, now that you think about it, your brain is kind of speeding up a bit. It's getting harder and harder these days to shut down at night and just go to sleep. There's so much to do, so much to think about.

Being friendly, feeling sociable, thinking creatively, talking a lot—those aren't necessarily bad things in and of themselves. But if they're combined with any other of your early symptoms, or if they're in stark contrast to your "normal" personality, then they're at least noteworthy, something you should bring up with your clinician sooner rather than later.

**Libido Increase** A lot of the signs of an oncoming manic episode are subtle. And a lot of them are pleasurable, especially when they're still at a relatively low level. So not only are they hard to pick up, they're hard to *want* to pick up. Libido definitely falls into this category.

Nobody's going to tell you that having a strong sex drive is a bad thing. But there is usually a very clear difference between a strong sex drive and a sudden obsession with sex, no matter what the personal cost. And it's easy to differentiate between the two.

For instance, wanting to have sex with your partner is one thing. Feeling driven to have sex with your partner or, more tellingly, to have sex with someone outside your relationship, or with someone you barely know, is another thing entirely. And it's especially telling if you're not normally that way between episodes—or if the people around you comment on your changed behavior.

Nobody's saying that you can't have sex with your partner without worrying that you're spiraling into mania. But if there's a noticeable change in frequency, compulsion, and especially, safety and responsibility in relation to sexual activity, then you might just want to heed it as a potential warning sign, if only to use it as a prompt to take a look at your other behaviors, and see if they, too, are telling you something about changes in your overall mood.

**A Manic Intervention** In the process of developing their Coping Inventory for Prodromes of Mania, Wong and Lam tried out the tool with 206 people with bipolar disorder. "Since the appearance of *prodromal symptoms* of mania may precede the full syndrome by weeks, their early detection and intervention are particularly important if mild changes in mood states are not to spiral into more severe and prolonged conditions," they wrote in the paper describing their inventory, which was published in the *Journal of Affective Disorders*.

## PsychSpeak

Prodromal symptoms are the signs of illness that appear during the *prodrome,* which is the period of time between the first recognition of a disease's symptoms and when it reaches its most severe form.

What they found was that although everyone has different ways of coping with the onset of mania, some generalizations can be made. For instance, the most frequently used coping mechanism in their study was "stimulation reduction"—basically, avoiding situations that might make symptoms worse. Next came "problem-directed coping," in which the people in the study actively worked on beating back their symptoms by a variety of methods including monitoring and restraining their behavior, distracting themselves, or even consciously trying to slow down their speech or thought processes. There were several people whose main coping style was simply to seek professional help, whether in the form of seeing their doctor, taking their medication, or threatening themselves with the possibility of hospitalization as a way to swing themselves into action. And, finally, there was denial—or non-coping, as it were—in which people basically ignored the signs and symptoms or comments of others and went on as if nothing were wrong.

Now, those are the strategies patients have come up with on their own, or in conjunction with their clinicians, to deal with their symptoms and the impact their disease is having on their lives. But there are also ways in which the clinician can intervene—by being more aggressive or outgoing, getting the people who have bipolar disorder to learn how to help themselves. For instance, one prestigious study that came out of the United Kingdom and was published in the *British Journal of Medicine* monitored the effect of using patient education as a prevention tool. In the study, researcher Alison Perry and her colleagues looked at how effective they could be in preventing relapse simply by teaching their patients to identify its early symptoms and giving them fail-proof ways to seek prompt treatment.

"Simply" might be an understatement. The education and the emergency plan put into action by this team were almost precisely what you would think of when you consider a perfect-world scenario. Each study patient sat down with a psychologist and worked on identifying his or her own precise prodromal symptoms of mania or depression. The patients kept diaries they used to distinguish between true harbingers of disease and normal mood variations. "Three symptoms or life situations which reliably occur early in the manic or depressive prodrome constituted a warning stage for the patient to increase monitoring from weekly to daily," the researchers explained in their paper. "Three further symptoms or life situations occurring later in the prodrome constituted an action stage to seek help from a health professional of the patient's choice."

Perry and her patients put their action plan together early on, well before a crisis might arise. The researchers and patients picked who their health professionals would be, and arrangements were made such that at least one of those clinicians would be available at all times. The entire plan—the warning symptoms, the action plan, and emergency contact information for the clinicians—was then printed on a card that was laminated and given to the individual patient so he or she could refer to it whenever necessary.

All this was compared to what they called "routine treatment" in which patients were given the normal therapies—pharmaceuticals, mood monitoring, support, education, inpatient care when necessary—but without the focus on specific prevention techniques.

After 18 months of follow-up, the researchers found that there was a highly significant difference between the amount of time it took for the so-called experimental group—the people who had had the extensive education and emergency planning—to relapse into mania and the time it took for the routine-treatment group to relapse. To be more specific, 25 percent of the routine-treatment group relapsed into mania within 17 weeks of their initial episode, while it took 65 weeks—well over a year—for 25 percent of the experimental group to relapse into mania.

The difference in the time it took for the patients to relapse into mania spilled over into their everyday functioning as well, the researchers noted, with the experimental group reaping benefits in both social functioning and employment due to their less-frequent leaps into mania.

The differences between groups in the amount of time it took to relapse into depression was not statistically significant.

The British group's findings were replicated and even somewhat expanded upon by a group from Barcelona, Spain, who published a paper in 2003 in the *Archives of General Psychiatry*. Like their colleagues, they found that group psychoeducation on the signs of relapse was able to decrease the number of relapses experienced by people in the study as well as increase the amount of time between mixed episodes and episodes of mania, hypomania, and—in this particular study—even depression.

## Heeding Warning Signs of Depression

You'd think it would be easy to recognize the early stages of depression—especially if you've ever been depressed before. After all, you're not dealing with the same issues as you are with mania—the denial, the lack of insight, the allure. But the truth of the matter is that the signs of depression are actually more difficult to pick up on reliably, possibly because they are so broad and nebulous and hard to wrap your hands around.

Mania is unusual—the energy, the grandiosity, the outlandish behavior—and even its early symptoms have a sort of "look-at-me, pay-attention-to-me" flavor. Depression, on the other hand, is usually just more of the same, business as usual. It doesn't excite you or energize you or call attention to itself. It just creeps in slowly, stealthily, until it has eclipsed almost everything else in your life and left only numbness and pain and emptiness.

Still, it's worth keeping an eye out for whatever your early symptoms of bipolar depression might be. It's still difficult to treat bipolar depression, but at the very least, if you know what's coming, you can start to put into action some of the more effective coping strategies.

For instance, Tina, a 34-year-old mother of two who was diagnosed with bipolar II 3 years ago, says that simply knowing where her symptoms are coming from can help her grab hold of them and take control. "Before I slip into depression, I start getting angry at everything, and I get where everything irritates me," she says. "It feels like anger, but it's really the first step into depression."

191

**Q&A** *What sorts of early depression symptoms should I be looking for?*
It's hard to say on an individual basis—your depression symptoms might differ from the next person's depression symptoms so significantly that you'd think they weren't the same condition. Still, there are some trends. When researchers from the United Kingdom conducted a literature search on reports of prodromal symptoms, they found eight studies that had looked at bipolar depression. The most frequently noted symptoms included the following:

- Mood changes of any magnitude (48 percent)
- Slowed-down or speeded-up movements as a consequence of mood (41 percent)
- An increase in anxiety (36 percent)
- Increased or decreased appetite (36 percent)
- Suicidal thoughts or feelings (29 percent)
- Sleep disturbance (24 percent)

*(From "A Systematic Review of Manic and Depressive Prodromes,"* Journal of Affective Disorders, *May 2003)*

As it did for mania, a review study of prodromal symptoms of bipolar depression looked at how long it normally takes to go from the first depressive symptoms to depression's peak—or trough, as the case may be. They found that although the average number of days from warning to full-blown depression was actually less than that for mania—somewhere between 11 and 19 days after the first symptoms appear—the range of how long it can take was almost three times as large as it was in mania. In fact, they found that the prodromal period in depression can stretch anywhere from 2 days to a full year.

**Sadness or Anxiety** Depression can be stereotypical, filled with bouts of crying for no reason you can express accompanied by a deep, unending feeling of grief or sadness. But it can also be anxious or worried—or even just plain tired and numb.

It can be difficult to differentiate between anxiety that comes out of an actual anxiety-provoking event and anxiety that comes out of the bottom of your soul and is a sign of an oncoming depression. That differentiation becomes a lot easier as time goes on. A "normal" feeling of anxiety will ebb as the situation that caused it resolves itself. On the other hand, anxiety that's coming out of an incipient depression will simply feed on itself. It might have had an initial cause, but now it's on its own, cycling back and forth and back and forth. You're having panic attacks without any trigger that you can find, and you're jumpy and nervous all the time. This, my friend, is a sign. Make no mistake about it.

**Lethargy and Numbness** The early stages of depression can feel like you're coming down with a flu. You're tired all the time, you ache inside and out, and you have no energy. Food? Who needs it? Sex? Who wants it? God, everything about your life is just so ... boring.

This is one of the parts of depression that just sort of feeds on itself. The more lethargic you become, the more you pull back from your normal activities. And that, in turn, feeds the apathy you're already feeling. Soon, you find yourself not only uninterested, but almost physically incapable of getting out of bed and going to work, or seeing friends, or even getting dressed. Catching this in the early stages, when the cycle can still be broken, is critical.

**Negative Thoughts and Feelings** One of the most insidious parts of depression is the way your brain turns on itself, almost like an emotional autoimmune disease. Despite the fact that it's well known that depression is biological in nature, its symptoms include an ongoing cycle of self-blame and self-hatred. You're likely to be feeling guilty about things that have happened in the past or things that are happening right now. In fact, you're likely to be feeling guilty about being depressed. Talk about vicious cycles.

# Go, Dog, Go

Tina has bipolar II, heavy on the depression. She has attention deficit disorder. She has all the signs and symptoms of seasonal affective disorder. She has had postpartum depressions after the births of her two children.

But Tina also has Depakote and antidepressants to try to keep her moods stable. She has a husband who keeps a close eye on her. And above all, she has Kita. Kita is an American Staffordshire Terrier and is Tina's secret weapon against depression. That's because Tina has trained Kita as a psychiatric service dog.

"She's a barometer of my moods," Tina explains. "She responds to and reflects my moods right back at me. If I get where I'm angry or depressed, she is in my face ... She will do anything to nudge me out of myself."

Tina recalls one day in particular, when she was starting to sink into a depression and had become irritable and angry. "I actually raised my hands to the kids, I was so angry," she says. "And that's not how I am usually. Anyway, Kita physically put herself between me and the kids, started shoving a ball into my stomach, chasing her tail around and around ... She wouldn't let me focus on anything but her. I kept telling her to go away, to go sit down, but she wouldn't. Finally, I focused on her like she wanted me to, and when I did that, I realized what had almost happened. I said, 'Okay, Kita, it's okay.' And only then did she go over to the couch and curl up."

If Kita can't get Tina to snap out of whatever mood she's in, she's been trained to go and get help. "If I start crying, she's right next to me. If I ignore her, she'll whine and lick my face and shove her nose into me. If I still don't pay attention, then she knows she has to go get [my husband] Rick; she'll go find him and start whining and then she'll lead him to me."

All this, Tina admits, is simply a matter of taking Kita's normally nurturing personality and honing it using some basic training techniques. It wasn't easy at first; there aren't that many psychiatric service dogs out there. But Tina had some ideas about what she could do, and she had some experience with service dogs, having trained one for her aunt, who has severe arthritis.

Kita still has a way to go in her training. But she's already been a real lifesaver for Tina. Not only is she able to pick up on and mirror Tina's moods, but she also helps Tina remember to take her medication. "Nowadays I set up a timer that goes off twice a day when it's time for medication," Tina explains. "And I keep my pills and a little freeze-dried liver treat for Kita together. Kita's learned that when it's pill time for me, it's treat time for her. About 5 minutes before the alarm goes off, she'll start bugging me until I realize it's pill time. When the alarm goes off, she runs to the pills and sits there until I take them. Then she gets her treat."

Of course, Tina notes, Kita is just one part of the support system she has built up. But she's a very important part.

"Kita's always in the same room with me," Tina says. "If I let her, she'll even lie outside the shower door when I'm taking a shower.

"She's my dog. She'll take commands from other people and be with other people, but she's my dog. And she's exactly what I need."

*For more information about psychiatric service dogs, including how you can get and train one, visit the Psychiatric Service Dog Society at www.psychdog.org.*

At their worst, these thoughts can push you in the direction of suicide; they can make you feel so hopeless about yourself, and so sure of your inherent lack of worth, that you can find no reason to continue to inflict yourself on the world. This, of course, is your disease talking. Luckily, it's also a place that you normally don't get to until you've been depressed for some time. Still, should suicidal thoughts of any stripe start to creep into your mind at any point—whether or not you think you're having an "episode"— it's time to put the emergency plan into action. In fact, it's time to not only do that, but to call a suicide hotline such as 1-800-SUICIDE (1-800-784-7433) as well.

## Interventions in Depression

Although the initial studies of the effects of education and planning for emergencies on relapse rates were unable to show much of a response in dampening depression, later studies have refined the technique and have a more positive message for people at either pole. Researchers in Barcelona showed that group psycho-education, as they call it, not only reduced the number of people who relapse into depression, mania, hypomania, or mixed episodes, but also reduced the number of episodes in those who do relapse and lengthened the amount of time between relapses.

Another form of psychotherapy that seems to have an impact not only on acute phases of the disorder but also on attempts at prevention is family-focused therapy, or FFTs (see Chapter 8). David Miklowitz, Ph.D., a professor of psychology and director of the clinical psychology program at the University of North Carolina at Chapel Hill, was one of the people who created this particular technique. His impetus, he says, came out of studies— some of which were his own—that showed that living in a stress-ful family environment makes schizophrenics more likely to relapse, and that working with the family to change the home environment and attitudes toward the family member who is mentally ill improves the patient's chances of staying healthier for longer periods of time.

When Miklowitz and his colleagues tried the same sorts of strategies with bipolar adults and their families, they found that teaching family members to focus on expressing positive attitudes and emotions and to avoid criticism and negativity helped their patients avoid relapse for longer and relapse less frequently. The training—called family-focused therapy, or FFT—was also linked to a decrease in symptoms of depression, although it didn't seem to decrease manic symptoms.

Some clinicians suggest that another way to keep bipolar disor-der from swinging out of control is to attack it from its flanks. For instance, bipolar disorder seems to have intimate ties to the use and abuse of alcohol and drugs (see Chapter 10). There are even some researchers who think that using these substances can either bring on or predispose you to bipolar disorder. And if that's the case, they argue, then actively working to prevent drug and alco-hol abuse in those at risk for or recently diagnosed with bipolar disorder might either reduce the incidence of this mental illness or at least keep it from turning unusually ugly.

## What You Can Do

If there's any part of your disorder in which you can—and should—take an extremely active role, it's in trying to prevent relapses from occurring, or at least trying to reduce their incidence. That's because relapse-control isn't just about medication—although medication certainly has a role. It's also simply about you knowing yourself and your patterns and keeping an eye on when things start to sway or swing in an unusual way. A lot of the techniques here might seem simplistic, but they work. In fact, they can work quite well if you're willing to really commit to them.

☐ Keep an ongoing mood chart or mood journal.

☐ Create a list of your prodromal symptoms, both for mania and for depression. Give a copy to at least one other person who can watch for outward signs of your disorder while you patrol your internal corridors.

☐ Talk with your clinician or physician about an emergency plan for when you begin to notice the signs of oncoming mania or depression. Keep one copy for yourself, give another to your doctor, and give one or more copies to people close to you—family members, friends, your partner—who can help you if you're not able to help yourself.

☐ Talk to your clinician about providing you with either a prescription or a small supply of rescue medication for emergencies.

☐ Be sure you have 24-hour emergency contact information for more than one clinician so you can implement your emergency plan whenever or wherever necessary.

☐ Be aware that using recreational drugs or alcohol is going to predispose you to relapse—and that substance use is going to make bipolar relapses harder to stop or treat when they do occur.

☐ You're better off crying wolf a few times than ignoring potentially meaningful signals of an upcoming change of mood. After all, wouldn't you rather have your doctor pat you on the back and tell you that you're fine than visit you in the hospital and up your medication?

☐ Realize that your disorder is biological in nature and, thus, that you can't necessarily cure yourself, or even keep yourself safe from any and all recurrences of your symptoms. If you have a relapse, do not beat yourself up. It's just the nature of your beast. But do sit down afterward with your support team—your clinician, your family, your friends—and discuss how and whether your emergency plan worked. You might want to make a few changes so things go a little more smoothly next time.

# Part 3

## Taking Back Your Life

Stabilizing your moods is only half of your battle against bipolar disorder, and it might even be the easier half. Now you have some real work to do. You have to learn to avoid temptation, and you have to fix the problems you and your disorder have created in your life. To do this, you're going to need some support. In Part 3, you'll find strategies with which to tackle all these tasks. Follow them, and take back your life.

# The Sirens' Call

At sea once more we had to pass the Sirens, whose sweet singing lures sailors to their doom. I had stopped up the ears of my crew with wax, and I alone listened while lashed to the mast, powerless to steer toward shipwreck.

—Homer, *The Odyssey*

**A**lcohol. Drugs. Sex. Death. If you are living with bipolar disorder, any or all of these may be the Sirens that sing to you as you pass by. But tempting as they may be, you need to stop your ears with wax, lash yourself to the mast, and continue on straight ahead. To heed the Sirens' call is to invite death and destruction; to pass them by is to embrace life.

It's not easy, giving up what you might consider to be all the "fun" things in life. Like Odysseus, you'll probably struggle, scream, and demand to be released. But once you're beyond earshot, your head will clear, and you'll see just how much you've gained by letting go, by getting safely past it all.

## Substance Abuse

You're feeling a little hyper, so you have a drink or two to calm yourself down. You're feeling a little down, so you do a few lines of cocaine to help bring yourself back up. Or maybe the decision isn't quite this conscious. Maybe you just like to get high, to get stoned, to escape. Maybe you abuse drugs and alcohol, using large amounts on a daily basis, to the point where they interfere with your life. Or maybe you don't; maybe you just have the occasional drink or pop a couple pills at a party.

No matter what you do, if you're bipolar and you're using drugs and alcohol, it's a problem. And most likely it's not a minor problem—not by a long shot.

Still, if it makes you feel any better, you're certainly not alone. The numbers depend on whose papers you're reading, but in general, if you have a bipolar I diagnosis, the odds are about 60:40 that you're seriously using and probably abusing drugs or alcohol. And if you have a bipolar II diagnosis, you only drop to around 50:50. Those are the highest rates of *comorbidity* for any of the major clinical psychiatric diagnoses—the so-called Axis I diagnoses—in the American Psychiatric Association's *Diagnostic and Statistical Manual of Mental Disorders (DSM)*.

**PsychSpeak**

**Comorbidity** is a state in which two or more medical conditions exist simultaneously and usually independently of one another.

"We don't yet fully know how to identify the 6 of 10 patients who are going to have this and the 4 who won't," says Joseph Goldberg, M.D., director of the Bipolar Disorders Research Clinic at the Payne Whitney Clinic in New York. "What's protective? Who can safely drink? For whom is it an especially high risk factor? I think we have to assume for the time being that everyone with this diagnosis is at an enormously heightened lifetime risk."

And that's only the start of the problem. After all, the most recent version of the *DSM*—the *DSM-IV*—says bipolar disorder can only be diagnosed when such things as drug use or alcoholism can't otherwise explain the mood episodes. So those statistics given earlier are undoubtedly an underestimation. It's impossible to say how many more people out there are actually bipolar but don't get the diagnosis because they were first alcoholics or drug addicts.

Even with this underestimation, the use and abuse of substances by people who have bipolar disorder is puzzling—it occurs at such a high rate that you can't help but wonder how the two might be connected.

There are actually a number of theories on the link between bipolar disorder and substance abuse. Perhaps they have the same biological roots. Or maybe bipolar disorder is a risk factor for substance abuse. It's also possible that substance abuse actually causes bipolar disorder, at least in some cases. (In that instance, the bipolar disorder would sometimes be the result of the effects of the substances on your body, rather than a disorder in its own right.) Finally, there's a chance that substance use and abuse is simply an attempt at self-medication, a way to drive away sadness or calm agitated nerves.

Logical as that last supposition might seem, the truth is that patterns of substance use don't seem to back it up. If you're depressed and self-medicating, you'd be expected to use drugs that would bring you up. But instead, the substances of choice in depression tend to be "downers"—things like alcohol and barbiturates. And in mania, the opposite occurs. When you're manic, it seems, you're more likely to be drawn to cocaine or amphetamines or Ecstasy than you are to something that will help to bring you back down to Earth.

**Alcohol** Alcohol is perfectly legal (for those of you over 21), and it's certainly everywhere. But if you're bipolar, that's not necessarily a good thing.

Alcohol use is serious business for a person with bipolar disorder. A 2001 study done by Susan McElroy, M.D., professor of psychiatry at the University of Cincinnati College of Medicine, and colleagues from the Stanley Foundation Bipolar Network—an ongoing, multinational study of bipolar disorder—found that alcohol is the substance of choice in about a third of the people with bipolar disorder who have a substance abuse problem.

"I wasn't a stumbling, falling-down drunk," says Jacqueline Castine, who has been sober now for more than 16 years and who wasn't diagnosed with bipolar disorder until almost 10 years after her sobriety. "But in the end, it was three, four glasses of wine a night to get the brain to stop, because it felt like a mouse on a treadmill."

But of course, not everyone who drinks winds up with an alcohol abuse problem. So how much *can* you drink if you have a bipolar diagnosis? Once again, there's no simple, reassuring answer. For one thing, there's no data showing where the threshold is between alcohol use and alcohol abuse; it's an individual, ever-shifting line in the sand. Also, there's good evidence that alcohol plays a role in either bringing on or exacerbating your bipolar symptoms, most likely at levels well below those that would earn you the label of alcoholic. Still, just how much alcohol you can drink before it starts to hurt you remains up in the air. That's why a number of clinicians say that the best way for someone living with bipolar disorder to approach alcohol is not to approach it at all.

One thing clinicians do know is that the link between alcoholism and bipolar disorder is most certainly real. In fact, a 1988 paper in the *Journal of Studies on Alcohol* found that alcoholism occurs alongside mania 6.2 times more frequently than chance would predict.

## GET PSYCHED

"Have some fun. Don't take this to mean go out and get liquored up. At this point in your life, the one thing you don't need is drugs and alcohol. Not only can they interfere with your medications, but folks with bipolar disorder can experience a true loss of control when they are high or drunk. When I say have fun, I mean that you should do things you like to do." –*Shay Villere, in* The Bipolar Disorder Manual

George Winokur, M.D., a renowned expert in the field who passed away in 1996, conducted a number of studies on the ties between alcohol and bipolar disorder. In one such study, Winokur and his colleagues found that the rate of alcoholism in men without the disorder was around 16 percent, while men who had been diagnosed with mania or schizoaffective mania had a 73 percent rate of alcoholism. It doesn't take a Ph.D. in statistics to recognize that that's a significant difference in rates.

And yet Winokur roundly rejected the idea that alcoholism and bipolar disorder are comorbid, at least not in the strictest sense of the word. In his writings, he noted that under the general definition of comorbidity, someone with both alcoholism and bipolar disorder is said to be dealing with two separate, unrelated diseases that just happen to be occurring at the same time. In Winokur's eyes, that seriously minimized the connection between these two syndromes. Bipolar disorder and alcoholism, he noted, are too closely related to be considered separate; they likely have some sort of back-and-forth, cause-and-effect relationship.

That's not to say that everyone who is an alcoholic must also be bipolar, or that everyone who is bipolar must also be an alcoholic. It's simply to say that, in Winokur's view, when alcoholism and bipolar disorder travel together, it's because they have an intimate relationship with one another and aren't actually two separate disease entities.

**Q&A**

*Can alcohol abuse actually cause bipolar disorder?*

"Data support the possibility that alcoholism plays a role in precipitating mania ... Thus, for individuals who are biologically vulnerable to bipolar illness, alcoholism may be an important trigger—similar to antidepressants, sleep deprivation, or changing time zones." —*George Winokur, M.D., "Alcoholism in Bipolar Disorder," in* Bipolar Disorders: Clinical Course and Outcome, *American Psychiatric Press, 1999*

Alcoholism in bipolar disorder actually "looks" different that it does when it occurs on its own. For instance, bipolar-related alcoholism hits women particularly hard. In fact, another study coming out of the Stanley Foundation—this one headed by Mark Frye, M.D., from the University of California, Los Angeles—found that while men with bipolar disorder are not quite three times as likely to abuse alcohol as are men in the general population, women with bipolar disorder are well over seven times more likely to abuse alcohol when compared to women in the general population. (This is despite the fact that the men still abused alcohol in higher numbers than the women overall.)

"We're often told, and we often appreciate, that men tend to often have higher rates of alcohol abuse or dependence compared with the general population," Joseph Goldberg told participants at a symposium presented at the American Psychiatric Association's 156th Annual Meeting in May 2003. Because of that, he explains, the rates in bipolar men, although higher, are not as striking as the rates in bipolar women, who are not as likely to abuse alcohol when they are mentally healthy. "That means that women with bipolar disorder are an especially high-risk group in our society for developing drug or alcohol abuse," Goldberg says.

And Frye has shown that bipolar alcoholic women are likely to be sicker than those without the alcohol component to their illness. They're more likely to have dysphoric manias, more likely to have more depressive episodes, and more likely to cycle rapidly. In fact, rapid-cycling and mixed episodes (see Chapter 2) appear to be more common in people with any kind of substance problem. Put more concisely, substance abuse seems to go hand in hand more often with rapidly cycling or mixed bipolar disorders than it does with normally cycling, purely manic bipolar disorder.

In 1998, the National Institute of Mental Health (NIMH) published data from a 15-year study of depression in which they found that people who were depressed and who abused or were dependent on alcohol had a much worse outcome than did depressed people who did not drink heavily.

Alcohol abuse makes treatment more difficult as well. Although the jury still seems to be out on whether antidepressants have a place in the treatment regimen for bipolar depression, it's becoming more and more clear that it is a definite no-no if you are in a bipolar depression and are using or abusing alcohol. One of Goldberg's studies shows that if you're bipolar and abusing alcohol, you're seven times more likely to become manic if given antidepressants than you are if you don't have an alcohol problem.

Goldberg has also found that if you have a mixed-state episode, you're both more likely to abuse alcohol or drugs and are going to be much harder to treat. And worse yet, your risk of suicide rises.

"In our sample at Cornell," Goldberg reported, "we found that mixed-state manic patients with alcohol comorbidity were four times more likely to be suicidal. So, above and beyond the depression symptoms, alcohol does further raise the risk for suicide attempts or behaviors and poor outcome."

Likewise, the McLean-Harvard First-Episode Mania Project noted substance use comorbidity in 60 percent of patients with mixed-episode bipolar disorder, but in only 27.2 percent of people who had what is known as "pure" mania. And they, too, found that bipolar women were more likely than bipolar men to abuse some sort of substance. In addition, they noted, "patients who abuse alcohol or drugs are less likely to recover by 6 months or will take a longer time to recover than those who do not abuse alcohol and drugs." And they take a significantly shorter time to relapse back into mania, even if they do eventually find their way to recovery.

Still, an ongoing study Goldberg and his colleagues are conducting provides hope that both alcohol abuse and bipolar disorder can be controlled. In this study, olanzapine (Zyprexa) appears to be able to reduce both mood symptoms and drinking behavior in the first month of treatment. "The good news here, the optimism," Goldberg says, "is that we may well have treatments that are broad enough in their spectrum of activity that we can hit some of these additional symptoms when we think about breadth of spectrum of activity."

In addition to medications, a variety of different psychotherapeutic approaches, as well as any number of different support groups and organizations, can help you deal with both of your disorders. With so many of the same issues involved in both alcoholism and bipolar disorder—things like mood swings and denial and a lack of insight into

## GET PSYCHED

"I have been active and involved in a 12-step program. That program is a blueprint for living. I would like to see more people with mental illness not just go to support groups, but become involved with the steps. The steps kept me alive when I was sober and not yet well." —*Jacqueline Castine, living with bipolar disorder and alcoholism*

the problem—the tools you use to beat back one are probably going to be quite useful in your battle against the other as well.

There is also some hope to be found in increasing evidence that alcoholism associated with bipolar disorder dissipates over time. In fact, in another of Winokur's studies, only 1 of 131 bipolar patients were actively alcoholic after 10 years of follow-up. The rest had stabilized both their mood and their alcohol use.

# Drugs

Studying and dealing with drug use in bipolar disorder is, in many ways, more difficult than dealing with alcoholism. For one thing, due to the illegality of most substances of abuse, there's the tendency of drug users to be more secretive about their drug use than are alcoholics.

Still, rates of drug use in bipolar disorder are quite high. McElroy has found that, after alcohol, the drugs of choice for people ultimately diagnosed with bipolar disorder are as follows:

- Marijuana (16 percent)
- Stimulants (9 percent)
- Cocaine (9 percent)
- Sedatives (8 percent)
- Opiates (7 percent)
- Hallucinogens (6 percent)

All this begs the question; which comes first, the mania or the substance abuse? This chicken-and-egg conundrum was actually addressed to some extent in the McLean-Harvard First-Episode Mania Study, a program that studied 166 people with bipolar disorder for between 2 and 4 years. One of the findings of this study was that 17 percent of the patients experiencing their first bipolar episode also had a drug or alcohol problem, a number that is much, much lower than the percentages found when people at all stages of the disorder are studied. This, some researchers have noted, seems to indicate that the bipolar symptoms precede the substance abuse, at least in some majority of cases.

"Patients will sometimes begin using drugs at the inception of a mania or near the end of a mania, maybe to stave off what they perceive as an impending depression or perhaps to sustain the euthymia," Goldberg says. "This gets at the interplay of mood and drug use in patients' perceptions. They want to feel well, and the fear of becoming depressed again seems to be a very powerful driving force for many patients."

But self-medication simply isn't the answer. The whole concept of self-medication starts to fall apart when you realize that although cocaine can lift you out of a depression, it can only do so for a really short period of time. And the lift you get tends to look a lot more like mania than like stability. Take away the cocaine crutch (or the amphetamines, or the acid, or the Ecstasy), and you're going to crash. Hard. Really, really hard. The depression hasn't gone away; it's just been there, waiting, for the drugs to lose their grip on your brain.

In addition, data show that if you're abusing drugs or alcohol, you'll take longer to recover from a manic episode—and you're more likely to relapse in those first months after the episode—than someone who is just as sick as you but doesn't have the drug component.

Adding drugs and/or alcohol into the mix also changes the way you are likely to respond to treatment. Goldberg's studies have found, for instance, that lithium doesn't work as well for people who are substance abusers in addition to being bipolar, but divalproex (Depakote) in combination with carbamazepine (Tegretol) seems to really do the trick.

The connection between the two, it's thought, might also be linked to the kindling theory of bipolar disorder (see Chapter 4). The idea behind kindling in bipolar disorder is that although your very first episodes might have an outside "cause," at least some of your subsequent episodes will probably come on spontaneously, simply because the neurons have "learned" how to produce mania. In other words, they've been kindled. And kindled neurons are not only more likely to repeat their original performance, they are also likely to do so more frequently, leading to rapid cycling.

In keeping with that metaphor, you can think of alcohol and other substances of abuse as the initial sparks that start the bipolar fire in your brain. Intoxication and withdrawal from drugs or alcohol undoubtedly mess with your brain cells. It's possible that one way they do so is by kindling them and setting you up for a lifetime of mood swings and medications.

Finally, don't ever assume that just because you're feeling better, you're no longer vulnerable to the effects of drugs and alcohol. Nothing could be further from the truth. The one way to destabilize your recently stabilized disorder—to take your regulated neurotransmitter levels and kick them off-kilter once again—is to start using substances that raise and lower their levels. Not to mention that many of the drugs used for bipolar disorder do not mix well with alcohol, and substance use while on psychotropic medications can lead to all sorts of previously avoided side effects.

"Drug abuse doesn't really do anything good for you, by and large," Goldberg says. "It buys you more likelihood of unmasking the illness; the concept being, if you have the genetic predisposition, it will express itself sooner. There's a much greater likelihood of suicidal thoughts, actions, attempts, and completions in bipolar patients with drug or alcohol abuse, and we know that suicide risk remains enormously high in bipolar patients."

# Sex

The links between drugs and alcohol and bipolar disorder might be somewhat murky and debatable, but when it comes to the question of the sexual promiscuity that's so often associated with the disorder, there's absolutely no question about the relationship. Bipolar disorder—and in particular, mania—is the direct cause of the sexual exploits and escapades that are so often part of its repertoire. In fact, the link is so clear that sexual promiscuity is actually an official "symptom" of mania and, thus, of bipolar disorder. It's even more prevalent—or perhaps simply more noticeable—in children with the disorder, who often show such extreme sexual behavior that social services might be brought into the picture before a diagnosis can be made (see Chapter 15).

This so-called *hypersexuality* isn't just about feeling good. Like most of mania's symptoms, it's also about needing a release for all that energy; about being unable to control impulses; and about wanting, striving, and reaching for more and more and more. One of the things you look for as a sign that you're getting manic is an increase in goal-driven behavior—things like trying to start a business when you've never even put together a business plan, or going out to run a marathon when you've never run a 5K. Sex can become another one of those goals; you might start to subconsciously see each person you sleep with as another goal reached, an affirmation that you're a success. That sort of ego-pumping can be an aphrodisiac in and of itself, setting up a cycle in which your sense of self, your self-worth, is tied up in the next sexual conquest. Soon enough, you find yourself addicted to sex.

> **PsychSpeak**
>
> **Hypersexuality** is excessive sexual activity, desire, or interest.

"When I was younger, I was scared to death of girls," says my father, Jack Oliwenstein, who has had symptoms of bipolar disorder since childhood, despite not being diagnosed until the age of 59. "They were a big issue to me. Could I be attractive to women? Then, could I be attractive to more than one at a time? When I found out I could, there were times when that made me think more highly of myself. I would get manic, and I would run on the edge of the knife. It wasn't until much later that I would think, *Why did I want to be with that person? Why did I take such a chance with that person?*"

An increased sexual appetite might not seem like a bad thing at first, but like many of the other impulsive behaviors that go along with bipolar disorder, this one also has its consequences. And to make matters worse, the disease itself often renders you incapable of recognizing, or even considering, those consequences. In fact, one of the ways you know you're hypersexual is that you act in a way that is completely out of character for you, sexually, without concern for the consequences.

One problem is that mania's impulse toward sexual gratification rarely begins and ends at home. And as anyone who's ever been in a committed relationship knows, cheating almost never makes your marriage or any other relationship stronger. In addition, mania-driven goal-seeking can become all-encompassing. Rarely does all that excess sexual energy allow you to slow down and consider the consequences of your action. And when it comes to sex, that can lead to some pretty serious—even deadly— side effects.

**WEB TALK:** You can find help for hyper-sexuality from the National Council on Sexual Addiction and Compulsivity at:

**↑ www.ncsac.org**

For another thing, if you're living with bipolar disorder, you're much more likely to engage in so-called "risky" sexual behaviors than are your nonbipolar friends and relatives. You're more likely to have sexual contact with someone you don't know very well, someone whose sexual history you don't know. You're more likely to skip using condoms or, for that matter, any form of birth control, adding the risk of pregnancy to your risk of sexually transmitted disease. In fact, any number of studies have shown that people who have a psychiatric disorder such as schizophrenia or bipolar disorder are significantly more likely than people without the disorder to have one-night stands with people they met that same day and to be pressured into sexual relations, even when initially unwilling.

There is no real "treatment" for sexual promiscuity in mania besides stabilizing your mood. Once you've returned to your baseline mood—your "normal" mood, where you're neither depressed nor manic—your impulse control will return, and you'll be able to make much more reasonable and reasoned choices about your behavior, including your sexual behavior. Until that happens, perhaps the best you can do is to be aware of the danger … and lash yourself to the mast until you're out of earshot of the Sirens and their alluring song.

## The Dance of Death: Suicide

The statistics on bipolar disorder and suicide are unrelentingly grim: the risk that you will attempt or commit suicide if you're bipolar is anywhere between 8 and 20 percent, with the smart money going for the higher end of that range. Put another way, if you're bipolar, then you're between 10 and 20 times more likely to commit suicide than your nonbipolar friends and neighbors. You're also more likely to do it "successfully." Suicide attempts outnumber suicide deaths no matter what the diagnosis, but people with bipolar disorder are twice or even four times as likely to die by their own hands as are those without bipolar disorder.

Some people speculate that the reason people with bipolar disorder have such a high risk of suicide is that their mood-switching might actually give them the "energy" to act out suicidal thoughts. Jonathan Stanley, assistant director of the Treatment Advocacy Center in Arlington, Virginia, echoes those beliefs when he recalls his first depression at the age of 18 and the thoughts of suicide that plagued him. "The depression was horrendous," he says. "Have you ever been in a car and have to go to the bathroom, where you get that feeling that your bladder is about to burst? I would get that experience lying in my bed, and I still wouldn't get up and go to the bathroom, because getting up and crossing the room seemed like too much effort. I also thought all the time about killing myself. But if going to the bathroom is too much effort, well … I truly believe that's the only thing that saved me."

When bipolar experts Frederick Goodwin, M.D., and Kay Redfield Jamison, Ph.D., reviewed 31 studies that included almost 10,000 patients, they found some studies that showed as many as 60 percent of deaths in people with bipolar disorder could be attributed to suicide. But when those 31 studies were statistically weighted and averaged, the overall rate of death that actually could be pinned on suicide was just under 19 percent.

Suicide is such a significant problem in bipolar disorder—more so than in most other mental illnesses, including schizophrenia—that bipolar disorder ranks sixth on the World Health Organization's (WHO) list of years of life lost to death and disability in people worldwide between the ages of 15 and 44. (The first five are unipolar depression, tuberculosis, road accidents, alcohol use, and self-inflicted injuries.)

The Stanley Foundation Bipolar Network's studies into the factors associated with attempts at suicide have found that there is definitely a subgroup of people with bipolar disorder who are at greater risk than others. These are people who ...

- Have a family history of drug abuse or suicide (both attempted and completed).
- Have more early traumatic stressors such as physical or sexual abuse and more recent traumatic stressors such as the death of a significant other or the lack of support during crises in their illness.
- Are more likely to have an anxiety disorder as well.
- Are hospitalized more often for depression.
- Have suicidal thoughts when depressed.

But although the statistics are bleak, the prospects are considerably brighter. Day by day, month by month, researchers are starting to figure out how to reduce the risk of suicide. They're starting to understand what drives people to suicide—both emotionally and biologically. And they're even starting to figure out how to intervene.

For some time, the main approach to suicide prevention has been to cut the impulse off at its roots—roots that tend to be tangled up in either unipolar or bipolar depression. That's why antidepressants are considered to be important tools in the prevention of suicide.

That supposition was thrown into turmoil in early March 2004, when the U.S. Food and Drug Administration (FDA) issued a public health advisory asking the pharmaceutical companies that manufacture the antidepressants Prozac, Zoloft, Paxil, Luvox, Celexa, Lexapro, Wellbutrin, Effexor, Serzone, and Remeron to add warning statements recommending "close observation of adult and pediatric patients treated with these agents for worsening depression or the emergence of suicidality."

The ensuing media frenzy only served to obscure the fact that the FDA's advisory admitted that they had yet to conclude that the drugs actually do raise the risk of suicide and that most of their concern was centered on the use of these medications in children and young adolescents. In Great Britain, doctors are being asked to refrain from prescribing these particular drugs—called selective serotonin reuptake inhibitors, or SSRIs—to anyone under the age of 18.

In any case, says S. Nassir Ghaemi, M.D., director of the Bipolar Disorder Research Program at Cambridge Health Alliance, antidepressants aren't necessarily the best drug for treating bipolar patients in the first place—and the FDA agrees. In fact, in its health advisory, the FDA stated: "Because antidepressants are believed to have the potential for inducing manic episodes in patients with bipolar disorder, there is a concern about using antidepressants alone in this population."

For that reason and others, Ghaemi and his colleagues in the field prefer to prescribe bipolar disorder's oldest and most faithful friend, lithium, which they believe is better at both treating the disorder and preventing suicides. As Ghaemi notes, it's the only drug right now that has clinical evidence that it can reduce suicide rates in people with bipolar disorder (see Chapter 6). At least one analysis of the data on bipolar disorder, lithium, and suicide has found a reduction in risk of about 13-fold in annual attempts and completions of suicide for bipolar patients on lithium versus those not on lithium. And most recently, a study by Goodwin and colleagues that was published in the *Journal of the American*

*Medical Association (JAMA)* compared the risks of suicide attempts and deaths by suicide in more than 20,000 people with a bipolar diagnosis who were taking either lithium or divalproex (Depakote). They found that people taking Depakote are 2.7 times more likely to die as the result of a suicide attempt than people taking lithium, and that the Depakote-takers are 1.7 times more likely to make a nonfatal attempt and 1.8 times more likely to wind up in the hospital because of a suicide attempt.

"This evidence of lower suicide risk during lithium treatment should be viewed in light of the declining use of lithium by psychiatrists in the United States, particularly among recently trained psychiatrists …" the authors wrote. "If lithium does have an anti-suicide effect not matched by currently available alternatives, then current prescribing patterns should be reevaluated. At the least, use of lithium to treat mood disorders should be an essential component of training in psychiatry."

## you're not alone

## Why?

"In 1994, two days after returning from a happy family vacation, my 57-year-old mother put the muzzle of a handgun to her left breast and fired, drilling a neat and lethal hole through her heart—and, metaphorically, through our family's as well.

"It was around midnight on a Saturday night in July, the time of year, I was later surprised to learn, that has the highest incidence of suicide in the Northern Hemisphere. My stepfather was at home but didn't hear the single shot because he was taking a shower in a bathroom at the other end of the house. When he returned to their bedroom, she was crumpled on the carpet in her pajamas, almost gone. She tried to say something to him before she died, but he couldn't make out what it was. The emergency medical technicians arrived to find a patient, but not the one they expected: my stepfather nearly died himself that night from the shock, which all but overwhelmed lungs already compromised by emphysema.

"Through it all, I was asleep in my apartment 200 miles away. I was awakened at 2 A.M. by a call from my building's front desk, telling me that my sister-in-law was downstairs and wanted to come up. My first words to her when I opened my door were, 'It's Mother, isn't it?'"

"Our family has too much company in suffering the agony of having a loved one die by suicide: annually, 30,000 people in the U.S. take their own lives. That is roughly half again the number who died of AIDS [in 2002]. Why do they do it?

"Like an estimated 60 to 90 percent of U.S. suicides, my mother had a mental illness. In her case, it was manic-depression, also called bipolar disorder. Unless they are taking—and responding well to—the appropriate medication, manic-depressives oscillate between troughs of despair and peaks of elation or agitation. Most who end their lives have a history of depression or manic-depression, but people with severe depression differ in their propensity for suicide.

"Scientists have been uncovering behavioral tip-offs and are also exploring clues to anatomical and chemical differences between the brains of suicides and of those who die of other causes. If such changes could be detected in medical imaging scans or through blood tests, doctors might one day be able to identify those at highest risk of dying by suicide—and therefore attempt to prevent the tragedy from occurring. Sadly, that goal is not immediately in sight: many who have suicidal tendencies still end up taking their own lives, despite intensive intervention.

"The question of what drove my mother to her desperate act that humid night is the second most difficult thing I live with. Scarcely a day has gone by that I haven't been pierced by the anguish of wanting to know exactly what prompted her suicide on that particular night as well as the crushing guilt over what I could have done—should have done, would have done—to stop her. The hardest thing I have to live with is the realization that I will never know the answer for sure." —From "Why: The Neuroscience of Suicide," by Carol Ezzell, in Scientific American, February 2003

## What's Really Going On: The Craving for Stimulation

It's tempting to blame all the self-destructive behavior—all the drinking, drugging, and carousing—on the bipolar disorder. If you're bipolar, you've undoubtedly trotted out the old "My bipolar disorder made me do it" excuse once or twice, or at least you've considered doing so. But is it a valid excuse?

Roger Weiss, M.D., clinical director of the Alcohol and Drug Abuse Program at McLean Hospital in Belmont, Massachusetts, and his colleagues found that "nearly all" people in their 2004 study of bipolar disorder and substance abuse say they abuse substances to medicate one or another of their mood symptoms. (Depression was the main reason this group gave, with racing thoughts being the next-most-frequent reason to self-medicate with drugs or alcohol.) In fact, nearly 67 percent of the people in the study said they found their substance use did indeed improve at least one of their bipolar disorder symptoms.

These are the same people, the researchers found, who are more likely to get better when using a form of therapy that they developed called *Integrated Group Therapy* (IGT), which was designed specifically to address the issues of co-occurring substance abuse and bipolar disorder. "The treatment uses an integrated approach by discussing topics that are relevant to both disorders and by highlighting common aspects of recovery from and relapse to each disorder," Weiss and colleagues wrote in a 1999 paper published in the *Journal of Substance Abuse Treatment*.

And it does seem to work, at least according to the initial studies that have been conducted. For instance, in a May 2000 study, Weiss and his colleagues found that IGT gave people with bipolar disorder a significantly greater chance of staying straight and sober for 2 or 3 consecutive months as compared with a group that didn't receive any group psychotherapy at all. It's a promising start, Weiss notes, but the therapy still needs to be compared with other group treatments.

"The notion of self-medication is a very controversial one," Goldberg has noted. "It's something that in some ways is very appealing conceptually. It fits, it makes sense: 'If only my moods were better, then I wouldn't drink.' It kind of shifts things away from any intrinsic aspects about the substances themselves; the implication is that if the doctor can do a better job treating my mood, I wouldn't be using drugs or alcohol."

In reality, however, it just isn't that simple. For instance, if you were really self-medicating depression, you'd assume that when you're depressed you'd be more likely to use a stimulant of some kind. And if you were really self-medicating mania, you'd assume that when you're manic you'd be more likely to use something to bring you down. But this is not necessarily the case, Goldberg points out.

"Stimulant use has been shown to be more common in mania than in depression in some studies; misuse of alcohol has been associated with depression in some studies or comparable across mania and depression," he notes. "I don't think we can simplify it and say uppers went down, downers went down, or downers went up."

To complicate things further, patterns of substance abuse aren't necessarily in synch with mood cycles. In other words, while you'd think that drug-taking and alcohol-imbibing would fall into lockstep with other signs of mania such as sexual promiscuity or spending sprees, that isn't necessarily the case.

In the end, what might be more important than proving whether self-medication is fact or fantasy is understanding just what drives people with bipolar disorder to use and abuse these substances and to put their lives at risk with sexual promiscuity and suicide attempts—and then figure out how best to intervene before the ultimate damage is done.

## What You Can Do

If you can stay clean and sober, you'll be giving yourself the chance to get your moods stable. If you can control your manic sexual impulses, you will have a much better chance at establishing—and keeping—a real, strong relationship. And if your moods are in check and your relationships are strong, your suicide risk plummets. In other words, refusing to heed the Sirens' call might just save your life.

- ☐ **If you're feeling suicidal, get help right away. There's no such thing as overreacting to thoughts of suicide. Call 911 or 1-800-SUICIDE (1-800-784-2433).**
- ☐ If you're prone to sudden suicidal thoughts or feelings, keep yourself out of temptation's way. For instance, keep only a small amount of your medications around, and don't keep weapons in your house.

☐ Abstain from drug and alcohol use. If you are bipolar, do not drink or use drugs, no matter how casually. It's an invitation to disaster.

☐ If you already have a real drug or alcohol problem, do something about it. Join a 12-step program such as Alcoholics Anonymous or Narcotics Anonymous, and start taking steps toward sobriety. You'll likely find these programs help you take steps toward mood stability as well.

☐ You can also help yourself avoid using or abusing substances simply by being aware of the circumstances that lead to the abuse. Do you have certain friends with whom you often drink? Find something else to do together. Are there certain social situations that lead inevitably to drug use? Try to avoid those events. Are you trying to self-medicate? Talk to your doctor about adjusting your medication to better relieve your symptoms.

☐ If you're experiencing symptoms of sexual addiction or compulsiveness, talk to your doctor. Or if you'd prefer, seek out a 12-step or other self-help group for strategies on how to get a handle on the situation before it gets a handle on you.

# Beyond Burned Bridges: Fixing the Problems You Create

I t's the excesses that make bipolar disorder so very fascinating to so very many people. Face it: depression is not fun to watch. But mania ... mania can be titillating. Mania can be exciting. Mania can be fun.

And that's just from the outside. From the inside, it's equally exciting—at least while it's happening. But when the ride is over and the music stops, you're the one left holding the bag. You're the one who has to put the pieces back together, to try to make your life whole again. And you have to do it despite not always being quite sure what really happened in the first place.

Finding a way to repair the bridges that you burned—to fix the problems you yourself created—can either be overwhelming or extremely empowering. It's all about your attitude. If you look around at your life and see nothing but rubble, if you let your issues overwhelm you, if you wallow in guilt, then all these issues are likely to simply perpetuate more issues and more guilt and more depression. But if you look around at your life and see possibilities and challenges, then you've got a better than even chance of making something good come out of something bad. And isn't that the ultimate goal?

## Accepting Responsibility, Avoiding Guilt

Some months after former *New York Times* reporter Jayson Blair's career crashed and burned in 2003—a conflagration caused by 4 years of premeditated plagiarism and deliberate deceit—he revealed that he had been diagnosed with bipolar disorder. To many of those who also suffer with the disorder, this wasn't a particular surprise—the grandiosity, the sense of invulnerability, and the impaired judgment it takes to methodically lie for months and years on end are all glaringly manic symptoms.

When his book, *Burning Down My Master's House: My Life at* The New York Times, was published in 2004, Blair hit the talk-show circuit. And he was asked the same questions over and over again: *Aren't you just making excuses for yourself? Do you really think you've apologized enough? Do you really think you've been contrite enough?*

Blair's answers aside (as he told CNN's Larry King, "I've apologized in the book. I've apologized in interviews ... It seems to me some people would like me to crawl into a hole and disappear forever. That's just not in my nature."), his story brings into the spotlight some of the issues that almost every person with bipolar disorder has to grapple with at some time. How do you reconcile your disorder and your behavior? How can you take responsibility for the things you—or your disease—do, without letting the guilt of those actions eat you up inside?

For many people who've been living with bipolar disorder for some time, the answer is to simply do it. Take responsibility. Make amends to whatever extent possible. And then move on.

The truth is, there will be people whom you've hurt or wronged or scared so badly that they won't want to forgive you, or they won't be able to. Jacqueline Castine, whose bipolar disorder wasn't diagnosed until much later in her life, talks about a roommate she had when she was at the height of her mania, but was still undiagnosed and unmedicated.

"She was so freaked by my behavior in the end," Castine says. "She was so stressed that she didn't want anything to do with me ever again. That was a done deal. And I understand. I truly understand."

All you can do is offer an apology, if you feel an apology is needed. If the person can't accept the apology, you need to accept his or her decision. Recognize that actions have consequences, and sometimes apologies or even restitutions don't make everything better.

But it's also your job not to let others' opinions of you destroy your self-esteem. Your deeds—especially while you are ill—do not define you any more than your disorder defines you. In the paraphrased words of many people who have gone through extreme manias and lived to tell the tale, you can do bad things but not be a bad person, as long as you take responsibility—as long as you "own" your actions and take your emotional lumps and try to use them as a learning experience. If you can use your experiences to help yourself stay on your medication or overcome a substance addiction, then it was, ultimately, worth the pain.

> **GET PSYCHED**
>
> "All that stuff I did when I was manic and high? Only in the hospital did I have to reassess that and put it in my bucket and say, 'Hey, Jon, that's yours.'"
> —*Jonathan Stanley, living with bipolar disorder*

## Dealing With Legal Ramifications

It's not illegal to be mentally ill—but sometimes it might seem that way. Jails and prisons are rapidly filling up with mentally ill inmates as hospitals close their doors and insurance companies tighten their purse strings. And people with bipolar disorder make up more than their fair share of those inmates. In fact, bipolar disorder is six times more common in prison than it is in the communities in which we live. That certainly doesn't mean that if you have bipolar disorder you're going to wind up in jail, but it does mean that the issues you have with impulse control and anger when you're manic put you at greater risk than if you didn't have to deal with those symptoms.

"It is critically important that those with bipolar disorder recognize that they are suffering from a mental illness and seek treatment for it—the sooner the better," says Cameron Quanbeck, M.D., assistant clinical professor of psychiatry at the University of California, Davis. "Many do recognize that they are ill, but only after getting arrested and getting into other kinds of trouble. Those who don't recognize their illness often turn to alcohol and drugs, which only exacerbate their symptoms and can lead to aggressive and other criminal behaviors."

Dealing with these problems and reaching out to people with bipolar disorder who are at particular risk can be a real challenge. After all, some of the issues surrounding mental illnesses in general—and bipolar disorder in particular—are exceedingly difficult for people to talk about. Violence and criminal behavior are definitely right up there at the top of the list. The truth is that impulsive and grandiose behavior rarely allows you to consider what you're doing in mid-mania at any level, much less question its legality. Add inhibition-stripping drugs and alcohol into the mix, or throw in delusions and hallucinations, and you've got a true emotional and behavioral powder keg.

And when that keg gets lit, it can lead to a truly horrifying explosion. In a perfect world, someone who is violent and potentially dangerous because of a mental illness would recognize that illness and be treated voluntarily. In the real world, however, the illness is often unrecognized, and the person winds up incarcerated and getting little or none of the help she needs. Or she refuses to get help, even though everyone around her can see that the way she's headed leads to danger and disaster.

Several factors can tip the balance in terms of your potential for winding up "in the system." One of them is experiencing a psychotic mania. Another is substance abuse. Substance abuse is an issue for a majority of people with bipolar disorder (see Chapter 10), and among its repercussions appears to be an increased likelihood of finding oneself in jail or in some kind of legal trouble. Psychiatrist and bipolar disorder expert Joseph Calabrese, M.D., from Case Western Reserve University in Cleveland, reported at the 2003 annual meeting of the American Psychiatric Association that the use of substances such as alcohol, marijuana, and cocaine by people who have bipolar disorder dramatically increases their risk of winding up in jail. In fact, in his study of 81 patients with rapid-cycling bipolar disorder, those who had spent time in prison were 7 times more likely to also have a substance abuse problem than those who'd never been jailed.

In addition, a February 2004 study published in the *Journal of Clinical Psychiatry* by a research team led by Quanbeck looked at the similarities among 66 bipolar inmates in the Los Angeles County Jail. They found that at the time of their arrests, just over 74 percent of the inmates were manic, and an overlapping 59 percent were psychotic. Most had recently been released from the hospital when they were arrested, and a few had been doing outpatient treatment. And dovetailing with Calabrese's study, almost 76 percent of the bipolar inmates had a substance-abuse problem, compared to only 18.5 percent of a control group of people with bipolar disorder who had never been arrested.

"The results of this study suggest that manic symptoms place bipolar patients at significant risk for criminal offending and arrest," the researchers wrote.

But the problem of anger and violence in bipolar disorder neither begins nor ends in jail. It begins with the same basic emotional and neurological disturbances that all bipolar disorder is rooted in; in particular, it begins in the impulsivity and lack of impulse control that characterizes mania. And it takes off from there. In 2001, researchers from Australia and New Zealand published a paper looking at the impact of bipolar disorder on "caregivers"— friends and family members who either live with you or step in and take responsibility when you're sick (see Chapter 16). They found that almost half the caregivers they interviewed had experienced violence, or were scared that there would be violence, when their loved one was ill. A quarter of the group had actually experienced what could be called "serious forms of violence"—being threatened with a chain saw, for instance, or being attacked with a kitchen knife. Interestingly, it didn't seem to matter if the bipolar patient was male or female; they were equally likely to act out toward someone they loved when in the grips of mania.

## Q&A

*Are people who have bipolar disorder more likely to be violent than other people?*

"Studies have shown that people with mental illness who are in treatment are no more violent than anyone else. They've shown that people with mental illness who are not substance abusers are no more violent. But, when I look back at my life, I'm just thankful that I didn't hurt anyone when I was psychotic and unmedicated. As luck would have it, my delusion was such that I wasn't going to hurt anybody, but I just don't understand how anyone can say that people who are bipolar with psychotic tendencies are no more violent than anyone else when they have this risk factor that no one else has. And the studies back that up, no matter how much some advocates like to ignore them."
—*Jonathan Stanley, lawyer, assistant director of the Treatment Advocacy Center, living with bipolar disorder*

What good does knowing all this do you? For one thing, maybe giving at least a passing acknowledgement to the darker side of mania gives you a little better understanding of the look of fear in your partner's eyes when you forget to take your medication or when you start to slide into a manic episode. And maybe it gives you a renewed resolve to stick with your treatment program or kick a drug or alcohol habit.

In addition, it helps you understand why there is such disagreement, even among those in the mental-health advocacy community, as to the best way to balance civil liberties and safety. "I've always been a huge defender of liberal causes and an individual's rights," says Lynn Albizo, a lawyer and mental-health advocate. "But when you get into the system, you start to realize how absurd it is, this right for someone to be sick and live on the street and not get help when it's so clearly needed."

It was this sort of philosophical struggle that led the National Alliance for the Mentally Ill (NAMI) to create the Treatment Advocacy Center, or TAC, which works to advocate for laws requiring treatment for people with significant mental illnesses who are too ill to make rational decisions about treatment. They've been particularly successful in two states—passing Kendra's Law in New York and Laura's Law in California—and have also played a role in what Jonathan Stanley, TAC's assistant director, calls "less wholesale reforms" in a number of other states, including West Virginia, Illinois, Utah, Maryland, and Idaho. But there is more to be done, says Stanley, and they are pressing on, albeit cautiously. "We would be having real bipolar grandiosity if we thought we could walk into any state and enforce our will upon it," Stanley says.

There are, of course, many people who disagree with these sorts of activities and who work on the other side of the issue, trying to protect people with mental illnesses from laws that would commit them involuntarily or require them to submit to treatment against their will. One of the most prominent of these is the Bazelon Center for Mental Health Law.

**WEB TALK:** Find out what the Bazelon Center is doing to preserve the rights of the mentally ill at:

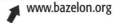 www.bazelon.org

One of the Bazelon Center's top initiatives is working to prevent what they call "unnecessary coercion" in the process of involuntary commitment. "The Bazelon Center opposes involuntary inpatient civil commitment except in response to an emergency, and then only when based on a standard of imminent danger of significant physical harm to self or others and when there is no less restrictive alternative," they said in a position statement on the subject. In addition, they oppose the very laws that the TAC is trying to enact, saying issues such as lack of insight and a possibility of future violence—both of which play a part in the TAC's argument for the necessity of these laws—are "not meaningful. They cannot be accurately assessed on an individual basis, and are improperly rooted in speculation."

Stanley believes that such arguments are short-sighted. "The violence issue is focal not to us, but to people like those at Bazelon," he says. "To their consternation, we actually do address the issue. Yet for us it is only a part of the tragic package of consequences that come with untreated bipolar disorder. So if you look at our fact sheets, you will find one on violence, but you'll also find ones on suicide, homelessness, criminalization, and victimization."

Where you stand on this issue—and on other issues such as providing appropriate treatment to incarcerated people with mental illness both while they are in jail and when they are first let out—is obviously a personal choice. But it is undoubtedly in your best interest to know what your rights are at this moment and to know what the laws are in your state. After all, they might one day affect you, as unpleasant as that might be to consider. And even if they don't, they're affecting people just like you every day.

If you're not happy with any of these laws or policies that might have an impact on your life or on the life of someone you love, get involved. Your voice can and should be heard.

## Dealing With Financial Ramifications

"I have no respect for money," my father once admitted to me. "At one point, I had almost a million dollars in a checking account, and to this day I don't know where it went."

To say that overspending is a not-uncommon problem for people in the midst of a manic episode would be a blatant understatement. It is, rather, almost symbolic of the disease, one of the stereotypes of mania.

Kay Redfield Jamison, who is an expert on bipolar disorder from both the scientific and personal points of view, describes in *An Unquiet Mind: A Memoir of Moods and Madness,* urgently buying, at one time or another, a dozen snakebite kits, 3 watches in just a few hours, and 20 books about penguins (in hopes of forming a colony). And then she recounts the aftermath: ruined credit and personal mortification.

"It is devastating to have the illness and aggravating to have to pay for medications, blood tests, and psychotherapy," she writes. "They, at least, are partially deductible. But money spent while manic doesn't fit into the Internal Revenue Service concept of medical expense or business loss. So after mania, when most depressed, you're given excellent reason to be even more so."

It might seem unfair that you can be held responsible for the financial havoc you wreak while so completely manic—or possibly even psychotic—that you can't even remember what stores you went to. And there's a chance that you could argue in court that you were incompetent to make financial decisions at the time of the purchases. There's also a chance—although it might only be slim—that you could win that argument. But would you really have won? Do you really want to argue that your disorder makes you incapable of making your own decisions, financial or otherwise?

There are undoubtedly situations in which this is precisely the right argument to make, but those are few and far between. For most people, whose mania ebbs and flows, being declared incompetent is a very last resort.

Another protective option is a court-appointed guardian. In the case of finances gone amok, a family member can petition the court to become your legal guardian. "You need to be very careful about doing this," says Albizo. "It's a mixed bag. What a guardianship is doing is taking away an individual's legal right to make decisions on his own behalf and giving it to another person. There is often, justifiably, a resentment until you come to the realization that this person is looking out for your best interests."

Because guardianships don't come and go with your symptoms, a better solution, Albizo says, is to try to work out something with your family members that enables you to have freedom but "acknowledges that sometimes you need help."

One thing you can—and undoubtedly should—do is to be sure your spouse or parents or siblings or close friends know how to

## PsychSpeak

**Durable power of attorney** is a document that gives another person the right to make legal and financial decisions on your behalf when and if you become either physically or mentally incapable of making them yourself.

spot the signs of an oncoming mania and get you out of harm's way—including financial harm. You might even want to give them permission to take away your credit cards and bankcards and checkbook in situations where they think you're no longer in control. In fact, if your moods aren't quite as stable as you'd like them to be, you might want to give them those sorts of rights legally, by voluntarily granting them a *durable power of attorney*.

**Credit Counseling** In general, credit card companies don't really care about your state of mind when you bought six business suits even though you're a stay-at-home mom or felt compelled to duplicate your entire CD collection in one weekend. All they care about is that you pay them back the money you owe.

Now, of course, here you are, reeling from an extended manic episode, and looking at the bills you created is probably giving you a financial hangover. There are, however, things you can do and people who can help you.

Before you do anything drastic like declaring bankruptcy, you'll probably be advised to talk with a credit counselor. In fact, laws are currently under consideration that would require you to talk to a counselor before you could file a petition for bankruptcy. But there's a catch: although there are dozens upon dozens of credit counseling and debt-reduction services out there, not all of them are completely trustworthy and forthright.

In 2003, the National Consumer Law Center (NCLC) and the Consumer Federation of America (CFA) came out with a report called "Credit Counseling in Crisis: The Impact on Consumers of Funding Cuts, Higher Fees, and Aggressive New Market Entrants." The report looked at what the two consumer agencies called a "severe threat" to consumers by "a new generation of credit counseling services." According to the report, the Better Business Bureau had fielded some 1,480 complaints about credit counseling agencies nationwide in 2002, as compared with 261 complaints just 4 years earlier.

*I'm thousands of dollars in debt, and I'm scared of what's going to happen to me. How am I supposed to find a good, honest credit counseling service?*

"It is virtually impossible to distinguish the honest, caring agencies from the rip-off artists by just looking at a TV ad or making a quick phone call. Don't just respond to television or Internet ads. Get referrals from friends or family, find out which agencies have had complaints lodged against them, and look at several agencies closely before making a decision." *–Travis B. Plunkett, legislative director, Consumer Federation of America, Washington, D.C.*

And so, before you embark on a credit counseling course to try to find your way out of a mania-induced financial morass, you might want to consider some of the tips put forth in "Credit Counseling in Crisis," including a list of "red flags"—practices that should make you suspect an agency might not be on the up-and-up. Some of those red flags include the following:

- **Fees that are more than nominal.** The CFA and NCLC suggest no more than $50 to set up a debt management or debt consolidation plan, and no more than $25 for monthly maintenance of that plan.
- **Commissioned employees.** These credit counseling services are almost all nonprofit organizations, and a nonprofit organization shouldn't be selling enough of anything to keep a commissioned employee in good financial shape.
- **A too-quick solution.** It should take way more than just 15 or 20 minutes for a credit counselor to get to know you and offer the right sort of plan for you.
- **No variety.** If a service can only come up with one way for you to get out of debt, it's probably just trying to make a buck off of you, rather than really understand your unique issues and needs.

Done correctly, however, credit counseling can make a huge difference in your ability to cope with the financial aftermath of mania. Even better, says Albizo, is to try to get the same sort of counseling through a mental health legal firm or agency, where they can refer you to someone who has a background in dealing with these issues in relation to mental illness.

**Bankruptcy** There are two "kinds" of bankruptcy: chapter 7 and chapter 13. Chapter 7 bankruptcy completely wipes out your debt, while chapter 13 provides a schedule for repayment of at least a portion of your debts. Both protect you from your creditors once the bankruptcy has been made official. Most people choose a chapter 7 bankruptcy, although there are advantages to chapter 13 that might apply in your case, such as being able to keep property that otherwise would be taken from you and liquidated to pay your creditors.

Many bankruptcy laws vary by state and by the judge's interpretation. For instance, in community property states (Arizona, California, Idaho, Louisiana, Nevada, New Mexico, Texas, Washington, and Wisconsin), your husband or wife will be considered equally responsible for your credit card debts, despite not having signed any of the receipts.

Bankruptcy stays on your credit record for 10 years. You have to wait 6 years to file for a second chapter 7 bankruptcy; chapter 13 bankruptcies, however, can be filed pretty much whenever you might need that protection.

Some debts, though, are not wiped out by a bankruptcy, including debts incurred by lying to or defrauding a creditor, child support, traffic tickets or criminal restitution, tax debts, and student loans. There are exceptions to every rule, however. In fact, there are cases on the books in which people with bipolar disorder have gotten their student loan discharged as part of their bankruptcy proceeding, especially when it can be shown that their disorder makes it difficult for them to work and that having to repay the loan would be an *undue hardship*.

## PsychSpeak

In legal terms, an **undue hardship** is an action that carries with it significant difficulty or expense to the extent that it would do more harm than good.

# Biting the Bullet

Jacqueline Castine knew what she had to do. "I was working in a ministry, and I believed that God was calling me to give away all my money," she says now with a sort of disbelieving laugh. "He was calling me to use my credit—my perfect credit—to bring the Boys' Choir of Harlem to Detroit."

Six weeks and debt totaling $42,000 later, Jacqueline realized something was wrong. "That's what it took for me to face the fact that I was really sick," she says. "The fact that it came around money was probably really critical. It was an area in which I always had so much pride and was always extremely careful and responsible."

Once Jacqueline was diagnosed with bipolar disorder and stabilized on medication—once her mania had mostly subsided—she realized she had to face the music. Because she is an alcoholic, she turned to her 12-step philosophy to help her through. "I took an inventory," she says. "I had to face how much money I owed. I knew I was too sick to be dealing with bill collectors, and I knew I couldn't pay it off. There was only one recourse: I had to file for bankruptcy."

It was, Jacqueline says, the most humbling experience of her life, bar none. Today, however, she sees it as a gift—a spiritual gift. "Part of what I needed to do to get better was to be humbled," she says. "This experience leveled me out, made me realize I was like everyone else."

Jacqueline is proud, however, that as scared as she got, as convinced as she became that she'd spend the rest of her life on welfare, she never gave up. "I cleaned houses, and I lived with my mother," she says. "And then someone asked me to be on a committee for the community mental-health center where I was receiving treatments. When one of the community advocates on the committee found out about my professional background—I'd done PR, sales and marketing, and writing—she said, 'I'm taking you in right now to meet the director.' I wasn't ready; I wasn't prepared. But she listened to my story, and she said, 'You have a job.'"

Today, Jacqueline is a community education specialist in public relations for the Oakland County Community Mental Health Authority. She's sober, and her moods are stable, but she's still working her 12-step program, and she's taking full responsibility for her own actions.

"I did a lot of letter writing, made a lot of phone calls. I knew I had hurt my children desperately, each in a different way. And there were many other people, too … I had to recognize how my illness had impacted them all. And now they've all forgiven me. They say they're just glad they have me back."

The process of filing for bankruptcy is quite involved: it includes the filing of papers and a court date (called a 341 meeting) in which you'll be questioned under oath about your finances. Trying to get through a bankruptcy without legal counsel is simply foolish. It can legally be done, but it is, to put it mildly, ill advised.

## Apologizing to the People You Care About

To get past your past, you generally need to start by figuring out what it is you've done, and to whom. This means being sure you know who it is you've wronged and what you did to wrong them. And it might be easier said than done, especially on the down slope from mania, when you haven't slept in weeks and may have little or no recollection of the days that have gone by. In addition, verbalizing a nonverbal "hurt" can be quite the challenge. There might simply be times when saying to yourself, "I've hurt my children," or "I just wasn't a very good friend," is the best you're going to be able to do. On the other hand, the more specific you can be, the better the chance you can make a truly appropriate apology. "I hurt my children by involving and scaring them when I was paranoid," gives you something you can apologize for. "I just wasn't a very good friend when Lola was sick because I was so focused on myself that I couldn't care for her the way she needed me to," gives you the chance to do things differently next time.

In other words, "owning" your misdeeds is a great first step, but it's what you do with those misdeeds once you have them firmly in hand that will make all the difference.

> **GET PSYCHED**
>
> "It's one thing to clean house, but if you just stick the garbage out on the porch, it does you little good. You have to put it out by the curb and watch the garbage men come and pick it up and take it away. That's what frees you." *–Jacqueline Castine, living with bipolar disorder*

Jacqueline Castine, who is living with both bipolar disorder and alcoholism, remembers making a list of people to whom she needed to make amends. It had 25 names on it. "There were just a whole lot of things I had done that were damaging to people," she says. She's worked to repay money, even years after the fact, to people she owes on a personal level, despite having declared bankruptcy. She's apologized to people whose feelings she hurt. She's even written letters to people at a company where she was once a consultant and where "I didn't produce as much as I should have."

Part of righting wrongs, Castine adds, is knowing when an apology is only going to make things worse for the person you've hurt. Should you contact people who've asked that you never speak to them again? Will that only reopen old wounds? Apologizing for hurting someone at the expense of hurting him or her again seems counterproductive, to put it mildly.

And then there's the question of people who don't know they've been hurt. Should you tell your spouse about the affairs you had while you were manic? She might need to know if there's a chance you're exposing her to a sexually transmitted disease, for instance. But if that's somehow not the case, then telling her becomes a delicate balancing act in which you have to consider both the benefits of making amends and the hurt that revealing your deception is likely to cause.

The most important thing about apologizing or "making amends" is that it's an active process. It is you taking charge of your own life. It is you doing something to make things better. And when you're dealing with a disease in which it so often feels as if things are happening *to* you, the chance to be in the driver's seat, to have control of your own emotional destiny, can be fulfilling and empowering and just downright exhilarating.

## What You Can Do

Bipolar disorder hasn't cornered the market on bridge-burning. Hurting people, making mistakes, acting irresponsibly—there isn't a single human being who could throw stones from inside these particular glass houses. But these sorts of human foibles are actually built into bipolar disorder. Mania is defined and diagnosed by the existence of impulsive, hurtful, sometimes even dangerous actions. And so it's something you need to be not only aware of, but also prepared for—and something you need to be willing to fix once it's occurred.

- [ ] Take responsibility for your actions without making excuses for yourself.

- [ ] Get support. You might want to join a 12-step or some other type of group if any of your burned bridges are the result of alcohol, narcotics, or sexual addiction. The things you'll learn there can be applied to other aspects of your life, too, including your bipolar disorder.

- [ ] Write letters, make phone calls, repay debts. Apologize.

- [ ] Accept the consequences of your actions, but live in the here and now. There's a huge difference between taking full responsibility for what you've done and beating yourself up for your past mistakes.

- [ ] If you've gotten yourself into money trouble, talk with a financial counselor about your options. It's easy to get angry at the credit card companies and collection agencies, but they didn't spend all that money. You did. Now you have to figure out how to pay at least some of it back.

- [ ] Bankruptcy is certainly an option, especially if the stress of trying to repay mountains of debt threatens your mental health. If you do decide to file for bankruptcy, do your homework—and then get a lawyer.

- [ ] Consider giving someone you trust a durable power of attorney so he or she can make financial decisions on your behalf should you no longer be capable of doing so. This keeps you in the driver's seat, because you, rather than a court, are the one selecting who will be in charge.

- [ ] Know your legal rights. Know your state's positions on involuntary commitment or on involuntary treatment.

# Lean On Me

**Y**ou've been given a diagnosis that scares you. You might have been hospitalized; you're probably taking some heavy-duty medication with some heavy-duty side effects. You might have burned a few bridges—lost a job, destroyed a relationship—during your most recent manic firestorm. You might have friends, even family members, who aren't exactly reaching out to you right now. You're feeling awfully alone.

But you're not alone. Chances are, those friends and family are more "there" for you than you think. And even if they're not, there's a community full of people who know where you are and how you feel and are willing to help get you through it, to wellness.

Support—be it from your family or your friends or simply from people who've been there and done that—is an often underappreciated and underutilized part of treating bipolar disorder. It is, however, critical to your recovery and to the creation of a future in which you are going to thrive.

## The Importance of Support

According to the Surgeon General's Report on Mental Health, published in 1999 under the direction of then–Surgeon General David Satcher, M.D., about 2 to 3 percent of the people in the United States are involved in some sort of self-help group at any given time. That doesn't even count the untold millions of people who take advantage of the support that can be found on the World Wide Web.

Of course, support isn't something you get only in a meeting room or while chatting online. Support can be your significant other, who lets you know when you're becoming a little manic. Or it can be your parents, who call twice a week to check up on you, although they never put it quite that way. Or it can be your best friend, who offers you a place to stay for a few days when you just don't think you can make it on your own.

Or it can be a more formal group led by someone who has been—and most likely still is—where you are. These groups, called peer-led support groups, have advantages that most of your friends and family don't—the people there are not only sympathetic, they're empathetic. They know how you feel, and they have some ideas about what you should—or should not—do about it.

"This whole angle of what consumers and peers can do for each other, the value of the peer part of the puzzle, was just not widely recognized," says Lisa Goodale, Peer Services Director for the Depression and Bipolar Support Alliance (DBSA). "Now, more and more people are showing hard evidence that peer-to-peer support really works."

Indeed, the benefits of self-help or peer support have been not only studied but scientifically sliced, diced, and filleted. Researchers in the field have shown, for example, that *peer-run services* seem to bring people into the realm of support who might otherwise remain completely socially isolated. They've shown that if you attend peer support groups, for instance, you're less likely to be hospitalized and more likely to feel better than you would if you didn't participate. They've shown that if you attend support groups populated with your peers, you're more likely to communicate better with your doctor, follow her instructions, take your medications, and cope with their side effects.

## PsychSpeak

**Peer-run services** are developed and led by people who have a mental illness for other people with that same mental illness. The peers participate fully in the group and are not treatment professionals.

Support groups can also help you feel less isolated; give you tons of practical and useful information on treatment options, finding physicians, and how to cope day to day; and provide you with somewhere to go or people to turn to in a crisis. In other words, they empower you. And when you're dealing with a disorder that's anything but empowering, that can make all the difference.

The so-called "peer providers" benefit as well. For one thing, they're right there in the midst of it all, getting the same support and social boost as everyone else. In addition, they're also getting a more unique perspective on the situation, watching people like themselves working their way toward health and gaining invaluable insight into how that can best be done. The sense of self-esteem they acquire as they watch people getting better because of their help is immeasurable, not to mention the ego boost of being asked to do work with significant responsibilities—work that requires people have trust in them.

These sorts of findings have energized not only the people living with all types of mental illnesses, but also the local, state, and federal agencies and groups involved in the mental health field. After all, a therapy for mental illness that is successful, accepted, and run by unpaid volunteers is not likely to engender much argument from either you or your insurance company.

There are, however, downsides to peer counseling and support—or rather, cautions that need to be kept in mind. Perhaps the most important is that although discussions of treatments and how they work might be fascinating, they should be looked at as food for thought, not as set-in-stone fact. Anecdotes are just that—stories. They reflect

## GET PSYCHED

"By responding and empathizing with the experiences of people with mental illness, peer providers have found that recovery does not spring from outside factors, but rather, is grounded in an individual's mind and body—in each person's hopes, needs, preferences, and choices." –From "Emerging New Practices in Organized Peer Support, 2003," National Association of State Mental Health Program Directors and the National Technical Assistance Center for State Mental Health Planning

one person's experience. They aren't scientific studies, and they aren't medical advice. Listen carefully, do some research, then go talk to your doctor. But don't make any big change in your treatment—don't make *any* changes, in fact—without first talking it over with some sort of medical professional.

Alexis Maislen, a 27-year-old student and writer who attends a weekly DBSA peer-support group, agrees. "One thing I'm cautious about is, I have to double-check everything people are saying. People can say dangerous things about not doing medication and doing alternative stuff, like aromatherapy and journaling and exercise. I've done that, and I've gotten manic; you need to do those things with medication."

Still, Alexis says, there's a lot to be gained from the experience, not the least of which is a sense of belonging and camaraderie and friendship. "I've made a lot of friends through DBSA. I find that it's good to have a network, and it creates that network. I think DBSA's good because it's peer run. Everyone's on the same level; there's no one in there trying to tell me how to feel."

**you're not alone**

Rachael Bender, a graphic artist and designer who owns her own company—Bender Consulting—was diagnosed with bipolar disorder only a year or two ago, after 11 years of searching for the truth behind her erratic and scary behavior. Within weeks of her diagnosis, Rachael had joined a support group in Fort Lauderdale, Florida, where she lives. It was a DBSA support group.

"I'm one of those people who, if they do something, they just jump right in and get involved," she laughs. "I was in the group for like two months before the local chapter president said, 'You should be a facilitator.'" (A *facilitator* is the DBSA's term for a peer or a consumer who keeps an eye on the meetings to be sure they stay within the organization's set of rules.)

Today, Rachael facilitates a once-weekly women's-only support group, a once-weekly friends and family support group, and a newly formed group for anyone with bipolar disorder. "Our chapter has 14 support groups right now," Rachael says.

The groups, she says, really run themselves. Her job is simply to get them started, keep them running if the conversation stalls, be sure everyone gets a chance to talk, and be sure nobody steps too far out of line. "A lot of times people with this illness are aggressive, especially when they're manic," she says. "I have to make sure there's no aggression, that it stays safe."

But aside from keeping a watchful eye, Rachael says, what she mostly does is participate. "We talk a lot about treatments," she admits. "We talk about what medications work for us, and we talk about our experiences with doctors. Unfortunately, what I've found is that there's a lot of really bad doctors out there. In fact, we're starting in our newsletter a list of doctors recommended by our members."

As it turns out, Rachael is not only facilitating three groups, but also is acting as the director of communications for the organization, publishing the chapter's newsletter.

Still, Rachael says there's no doubt that she gets as much, if not more, than she gives by her participation in the support groups. "Before I joined a support group," she says, "I felt so alone. I felt I was the only person who this happens to. Then, when you talk to other people, you realize how common this experience is. I always thought, 'Wow, I must be really sick.' You tend to think those are the really crazy people who are institutionalized. It's a very humbling experience to have that happen to you."

Still, says Rachael, there's a lot left to learn—for everyone.

"There's still such a stigma associated with mental illness. I think it's important to talk about it and show other people that it happens to perfectly normal people with great lives and good jobs. People like me."

## Building Support Systems

*Step one:* Reach out. You need to ask for help to get help.

*Step two:* Know that it might not be quite that easy.

Support comes in all shapes and sizes. Don't turn any of it away, and don't turn away from any of it. If you're going to get healthy and stay healthy, you're going to need help. Lots of it.

Start with your family. They're the people most likely to do whatever it takes to help you get your equilibrium back. And

## GET PSYCHED

"Over the years I've run the whole spectrum. I've been to my psychiatrist, I've had late night talks with my parents, I've spent four hours in my bathtub, I've hugged my dog, I've slept 12 hours a day ... whatever was needed to feel stable again."
—Shay Villere, living with bipolar, in The Bipolar Disorder Manual, www.mental-health-matters.com/articles/article.php?artID=550

they're the people you're most likely to want to lean on and feel comfortable leaning on.

Of course, not all people can count on their family to be there for them. The family might be dysfunctional. You might be estranged from them. Or perhaps this latest episode of yours pushed one or more of them over the edge and they've cut you off.

That's okay. That's what friends are for. Your friends might be willing to open their hearts or their homes to you at a time when your family swears they just can't do it again.

And if your friends flake on you? Don't despair. That's what the peer-led support groups are made for—and they're gaining in both number and momentum.

Take, for instance, the DBSA. This national organization for people living with either depression or bipolar disorder began as an organization with just five chapters, staffed almost entirely with volunteers. Today, there are 280 DBSA chapters around the country, with more than 1,000 support groups. "We serve more than four million people a year here," says Goodale. (See the following "Support for You" section for a list of other peer-group organizations.)

Peer support neither begins nor ends at support group meetings. The Surgeon General's report noted that mental health care "consumers" (as many advocacy groups refer to the people who use—or consume—mental health resources) not only run such groups, but also operate services and programs such as drop-in centers where you can go to get support or advice from someone who's been where you are. Peer-run employment and housing programs, crisis services, education and advocacy programs, and outreach programs are

**WEB TALK:** Learn about self-help groups from the National Mental Health Consumers' Self-Help Clearinghouse at:

↗ www.mhselfhelp.org/self.html

242

often staffed and run by the same people who use these services. It is, the report noted, a true win-win situation: "Consumer staff are thought to gain meaningful work, to serve as role models for clients, and to enhance the sensitivity of the service system to the needs of people with mental disorders. Clients are thought to gain from being served by staff who are more empathic and more capable of engaging them in mental health services."

**Support for You** The main reasons for putting together a support group—to have someone watching out for you, someone checking up on you, someone caring about what happens to you—are of particular importance in bipolar disorder, where lack of insight into your own behavior is often one of the first symptoms that things are going downhill.

> **GET PSYCHED**
>
> "There's a whole range of services coming to the forefront, each addressing the issue of recovery orientation in services. This means it's not just about getting symptoms to feel better, but to tell people, 'You can recover.' Not that everyone is going to be fine and dandy, but that you can get them better. And that may mean they might lead a whole lot better or a more meaningful life." –*Lisa Goodale, Peer Services Director for the Depression and Bipolar Support Alliance*

"I have a small support system of people who watch me, and who I check in with on a pretty regular basis," says Stephanie, a 40-year-old public relations writer living with bipolar disorder. "Everybody knows that if I don't get enough sleep, if I'm under enormous amounts of stress, I'm going to sway a little. So somebody will say to me, 'You're a little on the manic side. Maybe you need to take a sleeping pill or something.' And I may not like it— I think there's always an initial defensiveness—but I do it."

Regardless of how many friends and family members you have in your personal support system, you should consider getting involved in a support group, whether it's an online newsgroup, mailing list or chat room, or an in-person weekly meeting. The benefits are enormous, and the cost minuscule.

To start with, you can try getting in touch with any of the national mental health associations and asking about local chapters and whether or not they have an ongoing support group that you could attend:

- **National Alliance for the Mentally Ill (NAMI),** www.nami.org; 1-800-950-NAMI (1-800-950-6264)
- **National Mental Health Association (NMHA),** www.nmha.org; 1-800-969-6642
- **Depression and Bipolar Support Alliance (DBSA),** www.dbsalliance.org/; 1-800-826-3632

The Internet offers a variety of information and support options too numerous to list here. Here's just a taste of what's in store if you do a little looking around:

- **Usenet/News groups.** Search groups.google.com. Relevant groups include alt.support.depression.manic, alt.support. depression.manic.moderated, and soc.support.depression.manic.
- **groups.yahoo.com.** More than 650 groups are listed in its bipolar disorder category; just search on bipolar. Many are not active or even still in existence, but it's fun to browse and see all the options available to you.
- **www.bipolardream.com/groups.htm.** Bipolar Dream has a number of specialty support groups: a general bipolar disorder group; a group for people who have suffered physical, emotional, verbal, or sexual abuse in either childhood or adulthood; an ADHD group; an anger management group; a bipolar mates group; a dissociative disorders group; an eating disorders group; a newbies group; a rainbows group (bisexuals, gays, and lesbians with bipolar disorder); a suicide left-behinds group; and a young adults group.
- **www.harbor-of-refuge.org.** Online peer-to-peer support groups only for people with bipolar disorder who are "receiving appropriate medical treatment" for their illness.

- **www.manicmoment.org/support/support** the online presence of an e-mail support group for bipolar disorder. You can sign up for the e-mail group at the site, as well as use their real-time chat rooms, get information on bipolar disorder, and more.
- **www.thewindsofchange.org:** The Winds of Change Bipolar Disorder Support group has online support as well as articles and information about the disorder.
- **www.a-silver-lining.org:** A Silver Lining has a chat room, online bulletin boards, and mailing lists for people with bipolar disorder and is staffed by a group of peer volunteers.

If the support available on the Net isn't quite right for you, if there are no peer groups in your area, or if you just aren't comfortable with the choices before you, you might want to think about starting a peer-led group of your own. Find a couple other people with the same needs you have, sit down, and develop a plan. The National Mental Health Consumers' Self-Help Clearinghouse (NMHCSC) suggests you consider the following issues:

- The group's purpose
- The people you want to reach
- How you'll find those people
- How and whether you'll tie your group into other services in the community
- Where you'll meet

> **GET PSYCHED**
>
> "Empowerment happens when a person who is seen as the problem begins to see him- or herself as part of the solution." *—Saul Alinsky, in "Emerging New Practices in Organized Peer Support, 2003"*

For more information on how to get started, check out the NMHCSC website (www.mhselfhelp.org).

Keep in mind that, helpful as it is, sometimes support doesn't feel quite so supportive. After all, there's only a thin line between being helped and being controlled, and when you're already vulnerable and off-kilter, one can certainly feel like it's morphed into the other, even if it hasn't.

**Q&A** *I'm a little nervous about going to a support group meeting for the first time. What can I expect?*

"We start out every meeting by going around the room and each person saying their name and diagnosis. Then we open it up for topics you want to talk about. If there aren't any, then we pose a topic about how you deal with work, how you deal when you're depressed, how you talk to doctors. And then we just let the discussion go on from there." —*Rachael Bender, living with bipolar, DBSA facilitator in Fort Lauderdale, Florida*

"Sometimes I feel like I have a personal watcher," Stephanie says of her partner, Tina. "I feel like I'm going to be watched for the rest of my life, and I hate that. But I need it. I need someone who knows all the nuances of my little quirks that nobody else would notice."

**Support for Your Family and Friends** The challenges facing your family and friends are different than the ones facing you, but they are no less real, and they are often no less hurtful. The people who love you have to grapple with issues of guilt, fear, and concern. They have to learn when to protect you and when to let you make your own mistakes. They, like you, have to find a balance between blaming your disorder and helping you take responsibility. And they have to try to avoid some of the downfalls that plague many people who are "care-takers"—issues of anger, burnout, and losing themselves in your disorder. In short, they have to learn how to focus on and take care of themselves (see Chapter 16).

Many of the organizations mentioned in this chapter— especially the larger national organizations—will likely have some sort of support available to the people who are supporting their constituents. NAMI, for instance, has an entire "community" on its website (www.nami.org) devoted to the families of people with bipolar disorder; click on "Find Support," "Communities," "Shared Interests," and "Family." DBSA has both "real-life" support groups that cater directly to friends and family, as well as a friends-and-family e-mail forum on its site (www.dbsalliance.org).

Some organizations are even entirely devoted to the people who love and support you—or who at least care enough to seek help. Bipolar Significant Others is an e-mail list whose web presence—filled with information and links—can be found at www.bpso.org. The group was formed in 1995 as "an informal organization whose members exchange support and information about bipolar disorder by e-mail, and discuss issues related to the impact of the illness on families and intimate relationships." BPSO defines "significant others" as almost anyone in a bipolar person's life, from boyfriends or girlfriends to siblings, parents, and children. The only thing they ask is that the person joining the list not have a bipolar diagnosis him- or herself, "to protect uninhibited discussion."

A similar group, called Guides, can be found at bang.dhs.org/guides.

## Fighting the Stigma, Finding Acceptance

The stigma of mental illness is alive, well, and, unfortunately, thriving. "Even in this day and age, people still don't want to hear [about mental illness]," says Lynn Albizo, a mental health attorney whose mother and brother are both bipolars (see Chapter 4). "It's the dirty little secret that people don't want to hear about."

Sometimes stigma comes not only from without, but from within as well. "Before I was diagnosed, I would say to people, *manic* sounds like *maniac*," says Rachael Bender, who is now a DBSA facilitator running several of their peer-led support groups. "I would have never wanted to associate myself with that."

Even former Surgeon General David Satcher admitted, in his 1999 Surgeon General's Report on Mental Health, that stigma has a very wide reach. "Stereotypes and ignorance are omnipresent," the report stated.

"The lives of consumers are frequently set apart by angry or indifferent communities that reject, shun, and sometimes attack them," added a 2003 report on peer-support practices produced by the National Association of State Mental Health Program Directors and the National Technical Assistance Center for State Mental Health Planning. "Stereotypes of persons with mental illness as dangerous, unpredictable, or incompetent are pervasive. The belief that people with mental illness do not know what is in their own best interests persists in popular culture, while social isolation due to such discrimination and stigma erodes hope and diminishes individual dignity."

To take on what they perceive to be the cause of at least some of this negativity, NAMI created StigmaBusters, "a group of dedicated advocates across the country and around the world who seek to fight the inaccurate, hurtful representations of mental illness."

NAMI's StigmaBusters group issues regular e-mail alerts that inform all subscribers of media portrayals or language that is offensive to or further stigmatizes people with a mental illness. They then urge the StigmaBusters to contact the offending outlet (using the contact information provided in the newsletter) and let them know how they feel.

In addition, NAMI notes, StigmaBusters also "sends letters of appreciation and commendation to producers of TV or motion-picture films for their accurate portrayal of a character with a mental illness."

You can sign up on the NAMI website to become a Stigma-Buster: Just go to www.nami.org and click on "Take Action" and "Fight Stigma."

## Becoming an Advocate

The experience of living with a mental illness can be terrifying. But it can also be truly transforming, especially if you are supported by friends, family, and peers through the darkest of days and back into the light. It can make you want to pay back or pay tribute to the people who ensured your safe passage.

**PsychSpeak**

An **advocate** is someone who pushes forward an idea, pleads for a cause, or argues in favor of a particular point.

One way to give back is to become an *advocate* for mental health issues. Being an advocate is as simple as finding a cause about which you are passionate and throwing yourself into it as much or as little as you want.

Jonathan Stanley became an advocate for assisted treatment after an extreme psychotic break—which came on during a time when he was refusing to take his mood-stabilizing medication—almost destroyed his life (see Chapter 5). Lynn Albizo has dedicated her law career to mental health issues: advocating for changes to the involuntary commitment laws, representing people from both sides of the argument in "forced treatment" cases, and helping people get the services they need. That's often much easier said than done.

"There's the phenomenon that happens in hospitals sometimes," Albizo says. "The person with the mental illness suddenly has no credibility whatever. It's a really hard road to overcome that sort of prejudice once you're labeled this way. So they need someone to advocate for them."

To be an effective advocate, however, you don't have to devote your life to a career in medicine or the law or mental health lobbying. You don't have to quit your job and uproot your life and try to single-handedly save the world. You can be as involved or uninvolved as you'd like and still manage to make a significant difference. For instance, simply staying informed of the issues of importance in the field of mental health, determining where you stand, then voting for candidates at both the local and federal level who believe in what you do is a critical form of advocacy.

Want to take it a little bit further? You can ...

- Join and get involved with some of the national organizations that do advocacy work in this field, such as the

National Alliance for the Mentally Ill, the Depression and Bipolar Support Alliance, and the National Mental Health Association. Look for a chapter in your area if you want to get locally involved.

- Write to your senators and representatives at all levels of government, expressing your opinion on topics of importance to you.

- Advocate in person at the local or federal level by actually making an appointment to meet with the people who represent your interests. (There are many tricks of the trade in lobbying, however, so be sure to do your research before going out there. Most of the advocacy groups will be able to provide you with tips or even training if this is something you want to pursue.)

What things might you advocate for? One of the hottest topics right now is mental health parity, which seeks to ensure that the mental health insurance benefits being offered throughout the country are on equal footing with those being offered for physical health (see Chapter 5). In addition, you could join the fight against stigma both in the community and in the media (see the preceding "Fighting the Stigma, Finding Acceptance" section) or work to right discrimination in housing or employment. Or you could get involved at a slightly higher level and help organize, plan, and execute an advocacy campaign around a topic that energizes you, moves you, or gives you the passion necessary to fight the good fight.

**WEB TALK:** To make your voice heard on issues of interest to people with bipolar disorder, go to DBSA's Action Center at:

➤ www.capwiz.com/ndmda/home/

## Emergency Planning

No matter how religiously you take your medications, no matter how diligently you attend therapy sessions and support groups and Internet chats, you eventually might very well feel the danger signs sneaking up on you. You'll recognize them, because you've been there before and because you already know that the best defense against a full-blown relapse is an offense rooted in knowledge and self-awareness (see Chapter 9).

But recognizing the signs and symptoms and doing something about them are two entirely different beasts. Mania's insidiousness is in its tendency to lower your self-awareness so you don't know to reach out; depression's danger is in its tendency to make you not care enough about yourself to reach out.

That's why you need to have a sort of psychological emergency kit—a set of strategies you put together in advance. Then, when the need arises, the plan only needs to be set in motion. The bulk of that kit is going to be made of the people in your support system. You'll need to give them explicit instructions on what to expect, what you want, what you don't want, and more (see Chapter 9).

**WEB TALK:** The DBSA has a sample "Plan for Life" that lists emergency contacts and important health information: www.dbsalliance.org/info/PlanforLife.html

This information should be compiled while you're feeling well. You should talk to the various people on your "support team" about the roles you'd like them to play and find out if they're willing and/or able to do what you need of them. You should consider giving one person a durable power of attorney so he or she can make financial and medical treatment decisions on your behalf if you're no longer able to make them for yourself.

Putting together this sort of emergency or crisis plan might be one of the more difficult things you have to do, but it's important. It's empowering. And it's likely to make a huge difference in your mental health, and in your life, one of these days.

## What You Can Do

*No man is an island. Lean on me. You've got a friend. It takes a village.* Support is an integral part of the way people relate to one another in this world, whether they have a mental illness or not. Unfortunately, if you're someone with bipolar disorder, support can be difficult to find—and to keep. Keep trying. Keep reaching out. Now's the time to not only get the medical help you need, but to get the support you need to stick with therapy and find your way back to mental health.

- [ ] Reach out to people around you. Ask for help. Ask for support. Ask for them to simply keep an eye on you and to let you know if you seem to be acting in an unusual manner.
- [ ] Find a local support group and go to it at least a couple times to see if it's a good fit for you.
- [ ] If you're not comfortable attending a peer group in person, check out some of the options on the web, including newsgroups, e-mail lists, bulletin boards, and chat rooms.
- [ ] Once you've gotten comfortable in a peer group, consider volunteering to help others. The more you put in, the more you'll get out.
- [ ] Put together a crisis plan, including all your relevant medical information as well as your wishes about your treatment should you need to be hospitalized or if you're simply no longer able to make your own decisions.
- [ ] Contact your local representative, state senator, or even the White House with your concerns. Your voice won't be heard unless you use it.
- [ ] Let entertainment and media outlets know when they're portraying bipolar disorder or mental illness incorrectly, reinforcing stereotypes. And just as important, let them know when they're doing it right.
- [ ] Don't let the lack of a local support group keep you from reaping the benefits of support: Start a group of your own.
- [ ] Fight stigma, either by educating the people around you or by speaking up when you see an injustice.

# In the Workplace

F or so many adults, a job is more than a place to spend several hours each day. It's independence. It's a source of income that enables you to make your own choices about how you live, where you live, and what you do with your free time. It's a way of adding meaning and value to your life, a means of contributing to the world. And it's an identity. When someone asks you what you do for a living, you say, "I'm a lawyer," or "I'm a medical technician," or "I'm a store manager."

Bipolar disorder threatens to take that from you—to rob you of your independence and strip you of your identity. When the waves of mania and depression come crashing over you, maintaining your work ethic or making a deadline is one of the last things you can deal with. Next come the medications, with their uncomfortable and sometimes crippling side effects. When you're shaky and fuzzyheaded and too tired to stand up, doing your best work is a near impossibility. Soon, you're no longer a teller or a media consultant or a child-care provider. You're bipolar. In fact, with all the disorder takes from you, sometimes it might feel as if the only thing it gives you is a label, a stigma.

Yes, it can be difficult to keep your job, to keep your identity, when your moods and your energy levels fluctuate. It can be even more difficult when the job itself, with its stresses and its demands, contributes to those fluctuations. But the benefits of working are significant. It's not just about money, although certainly having some always helps. And it's not just about insurance, although that's a big plus as well. Really, it's about the emotional satisfaction you get when you're productive, when you're making a mark, when you're making a difference. Work that adds value to your life can actually help stabilize your moods. Work that fulfills you is worth fighting for. Here's how to do it.

## The Stigma of Mental Illness

Really, there are two basic issues when it comes to dealing with bipolar disorder in the workplace. One comes from within: it's the issue of how your moods and changes in those moods affect your ability to do your job. The other comes from without: it's about how and whether your condition changes the way your supervisors and your co-workers in general perceive you.

The truth is that bipolar disorder can affect your ability to do your best work, especially if your disorder isn't under control or if you lack insight about how everyday events interact with the unique inner landscape each one of us inhabits. Add to that the preconceived notions that many people carry about what it means to be mentally ill, and getting and staying employed becomes an uphill battle.

To illustrate that point, here's what 600 people with bipolar disorder told the Depression and Bipolar Support Alliance (DBSA) about how their condition, when it's not being managed correctly, affects their employment:

- The illness affects their ability to perform job duties (88 percent)
- Their career aspirations are lower (75 percent)
- They find it necessary to change jobs more frequently than their peers (65 percent)
- They find it necessary to change their careers or professions entirely (60 percent)

- They are treated differently than other employees (63 percent)
- They have quit working outside the home (58 percent)
- They have been passed up for promotion (65 percent)
- Their job duties and responsibilities have been decreased (48 percent)

How much of these outcomes is the result of the disease and how much is the result of what the people around you think about your disease is hard to say. Although it's easy to spot out-and-out discrimination, sometimes the stigma of mental illness plays itself out in much more insidious ways.

Say, for example, a co-worker of yours comes up with a great new idea. He's excited about it. He tells everyone who will listen, and they all clap him on the back and congratulate him on his insightful thinking.

Now, let's say you come up with an equally brilliant idea. You, too, are excited. You, too, prattle on about it to all comers. But you don't get clapped on the back quite so often, or quite so heartily. Over your head, or behind your back, people are raising their eyebrows. "She seems a bit ... manic ... don't you think?" they're saying to one another. Your idea gets pushed aside as grandiose thinking, the product of your bi-polar disorder.

None of this is easy. If you think it's hard for you to tell what's your disorder and what's just you—if you think *you* are second-guessing every minor mood swing, searching for signs of mania or depression—it's even harder for those around you, who aren't in your head and don't know what to think. It's especially hard if they've seen you when you're manic and when you're depressed and, therefore, know that it can—and does—happen.

> **GET PSYCHED**
>
> "I think the bipolar has given me a lot more perspective on life. I'm not as much of a workaholic as I used to be. There's more to my life than just work. Still, I've always been a very ambitious person, and I still am. I strongly believe that people who are bipolar have more ambition." –*Rachael Bender, graphic designer, living with bipolar disorder*

Still, the only way to beat back the stigma of mental illness—to make life both on and off the job easier for yourself and others with mental illnesses—is to confront it, be open about it, and show by example that people with bipolar disorder can lead productive, healthy, even joyful lives. The only reason we've come as far as we have in accepting mental illness is because of people who have come out of the psychiatric closet and drawn attention to their successes and their failures—people who've shown that although mental illness can be messy, difficult, and disruptive, it doesn't have to be scary.

No one can legislate how others feel about you and your disorder, but laws that protect you from unfounded and biased attitudes in the workplace are on the books. The Americans with Disabilities Act, or ADA, may very well apply to you. After all, bipolar disorder is a biological condition, and it certainly can and does disable.

**WEB TALK:** For more on the Americans with Disabilities Act, visit:

↑ www.ada.gov

The ADA, enacted in 1990, was designed to halt discrimination in employment, public services (like education—see Chapter 15), and more. The problem is, although most people in the mental health field are well aware of the level of disability psychiatric disorders can cause, the same can't necessarily be said of employers and the public in general. You might have to push a little to get the help you need to even out the workplace playing field so that you have the same chance of succeeding as do your co-workers. But it is possible, and it's getting just a little bit easier all the time.

## Q&A

*How do I know if I'm considered disabled by the Americans with Disabilities Act?*

"An individual with a disability is defined by the ADA as a person who has a physical or mental impairment that substantially limits one or more major life activities, a person who has a history or a record of such an impairment, or a person who is perceived by others as having such an impairment. The ADA does not specifically name all the impairments that are covered." *—From "A Guide to Disability Rights Laws," published by the U.S. Department of Justice, May 2002*

If all this talk about disability and discrimination is bringing you down, take heart in a study performed by the Center for Psychiatric Rehabilitation at Boston University. The researchers looked at the characteristics of people with mental disorders who were able to sustain employment for at least a year. They found that, overall, people with bipolar disorder have a higher occupational status, work more hours per week, and earn a higher salary than any of the other diagnostic groups. (People with schizophrenia had the lowest status, hours, and salary in the study.)

The point of the study, however, was to try to understand what makes some people with mental illness more successful at holding down a job than others. Among the things the researchers noted was that a huge majority of the people who remain employed over longer periods of time (2 years in one of the most recent of the studies of sustained employment) are taking psychotropic medications and are in some kind of psychotherapy. And when those stably employed people were interviewed, they said that having the support of a spouse or a significant other makes a huge difference as well. Finally, as with everyone else, education is a critical component in getting and keeping a job, as well as in advancing in that job or getting paid well.

It's not earth-shattering stuff, but it's good news nonetheless. Clearly, you can succeed in the workplace even if you have bipolar disorder. You just need to have the right tools at your disposal.

## To Tell or Not To Tell?

For many people, this is the ultimate question. And there is really no single, one-size-fits-all answer.

But there is clearly a trend. As a 2003 paper published in the *Journal of Vocational Rehabilitation* found, more than 86 percent of 350 people with psychiatric conditions who worked in either professional or managerial positions had disclosed their mental illness to their employer. That's not to say they wanted to do so. A full half of the "disclosers" said their hand was forced in some way or another, be it because of a hospitalization or because they experienced symptoms of their disorder while on the job and needed to explain them. Of the remaining 13 percent who didn't tell anyone at their workplace of their diagnosis, almost a quarter said their condition was probably suspected by at least some of their co-workers.

Still, half the people in the study said they didn't regret having been open about their condition.

Why tell? There are a lot of reasons, both personal and professional. "For some individuals with psychiatric conditions, *disclosure* relieves the stress in hiding information about oneself and provides the opportunity to be accepted," wrote Marsha Langer Ellison and her colleagues from the Center for Psychiatric Rehabilitation at Boston University in their study. "Disclosure may also educate others and address stigma."

Indeed, if you've become friends with one or more of the people you work with, you're likely to feel uncomfortable leaving this part of your life out of the picture. If you're having trouble controlling your moods, it might help to have someone at work who knows what to look for and who will alert you when you're spiraling out of control. Even if you're not having trouble gaining control, you might want to have someone at work watching your back in case of an unexpected relapse. And of course, you might find that talking about your disorder helps someone else to find her way out of a depression or gives her the impetus to get the help she needs for some problem or another.

## PsychSpeak

**Disclosure** is the deliberate informing of one or several people in your workplace or life about your psychiatric disability.

Finally, when the information is coming out of your mouth, you can control the message. You get to explain what people can and can't expect. You get to make sure everyone understands and that they are properly informed. If you don't tell, you take a risk that the information somehow gets around anyway—without your being able to control what's being said and discussed, and without your being able to make sure the information is correct and unexaggerated.

In addition, if you're feeling secure in your job and appreciated and liked by your co-workers or supervisor—in other words, if you feel as if you can trust the people you're going to tell—then telling can be a very positive experience. More than half the people in Ellison's study who disclosed their condition had no regrets about doing so—with most of these being people who made the choice to come clean rather than somehow being pushed into doing it.

Telling one person, of course, doesn't mean you have to tell everyone at your work. In fact, you probably shouldn't. Not everyone needs to know. Not everyone is likely to respond well.

For instance, most people in Ellison's study were much more likely to tell their supervisors about their struggles with mental illness than they were to tell their subordinates. They also were more likely to talk to co-workers than they were to talk to clients or customers.

There are times when the choice of whether or not to tell your employer is taken out of your hands. If you need to have certain accommodations made for you because of your disorder, it's certainly your employer's right to know the reason why you need these accommodations. And if your insurance claims are handled within the company, the people who deal with benefits will know simply by handling your paperwork. In that case, it might be better for them to hear the words from your mouth, because you're more likely to be able to pass along information, allay fears, and bust myths.

**WEB TALK:** Check out the Canadian Mental Health Association's Mental Health Works for information on mental illness and workplace issues:

www.mentalhealthworks.ca

Be that as it may, there are also many reasons to keep your mental health history to yourself. You might simply be a private person who would rather not have your personal life on display or open for discussion at your office. You might work in a competitive field, where this sort of information might be used against you, however subtly.

Even if you know for certain that you'll want to talk to your employer or co-workers about your bipolar disorder, you still need to decide when the time is right to disclose the information. Are you better off getting it out there as soon as possible—during the interview process, even? Or are you better off waiting until you've been able to prove yourself at the job, so the people whom you take into your confidence learn to see you first and your condition second?

Again, there are no clear answers. There are both benefits and risks to coming clean early on, just as there are benefits and risks to holding back for a while.

At least one study posits that people who talk about their mental illness during a job interview tend to do better on the job than those who choose to wait or not to disclose at all. On the other hand, there have also been studies that have heaped on evidence showing that disclosure's risks—being stigmatized, discriminated against, or held back—are also quite prevalent and don't simply represent paranoia on the part of the psychiatric community. Some specialists in the field of *psychiatric rehabilitation* have interviewed employers and found that, as you might suspect, they tend to have a wide variety of concerns about hiring someone with bipolar disorder or some other mental illness. And more studies have quantified these results, providing evidence that if you divulge information about a mental illness during an interview, you're less likely to be seen as a good candidate and, thus, less likely to be offered the job.

## PsychSpeak

**Psychiatric rehabilitation** is services designed to provide skills and support to people whose ability to function on one or more levels is affected by a mental illness.

In Ellison's study of 350 employees and their decisions to disclose or not, a third of the 303 disclosers said they'd done so during the application process. Another 16 percent said they began talking about their disorder to at least one person in their workplace during their first year of employment, while 24 percent said they waited more than a year.

# In and Out

Stephanie is not the kind of person to care what other people think. But even if she had been, the Tourette's syndrome she's lived with since she was a child—with its eye rolling and facial grimacing and throat clearing—would have knocked that right out of her. And if that hadn't done the trick, coming out as a lesbian would have finished it off.

So it is both sad and telling that there is one secret Stephanie still works to keep from her boss and her co-workers: her bipolar disorder diagnosis.

"I feel the stigma is too much to bear," she says. "Tourette's syndrome, being a lesbian, those I can handle. But bipolar? Whew ..."

Stephanie was diagnosed only a few years ago, when she was 37, although she'd had symptoms since childhood. "My mother knew I was a very angry child," she recalls. "She used to threaten to take me to a psychiatrist to see what was wrong with me—not to help me, but to see what was wrong with me. I think that's where I started to get the idea that mental illness just isn't acceptable."

Since her diagnosis, Stephanie has managed to find the right medications, and that has given her a fairly good grip on stability. She's worked steadily these past few years, aside from a couple layoffs that had nothing to do with her diagnosis, and today is a public relations writer with a high-powered Wall Street firm.

Still, she's worried that she would not be as successful in her life if she were to let the world know about her mental illness.

"I purposely asked to not be put on lithium or Depakote, in case I ever have to undergo workplace drug screening," she says with a quick, gruff laugh. "I can explain away the other meds I'm on as a Tourette's kind of thing without having to talk about the bipolar."

Stephanie says all she has to do is look around to realize that it's still not safe to be open about mental illness in this society. "Mental illness in general is so misunderstood," she says. "When I first came to New York, I used to work with the homeless mentally ill, and it was so difficult. There was so much stigma."

Still, Stephanie isn't quite as closeted about her bipolar disorder as you might think. She is, after all, a writer, and she does feel a need to help destigmatize her illness. "There is stuff in the public domain that I've written about bipolar disorder," she admits. "It's not a complete secret and shock to anyone who would care to look. I'm just not going to put it out there for them, that's all.

"I do think people need to know that you can function with bipolar disorder. Of course, not everybody can and not everybody can all the time. But most of us can live a useful life and contribute to society. I'm not really that different from somebody else who's not bipolar. We're all just people trying to hold it together."

In any case, disclosure is generally your choice—not your employer's. It is illegal for an employer to ask you directly about a mental condition during the interview process. In fact, employers can't even legally ask once you're an employee, either. You are, however, obligated to reveal at least some information about your disability if you're going to ask for reasonable accommodations under the Americans with Disabilities Act. Still, even in that instance, the only thing required of you is to give enough information so your accommodation can be considered and implemented. And you only have to tell those people who actually need to know: That might be anyone from a co-worker to your boss to the company's personnel office.

No matter what you decide, there's always the possibility that your hand ultimately will be forced. It's possible that someone in your office might find out about your condition through other channels—anything from a lithium prescription that needs to be cleared by your in-house insurance to a co-worker who runs into you at a mental health advocacy rally. Still, that shouldn't affect your employment: firing you (or demoting you, cutting your salary, or passing you up for a raise or promotion) would then become a clear case of discrimination and would wind up in court if you so chose.

Not disclosing your illness is neither illegal nor wrong; don't let anyone tell you it is. You might not be able to control a lot of things about your condition, but who knows what about you and your moods is one of them.

## Finding—and Keeping—a Job

One of the best ways to hold on to your job while still dealing with the ups and downs of your disorder is to be sure you have the right kind of occupation in the right kind of field in the first place. The chance of your doing well as an obstetrician who is on call at all hours of the day and night is much slimmer than if you're a radiologist with set hours. You're more likely to run into problems as a flight attendant or pilot constantly crossing time zones than as a bank teller with a regular shift.

There are questions that you, as a person living with bipolar disorder, need to ask yourself, questions that might help you decide if a profession or a particular job is the right one for you. Can you do your work on a set schedule, or are you going to have to sometimes put in long hours and get up unusually early to meet deadlines? How much stress will the job put on you—and how much of a trigger is stress for you?

Rachael Bender, who has been bipolar since she was in her teens, says that having her own business has been a sanity-saver for her. "I started my current business, Bender Consulting, about 2 years ago, but I've been working for myself for about 5 years," says the 26-year-old graphic designer. "It's been a blessing with this disorder, because when I first went on Depakote I was tired so much, sleeping 10 to 11 hours a day, and I was incredibly un-productive. If I had had a traditional job, that just wouldn't be acceptable. I probably wouldn't have been able to work at all. It can be really hard to find a job that can work with the hours you internally have, especially if you're on medication."

If you didn't already have a profession or a set of occupational goals when you were diagnosed with bipolar disorder, you might feel a bit overwhelmed at trying to learn how to live with your mental illness while at the same time trying to decide what it is you want to do with your life. There is, of course, help, in the form of books, websites, and job counseling programs. And you might also qualify for vocational rehabilitation, which is like psy-chiatric rehabilitation, but focuses on your job and often includes the input of a "job coach," whose role is to help you and advo-cate for you throughout the process—from choosing a career path to interviewing for jobs, to training for on-site tasks.

Qualifying for vocational rehabilitation is often based on the severity of your mental illness. For you to receive vocational reha-bilitation services, you'll probably have to be able to demonstrate just how your bipolar disorder is impeding your job search or handicapping you in your ability to carry out your assigned tasks. Exactly what you'll need to prove to qualify varies from state to state.

## Making Accommodations

Still, no matter what your profession, there are things you can do to help yourself—or rather, things you can ask for that will help make your job the best possible situation it can be. These are called accommodations—*reasonable accommodations*—and are actually required of your employer by the ADA.

What makes an accommodation "reasonable"? If the change you're requesting actually addresses a need you have because of your condition, rather than fulfilling your wish for the perfect job, it's probably reasonable. If it makes it possible for you to do just as well at your job as the next person, it's probably a reasonable request. If it doesn't cost your company an exorbitant amount of money to comply with your request, it might well be reasonable.

In other words, it's reasonable to ask to shift your work hours from 9 to 5 to 10 to 6 so as not to disrupt your normal circadian rhythm. It's probably not reasonable to ask to change your work hours from 9 to 5 to 11 to 3 because you don't feel like putting in a full day. It's reasonable to ask to take work home rather than having to put in long overtime hours; it's probably not reasonable to ask for a new computer to use at home simply because you're tired of your old one.

Other reasonable accommodations might include the following:

- Use of a job coach in the hiring process, the training process, or on the job itself, or all of the above
- Getting extra training to reduce the stress of on-the-job learning

### PsychSpeak

**Reasonable accommodations** are on-the-job changes in things such as scheduling or job requirements and expectations that help provide a level playing field on which you have as much chance to both become and remain employed as do your co-workers.

- Setting a regular schedule, even if the job might normally require constantly changing shifts
- Scheduling or eliminating overtime work
- Setting up a regular, frequent break schedule
- Setting up a private workspace to reduce distractions
- Taking extra time off for doctor and therapist appointments
- Taking an unpaid leave of absence when necessary

**GET PSYCHED**

"My job is absolutely tailor-made for me. I'm still a workaholic, more so than I should be, but because it's a mental health agency, there are some accommo-dations there for me if I need them." –*Jacqueline Castine, community education specialist in public relations, Oakland County Community Mental Health Authority*

Interestingly, accommodations given to people with mental illnesses tend to be much less costly than those given to people with physical disabilities. In fact, notes Kim MacDonald-Wilson, the Reasonable Accommodations Project Director at the Center for Psychiatric Rehabilitation, most costs are indirect—things like fewer hours on the job resulting in less productivity, or supervisors and peers who have to spend an increased amount of time working with their employees to help them get up to speed.

**Dealing With Cognitive Demands** Mania can set your thoughts racing so fast you can't keep up with them; depression can slow you down so precipitously that you barely have the energy to think. And the medications you take to treat your disorder can make a simple intellectual exercise feel like you're slogging through sticky mud.

So perhaps it's not so surprising that MacDonald-Wilson's study of 194 employees with mental health issues in Maryland, Massachusetts, and New Jersey found that the second most prevalent problem for the workers was being able to meet the intellectual challenges of their job without losing control of their symptoms. In particular, the workers cited having trouble with remembering office routines, following detailed instructions, and learning their myriad job responsibilities. In addition, other workers cited difficulty in solving problems or organizing their work and concentrating as hurdles they had difficulty getting over.

There are, however, a number of accommodations you can ask for if you find yourself in a similar situation. As noted earlier, a job coach can help guide you through the early days at work and assist you in figuring out new routines and skills. Or you can simply ask for additional training. You can ask your boss to put requests and assignments in writing if you're finding it hard to remember what you have to do. Finally, you can simply ask for more frequent feedback, be it in the form of quarterly performance reviews or informal weekly discussions. That way, any problems that might be developing can be nipped in the bud.

## GET PSYCHED

"Bipolar disorder can be a great teacher. It's a challenge, but it can set you up to be able to do almost anything else in your life."
—Carrie Fisher, actress, in Psychology Today, November/December 2001

With medications bogging you down and making a tough job even tougher, it might be tempting to back off your regimen to give yourself that hypomanic "edge." Don't do it. You might well get an initial boost in energy and creativity, but you'll almost inevitably wind up paying for it somewhere down the line—either in terms of full-blown mania and its destructive impulses and lack of insight, or in terms of a major depression and the effects that will have on your job performance.

**Avoiding Reactivity and Intrusiveness** Along with those newfound intellectual challenges that keep you hopping, you might also find yourself having difficulty dealing with social interactions on the job. The problem is that good old lack of insight that plagues all things manic. Transfer that inability to see what's going wrong to the workplace, and you have a recipe for some pretty uncomfortable interactions at the very least.

In some ways, when it comes to bipolar disorder, it sometimes seems almost as if your emotional reactions—to good things and to bad—get wound up just a bit too tightly. A positive comment can send your mood soaring, while even the slightest hint of criticism can make you anxious, depressed, or even paranoid.

This tendency to react (or rather, to over-react) to every compliment and every slight—real or imagined—can make the people around you uncomfortable. Controlling your reactions, however, can be extremely difficult, especially if your moods aren't completely stable. Indeed, the hardest part is breaking through the denial and lack of insight to recognize your overreaction in the first place.

This sort of hyperreactivity goes hand in hand with what is called social *intrusiveness*. Social intrusiveness is a sign of mania or hypomania—part and parcel with the rapid speech and racing thoughts. The same almost-physical pressure that makes it impossible for you to slow down your brain can also drive you to insert yourself into discussions and situations where you don't belong, blithely offering your opinions and thoughts without recognizing that your behavior is inappropriate.

The best way to deal with these symptoms before they become a problem at work is to talk to a co-worker or supervisor who knows about your bipolar disorder. Ask him or her to let you know when your reactions seem excessive or you begin to interrupt and intrude on your co-workers' meetings and discussions. That way, you can try to get control of both the symptoms and the impetus behind them before either swing out of your reach.

---

## GET PSYCHED

"I worked my way up from the mail room to become executive vice president of a major textile firm. I used to get scared and depressed, thinking, *What am I doing in the huge office with a secretary; I should be delivering the mail.* I was successful beyond my wildest dreams. I worked long hours, sometimes around the clock, and I loved it. I now know that it was mania, but at the time I was just so proud and excited by my accomplishments. It was like being on a 24-hour high." *—Jack Oliwenstein, living with bipolar disorder*

## PsychSpeak

**Intrusiveness** is the act of aggressively advancing yourself and your ideas without invitation or regard for the appropriateness of your meddling.

## Time Out

It can happen to anyone: You get laid off, you get fired, you quit. Unemployment is stressful under the best of circumstances, but when you're fretting about paying for your medication or keeping your mental health coverage on top of the normal how-to-make-ends-meet worries, your stress levels can intensify. And intense stress can undo all the work you've done to get yourself and your moods to a stable place.

Take a deep breath. First of all, if you think you were dismissed unfairly—if you think you were discriminated against because of your bipolar disorder—contact your local office of the Equal Employment Opportunity Commission (EEOC). You can find contact information for your local EEOC office at www.eeoc.gov.

WEB TALK: The National Center on Workplace and Disability offers resources to help people find jobs and understand their rights at:

↑ www.onestops.info

If the choice to leave your job was yours, or was caused by something other than your disability, then you probably don't have a right to file a grievance. You might, however, have the right to file for, and receive, unemployment.

And don't be ashamed to reach out for help in finding another job. The EEOC might be able to provide you with help finding a vocational rehabilitation center nearby.

Unemployment isn't the only thing that might put you on the vocational sidelines, however. There might be times when you experience a relapse, and no matter how much you want to keep working, you simply can't. You might need to be hospitalized, or you might need a recovery period, be it long or short. You might have to tweak your medications, or change them entirely, and you might need some time off until your symptoms and side effects settle down a bit.

Take time when you need time. You can use accumulated vacation or sick time at first, but if that runs out, talk to your employer about other accommodations. Remember, bipolar disorder is a disability. If you can't work because of your symptoms, you are no more or less entitled to disability benefits than your colleague who takes a leave for the birth of her child, or your co-worker who throws out his back and is on bed rest.

Depending on the length of your disability, you'll get different levels of benefits. Short-term disability generally covers you if you're laid up for a few weeks; long-term disability kicks in later on, paying you a percentage of your salary as long as a doctor—including your psychiatrist—signs off on a statement certifying your disability. If your company doesn't have its own long-term disability plan, most states have plans you can apply for.

You might also be eligible to collect that Social Security Disability Insurance (SSDI) that's been coming out of your paycheck every week. To find out about SSDI or apply for your benefits, call 1-800-772-1213 or visit www.ssa.gov.

Finally, you might be eligible for leave under the Family and Medical Leave Act (FMLA). FMLA provides for up to 12 weeks of *unpaid* leave each year for birth or caregiving or serious illness—either your own or that of someone in your family. When you come back to work from your leave, your employer is expected to have kept your job open, or to be able to find you a comparable one within the organization. If you're the spouse, parent, or sibling of someone with bipolar disorder and you need to take some time off to care for him or her during a crisis, FMLA might cover your job as well.

Because FMLA is such a complicated law, you'll want to get more information before applying: You can either call 866-487-9243 or visit www.dol.gov/esa/whd/fmla.

## What You Can Do

Taking on a bipolar disorder diagnosis does not mean surrendering your right to a job, career, or ambitions and aspirations. There are laws to protect you and agencies to assist you. Nobody's going to give you a free pass, but if you've got the drive and the talent, you'll find your way.

☐ If a potential employer asks you whether or not you have a mental illness, you can decline to answer. If he or she presses the question or refuses to hire you because you wouldn't answer, you have the right to pursue legal action.

☐ If you decide to talk about your disorder to your boss or co-workers, be sure to educate them about bipolar disorder. Ignorance breeds fear and stigma; knowledge breeds acceptance.

☐ Get to know the provisions in the Americans with Disabilities Act and how they can work on your behalf.

☐ If you think your ADA rights have been violated, contact the Equal Employment Opportunity Commission and file a complaint.

☐ Request accommodations if you need them. Don't expect your employer to come up with solutions on his or her own; you'll need to lay out your requests and explain how they'll benefit not only you personally, but your job performance and productivity as well.

☐ If you're really having trouble finding or keeping a job, consider using a job coach—someone to help you navigate the interview process and advocate for you on the job.

☐ Come up with on-the-job strategies to deal with your mood triggers. For instance, if you find yourself becoming stressed when a co-worker looks over your shoulder, get up and go to the restroom rather than let it get to you.

☐ Get yourself onto a work schedule, and stick to it. Structure is the key to keeping your mood stable.

☐ Take breaks as frequently as you can to keep stress levels low. Take every scheduled break even if you think you don't need one.

☐ Sometimes you'll have to make allowances for your disorder. You might need to take a medical leave if you feel an episode coming on, or you might need to take more time than you think you should to recover from an episode.

☐ Not everyone has a job he or she loves. If yours is "just a job," and not a passion, be sure you're also including time in your life for things you *do* feel passionate about.

# Part 4

## Thriving With Bipolar Disorder

Bipolar disorder is not your life, and your life is not bipolar disorder. But the two are inextricably intertwined. If you're going to move forward, to strive and to achieve in your life, you're going to have to learn to blend the two as seamlessly as possible. In Part 4, you'll learn some techniques for doing just that, for truly thriving with bipolar disorder.

# At Home

**H**ome. It's where you hang your hat, where your heart is. If you have bipolar disorder, you might spend time in hospitals, in doctors' offices, or on therapists' couches. But it's at home where you're going to do most of the actual *living* part of living with your condition. And that, as you may well know, is not always easy.

Watching your friends, family, or spouse cope with your diagnosis and with the ups and downs of your disorder can be difficult. It might take some time for them to really understand what's going on. If it's hard for you to consistently tell the difference between smiles and frowns that are a response to normal, everyday events and smiles and frowns that are inappropriate responses to what's going on around you, and are, thus, coming from your disease, imagine how hard it is for those who aren't inside your head.

In a perfect world, everyone would be able to make those judgments—and get them right 100 percent of the time. Then those people would stand behind you, supporting you and helping you find your own stability. But this is the real world. And in the real world, things aren't quite so tidy.

You might find yourself losing friends, clashing with relatives, or distancing yourself from your spouse. And in the midst of all this chaos, you might also find yourself considering starting a family of your own—but terrified of what that might mean for you and your children.

By giving you some idea of what you might be in for, I hope this chapter will help calm some of that terror. Or better yet, I hope it will provide you with strategies that will enable you to nudge your "real world" a little closer to your perfect one.

## Family Matters

Bipolar disorder might be your diagnosis, but it's not only your problem. The effects this mental illness can have on your family can range from mild to profound, but they do exist. And together or apart, you, your family, and your friends are all going to have to deal with the changes bipolar disorder brings to your lives.

Initially, at least, those changes are not likely to be positive ones. The Depression and Bipolar Support Alliance (DBSA) did a survey of its constituency in 2000 and then compared those results to information obtained in a similar 1992 study. When they tabulated the results, they found that, overall, the survey had some rather dispiriting things to say about family relationships and bipolar disorder. For instance, only 67 percent of the people responding agreed with the statement, "My relationship with my family is good," down 10 percent from 1992. Other statements included the following:

- "In general, my illness has decreased my family's expectations for my success": 73 percent agreed, up 8 percent from 1992
- "Most of my family members do not believe that my illness has had permanent damaging effects on our relationships": 63 percent agreed
- "My family has always been very involved in my treatment": 48 percent agreed
- "Most of my friends/family have a good understanding of what it means to have bipolar disorder": 41 percent agreed, down 9 percent from 1992
- "My illness has had a negative effect on my relationship with my children": 64 percent agreed
- "Most of my friends/family do not know about my illness": 27 percent agreed

Despite the issues and obstacles, your family can play an extremely important role in your disorder. They can be the eyes and ears you don't have when you're manic, or the push to get help you're missing when you're depressed. In fact, says S. Nassir Ghaemi, M.D., director of the Bipolar Disorder Research Program at Cambridge Health Alliance, the best way for a physician to evaluate someone for bipolar disorder or other mood disorders is to have him or her bring a family member along to the appointment. Family members are the ones who are more likely to have noticed subtleties in your symptoms that even you might not be aware of, or they might have insight into your psychiatric history you couldn't possible have. "Then I ask the family to feel free to call me any time the patient is developing mood symptoms of any variety," Ghaemi told *Psychology Today* in March 2002. "There's no confidentiality constraint against my ear being open. I can't say anything, but I can listen to what they say."

You can help your family, as well, if you keep the lines of communication open. You can teach them about the impact of mental illness and about how the disease doesn't change the value of who you are. You can teach them about compassion and effective communication. And you can teach them about acceptance and unconditional love. These are lessons that will benefit all of you.

**Asking for—and Accepting—Help** You know how important support is, especially support from family members. You could get through this without them, but it's so much easier if you've got people on your side. So why does it make you want to scream every time your mother offers to pick up your medication for you or your spouse offers to call to confirm your therapy appointment?

Actually, it's not all that surprising that you feel this way. You're a grown person. You've been fending for yourself for years. And now, suddenly, everyone's treating you like you can't take care of yourself. You're a little bit afraid of giving up your sense of independence, your sense of control over your own life. And if you're manic, you probably don't even think you need help.

What you're feeling is so normal, in fact, that scientists have actually studied it. In a 1999 paper, psychologists at the University of Colorado at Boulder stated that when a family member or someone in your "social network" starts playing a role in your health, you're actually more likely to start taking care of yourself *and* more likely to show signs of "psychological distress"—of feeling resentful or angry at the person helping you.

What you want—and need—is the best of both worlds. You need help; you need someone looking out for you. But you also need to retain your independence, or at least know that when you're more in control of your moods, you'll be able to be more in control of your life again.

It can be done, especially if you and your family can set some limits. If you need to hand over control of your finances, for instance, be sure anything you might sign or agree to specifies that you're asking for assistance while you're sick—and only while you're sick. Once your moods are stable again, and you've maintained that stability for some period of time, you want to be able to handle your own money matters. Or perhaps you need to move back in with your parents for a while, when you're deep in the throes of a depression. Tell them how much you appreciate their letting you stay and then set some goals for moving back out on your own.

Kay, a woman who's dealt with several family members who have bipolar disorder (see Chapter 16), says that the sort of help your family can give you may be lifesaving in the short term but can be debilitating in the long term if you don't work to get back on your own two feet.

"There's no such thing as too much support—until they get diagnosed and medicated and stabilized," says Kay, who has also facilitated support groups for people with bipolar disorder. "But when they get stabilized, they need to be encouraged; somebody has to push them to be who they are. A bird pushes her young out of the nest, and I think the family needs to do that, too. The people with the disorder need to be made to feel like the functioning people they are, not like they're disabled. They must fully understand their illness, accept that they have it, and take responsibility for running their lives."

**Dealing With Family Dynamics** It's become more and more clear over time that the reaction you get from the people closest to you can really make or break your recovery and your long-term prognosis. As David Miklowitz and colleagues have shown with their studies of family-focused therapy (see Chapter 8), it's simply that much harder to find your footing and regain your stability if the people around you are negative and unsupportive, critical of your choices or of your behavior, or smothering. If they're positive and supportive and empower you, it'll be that much easier.

That's not to say the negativity that tends to creep into families dealing with bipolar disorder is all their fault. After all, that same attitude tends to cling to your own depressive episodes and can be contagious, spawning its own destructive kind of dynamic. But really, what does it matter? Both logic and research support the idea that criticism, anger, or emotional overinvolvement—in other words, a high level of *expressed emotion* as it's been dubbed in the world of psychology and psychotherapy—is hurtful and harmful. In fact, Miklowitz has quantified that harm. He has reported that patients who had been hospitalized with mania were two to three times more likely to relapse within nine months to a year if they went home to families with high expressed emotion than if they went home to families who were supportive and positive.

**PsychSpeak**

**Expressed emotion** is a set of negative attitudes (criticism, anger, hostility, emotional overinvolvement) that relatives hold toward someone in the family who is psychiatrically ill.

Miklowitz has also seen this with his own eyes, as he told *Psychology Today* in 2002: "Imaging studies show that fear centers are activated in the brain when depression-susceptible people hear a family member criticizing them."

This sort of research makes a good case for the importance of family support and positivity. And certainly, if you and your therapist can work with your family to get them solidly on your side, you're likely to reap significant benefits. But if you can't, it's not the end of the world—or of your sanity. A good cognitive therapist can help you find ways to deal with your family's attitude and keep it from sabotaging your treatment.

## Friends to the End

Bipolar disorder takes its toll on your relationship with your family, and it can take its toll on your love life as well. So it's not particularly surprising to realize that it can take its toll on your friendships, too.

The DBSA survey backs that up. When asked if they believe they have difficulty maintaining long-term friendships because of their illness, 60 percent of the people with bipolar disorder said yes, up 8 percent from the 1992 survey.

What causes these problems? It's possible that some of the people who you thought were your close friends will be scared off by the changes in you when you're experiencing an episode of mania or depression, or will be frightened by your disorder and the labels they associate with it. Education and communication might help put things right again, especially if you're willing to devote the time and effort. But if they were just "social" friends or acquaintances, you're probably better just writing them off.

Friendships can also be scarred by your behavior during an episode. Maybe you were irritable and said some things you would never have otherwise said. Maybe you were depressed and kept blowing off plans. Maybe you felt like your friend simply couldn't keep up with you in your sped-up, king-of-the-world state and acted badly toward him.

If that's the case, now's the time—now that you're stable—to make amends. You can explain to your friend about your disorder and how the things you do when you're cycling are rarely related to how you actually feel about somebody. And you can apologize. Your behavior might not be entirely in your control, but you can still take responsibility for it.

**Q&A**

*How do I tell my friends about my disorder—and how much should I tell them?*

"When you explain it to them, keep it simple. Tell them that it means your emotions are intensified and that your highs are higher than most people but your lows are also much lower than most people … Make sure to keep things in a positive light. Don't go into the really horrible side of this illness unless you truly feel like enlightening someone. Most people don't need to know that suicidal thoughts are typical and that if things get too stressful you could pop. Just give them the basic facts and if they really want to research more, you can send them to the information Web page of your choice."
—*Shay Villere, in* The Bipolar Disorder Manual, *www.mental-health-matters. com/articles/article.php?artID=550*

Sometimes the schism between you and your friends will be one you'll feel the need to create, for your own mental health. For instance, if you're newly sober and stable, you'll probably want to avoid your old drinking buddies. Or if your friend is often critical of your behavior or overprotective or overly involved with your disorder, you might need to get a little distance from her. Other times, you might just want to slow things down a bit to help keep yourself on track, and that can mean pulling back on social events and seeing some of your friends much less frequently.

"Patients who, I think, rightly believe they need to markedly reduce the amount of stimulation they experience find themselves very socially isolated, having lost many of their social contacts, and many of the things that formed and shaped their social lives," says Ellen Frank, Ph.D., director of the Depression and Manic Depression Prevention Program at the Western Psychiatric Institute in Pittsburgh.

But then there are your "real" friends—the ones who don't enable you in your bad habits but who support you in your recovery. They're the ones who understand that your bipolar disorder is a disease like any other. They're the ones who want to help you through it.

These are the friends you need the most. They're the ones you can ask to keep an eye on you for signs of another episode without worrying that they'll smother you with concern the way your mother would, or dismiss you as self-absorbed the way your brother would. They love you, but they're objective enough and removed enough to tell you when you're stepping out of line. As Oscar Wilde once said, "True friends stab you in the front."

## Love and Marriage

The naysayers would have you believe that your bipolar disorder diagnosis was the death knell for your romantic life. But that is simply untrue. Yes, it's hard: Some statistics put the divorce rate for people with bipolar disorder as high as 90 percent, and there doesn't seem to be much in the way of studies of all the relationships that don't make it to the marrying phase.

More encouraging, but still somewhat distressing, are the results of DBSA's constituency survey, in which people with bipolar disorder were asked whether they feel they have difficulty maintaining long-term intimate relationships, including marriage, due to their illness. Sixty-five percent said yes, they did feel they had a hard time keeping their relationship vital and alive because of their disorder. In addition, a small survey of partners of people with bipolar disorder found that 62 percent would likely not have gotten into a committed relationship with their bipolar partner if they'd known more about the illness and its effects.

Still, making a relationship or a marriage work is by no means impossible, as any number of people who have been there and done that can tell you. And when it does work, everyone wins. Studies have shown that marriage and the support it brings also leads to stronger friendships and acquaintanceships, gives you closer ties to your community, and keeps your relapse rate low.

**The Dating Game**  As if dating isn't hard enough, dating when you're cycling is an exercise in futility. No fledgling relationship is going to be able to withstand the stresses of manic hypersexuality or the complete lack of interest that comes with depression.

But once you're stable, you have as much right to look for love as the next person. And although you might be inclined to be protective of your heart and your emotions, fearing what might happen if you experience rejection or any of the other hurts that can be spawned by a relationship, you need to realize that isolating yourself from the rest of the world pretty much guarantees that you'll fall back into your mood cycles. You need the support. You deserve to love and be loved.

Getting into a relationship does bring up some sticky questions, however, the main one being when to start talking about your disorder. Your gut instinct is probably to avoid it altogether—don't ask, don't tell is starting to sound mighty attractive, isn't it? But you know, or you should know, that way leads to nothing but disaster. Still, there are obviously some people who are giving it a shot. When the DBSA asked in its 2000 survey whether the people responding thought it was important to tell a person you're seriously dating that you have been diagnosed with bipolar disorder, 86 percent agreed wholeheartedly that you should. But that means that 14 percent think it's okay to keep it a secret, which is 5 percent more than felt that way in 1992.

**Staying Together**  Whether you're already married when your diagnosis hits, or you get married after you're diagnosed, bipolar disorder is going to make keeping your relationship strong a real battle. Communication, which is so important in making a marriage work, can be hard to maintain, especially when you're in the midst of a mood episode. And once that line of communication has been cut, it's hard to splice it back together.

In a study of spouses or significant others of people with bipolar disorder conducted by researchers in New Zealand, 90 percent of the 41 caregivers surveyed said their loved one was "distant" and "difficult to get close to" when having either a manic or a depressive episode.

Staying together seems to have a lot to do with staying healthy. In the New Zealand study, 80 percent of the caregivers said they had a close relationship with their significant other when the partner was emotionally stable or in remission. In fact, half of the group said they felt that, overall, their loved one's bipolar disorder had brought the two of them closer together. As one of the caregivers surveyed said, "He's more open with me now than he used to be. And I'm more nurturing than I used to be—I take care of him and listen more."

WEB TALK: For a peek at the good and bad of bipolar relationships from your partner's side, visit:
www.bpso.org/separation.htm

Still, most relationships that involve at least one person who's bipolar will hit some pretty rocky territory now and again. In the New Zealand study, 62 percent of the caregivers had been separated from their partner at some point because of issues brought up by the bipolar disorder. And in a larger study of psychiatric disorders in general, researchers from the University of Michigan in Ann Arbor found that bipolar disorder—and specifically mania—was far and away the toughest on marriage among the 14 different psychiatric disorders they studied (which included depression, panic disorder, phobias, anxiety, alcohol and drug abuse or dependence, and conduct disorder).

Using data from more than 5,800 people participating in the National Comorbidity Study, the University of Michigan researchers found that 9 of 10 people with a psychiatric disorder will marry by the age of 54 (the cutoff age for inclusion in the study), and about half of those marriages will end in divorce. People with bipolar disorder, they noted, are some 3.2 times more likely to get divorced than people who do not have a psychiatric illness. In fact, if you're bipolar, this study says you have twice the chance of getting divorced in your first marriage than do people with any of the other psychiatric disorders in the study.

One of the possible reasons for that—and one of the issues that pop up in many bipolar marriages—is the effect that the disorder, and specifically mania, has on sex and intimacy. No matter how much education he gets, it's going to be difficult for someone you love to understand how you could go off on some sexual escapade while manic, much less let the indiscretion just roll off his back. He might, if he's enlightened and extremely supportive, forgive you, knowing it's simply a symptom of your disorder. But he's going to be hurt, and he's going to have to find a place to put that hurt. And that can be hard.

The depression that usually follows mania doesn't help things, either. Even if he does deal with the manic symptoms, he's then going to be faced with your complete lack of sexual interest when you're depressed, which can be just as difficult to deal with and just as difficult not to take personally. Add to that the side effects of your medications—many antidepressants, for instance, have an impact on your libido—and there's a lot for the two of you to deal with. Your best bet? You guessed it: communication and the help of a good marriage or sex counselor.

## The Decision to Parent

Ah, parenthood. A daunting concept for anyone. And yet another opportunity for the naysayers to tell you about things they believe bipolar disorder removes from your list of options.

Once again, they're wrong. But once again, it will be hard. If you're a man, the decision is fairly uncomplicated, although certainly not simple: are you willing to take the chance—which weighs in at between 10 and 30 percent—of passing along your

> **GET PSYCHED**
>
> "I've proven that someone with bipolar disorder can live a pretty good life despite the illness. And besides, my kid will definitely have a father who knows what to look for."
> —Jonathan Stanley, living with bipolar disorder

disorder to your child? If you're a woman, it gets stickier. You're faced not only with decisions about how your choice will affect your child in the future, but with the ways in which it will affect you, your mental health, and your child's health in utero.

**What It Might Mean for You** Parenting means stress, and when you're bipolar, stress is dangerous. Parenting means sleepless nights, and when you're bipolar, lack of sleep is perilous. Parenting means pregnancy, and if you're a bipolar woman, that might mean reconsidering the medications you're taking and putting your stability in jeopardy.

Parenting means being responsible for someone else's mental and physical well-being at a time when you're having enough trouble being responsible for your own. It means curbing your impulses so you can provide a little stability. It means getting out of bed to cook dinner even when depression is overwhelming you.

But parenting also means love, both given and received, and doesn't love heal?

**What It Might Mean for Your Child** Bipolar disorder is at least partly rooted in genetics, so, yes, there might be consequences to your decision to have a child if you or your spouse is bipolar. For one thing, your child might wind up battling the same demons you're working so hard to overcome. But you need to put that in perspective, says Christine, whose bipolar mother committed suicide and who has been diagnosed with bipolar II herself. Christine recently weaned herself from lithium and is looking forward to trying to get pregnant—although that's not to say she hasn't struggled with the decision.

"I've actually been thinking about using a donor egg," Christine says. "Mood disorders are so common in my family—I worry about that. But then I think about how therapies are getting better all the time, and how it can be manageable now. And you just don't know what you're getting with a donor ... It's genetic roulette. Someone

284

else may not have the gene for bipolar, but who knows what else they might have?"

There are other issues as well, especially if you're a woman: the effect of your medications on your child's development both in and out of the uterus (see the next section, "Bipolar and Pregnancy"), the risk of postpartum depression and how that might affect your child's infancy, and the risk of recurrence throughout your child's life.

But if you know these things are coming, and you know, right now at least, you can control your disorder, you can prepare yourself and your child. And think about it: in so many ways, your child is going to be lucky. She's going to have the gift of you— with all your creativity and intelligence. And she's going to grow up in an environment that teaches acceptance, love, and the ability to see beyond the labels.

## Bipolar and Pregnancy

Everything changes when you get pregnant. Trying to keep your body from attacking this "foreign" object that's growing within it compromises your immune system. Your metabolism changes to accommodate the requirements of two living things rather than just one. And of course, your hormones go wild.

Because bipolar disorder is a biologically based condition, all this is going to have an effect on your symptoms and your moods. The question is, just how much of an effect will they have? And what will that effect be? The answers to those questions are only now beginning to become apparent.

Scientists already do know some things, however. For one, they know it's easier to deal with a planned pregnancy than an unplanned one—especially if the planned pregnancy is preceded by a discussion of how you'll want to handle treatment during gestation and after birth. For another, they know that the high rates of alcohol and drug abuse—not to mention high rates of smoking—among people with bipolar disorder might very well put your child at risk.

**The Hormone Honeymoon?** The virtual tidal wave of hormones pumped out during pregnancy can have some pretty intense and significant effects on your body. Researchers have shown that multiple sclerosis, for instance, seems to fade away to some extent during pregnancy, while rheumatoid arthritis comes roaring to life during those same 9 months.

What does pregnancy mean for moods? Most of the studies done to date seem to cancel one another out. Overall, it seems, you're probably no more likely to sink into depression or rev into mania during pregnancy than you are when you're not pregnant. At the same time, you're not any *less* likely to do so, either.

After pregnancy is an entirely different story. For women living with bipolar disorder (or any number of mood disorders, to be quite honest), the period right after birth is one of the riskiest times of their lives, often leading to postpartum depression or postpartum psychosis (see "Postpartum Depression").

**Medication Do's and Don'ts** Should you take medication during your pregnancy? And if so, which ones are safest for both you and your growing child? These are obviously difficult questions. No one wants your child to be exposed to harmful chemicals that might affect his or her development, but on the other hand, no one wants you to spend 9 months sinking into a major depression—eating poorly, not taking proper care of yourself, drinking too much, even contemplating suicide. In addition, it's still not clear how or in what ways the stress hormones produced during mood episodes affect the growth and development of a baby—or, for that matter, how the mood episodes themselves affect the growth and development of a baby.

Add to those questions the fact that there still aren't good answers about what psychotropic drugs can or will do to a developing fetus, and you've got yourself quite a conundrum.

In 2004, a group of very prominent experts in bipolar disorder and pregnancy—led by Yale University School of Medicine psychiatrist Kimberly Yonkers, M.D.—put together an in-depth review on the topic, which was published in the April issue of the *American Journal of Psychiatry*. Here is some of what they reported about the various drugs and their risks in pregnancy and beyond:

- **Lithium.** Your dose of lithium will probably need to be increased during your pregnancy, as your body ups its metabolism and the rate at which it excretes wastes. Some physicians advise that this level be dropped immediately when you go into labor so you won't have toxic effects once the baby is born.

  As for the baby, a physician database on babies born to mothers taking lithium has found a much higher rate of some very rare heart disorders and malformations. Lithium babies tend to weigh a lot more. And some babies who are exposed to lithium during labor come out "floppy"—that is, their muscle tone is low—and they might be a little blue in color.

- **Anticonvulsants.** Sodium valproate (Depakote) and carbamazepine (Tegretol) seem to have some fairly severe effects on the growth and development of a fetus. In studies of women with epilepsy, use of these drugs was associated with twice the risk of brain and spinal cord defects, abnormalities of the skull and face, low birth weight, and heart defects. Babies born to women taking Depakote show signs of withdrawal (irritability, difficulty feeding, low muscle tone) and occasionally liver toxicity or hypoglycemia.

  Lamotrigine (Lamictal) seems to be less dangerous to the fetus and has become the drug of choice for women with epilepsy who are in their childbearing years. Nonetheless, all the anticonvulsants do seem to raise the risks of miscarriage or stillbirth, so careful consideration and consultation with your doctor is definitely important.

- **Antipsychotics.** Studies of chlorpromazine (Thorazine) haven't turned up anything significant in terms of organ defects. There has, however, been some evidence of withdrawal symptoms and even a short-lasting version of the

287

so-called extrapyramidal symptoms (tremors, rigid muscles, spasticity, and more) that make these first-generation antipsychotics so difficult to use, and were the impetus for the creation of the atypical antipsychotics.

- **Atypical antipsychotics.** Very little data exist on the use of the atypical antipsychotics in pregnancy. So far, however, the main concern seems to be with the association of several of the atypical antipsychotics with diabetes and its risk factors. In particular, there is some evidence that olanzapine (Zyprexa) increases your risk of weight gain, insulin resistance, gestational diabetes, and preeclampsia (high blood pressure in pregnancy). "Weight gain, blood sugar levels, and blood pressure should be monitored carefully in patients who are taking olanzapine," the researchers recommended in their review paper.

If all that sounds unacceptably risky, recognize that there are other options for you, the main one being electroconvulsive therapy, or ECT. (For more on the specifics of ECT, see Chapter 8.) Unlike most drugs, there are almost no risks to ECT in pregnancy, and certainly none that can't be managed by preventive treatments. And in case you're wondering, the uterine muscles are of a type that generally do not contract during the electrically induced seizures of ECT. And in the very few cases in which contractions have been noted, they did not lead to premature labor.

There is one more option: you can discontinue medication during the period prior to and right after you conceive, or even throughout the pregnancy. Of course, this leads to a caveat that can't be stated strongly enough: You must do this in partnership with your physician or clinician, so that she can monitor you, and it must be done with an emergency plan in place, should you begin to relapse. The risks of medication in pregnancy pale in comparison to the risks of an uncontrolled and uncontrollable mood episode.

**Breast-Feeding** Finally, there's breast-feeding. Can you? Should you? When it comes to answering these questions, there's one certainty: the most critical time in terms of treatment is during the postpartum period, when the risk of a relapse shoots up (see "Postpartum Depression"). In fact, one study of lithium as a pro- phylactic treatment against postpartum disorders found that it reduced the rate of relapse from nearly 50 percent to less than 10 percent. So the question really is whether or not to breast-feed, rather than whether or not to take medication so you can breast- feed.

The American Academy of Pediatrics has said that women should use caution when taking lithium and considering breast- feeding; studies have shown that lithium makes its way into breast milk at about half the concentration found in the mother's blood. What the results of that exposure would be are still unknown. Depakote and Tegretol are found in lower levels in breast milk, leading the American Academy of Neurology to give a thumbs-up on breast-feeding for mothers on anticonvulsants. There haven't been any bad reactions noted in infants breast-feeding from moth- ers who are on Lamictal, the trade name for lamotrigene, but you'd probably want to be sure to keep an eye out for the appear- ance of the rash that can be so dangerous in adults exposed to this drug. Antipsychotic agents and even many antidepressants seem to also be relatively safe for breast-feeding, even though there are not many studies on the subject.

**Postpartum Depression** There is simply no way to work the numbers so this doesn't look as bleak as it is. If you're a woman with bipolar disorder—whether it's been diagnosed or not—and you deliver a child, you're nearly seven times more likely to be admitted to the hospital for your first bipolar episode and two times more likely to be admitted for a recurrent episode during the postpartum period than are women who are not pregnant. And if you decide to forego lithium treatment during this time— for whatever reason—you're three times more likely to be hit by symptoms during your postpartum period than the women who have not just given birth.

In another study of women with bipolar disorder, 20 of 30 women who had had a child had experienced a postpartum mood episode, all of which were characterized by depression rather than mania. And if they had a mood episode with their first child, then they inevitably had one after any subsequent pregnancies.

Clearly, this is no time to be slacking off on your medications. In fact, you and your doctor might want to talk about upping your doses or adding other agents to try to protect you from the worst of the postpartum effects.

## PsychSpeak

**Postpartum depression** is a mood disorder that begins after childbirth and usually lasts for at least six weeks. **Postpartum psychosis** is an extreme mental disorder that begins after childbirth and involves confusion, hallucinations, delusions, and sometimes suicidal or homicidal thought processes.

There are really three different forms of postpartum depression: the "baby blues," in which the symptoms, no matter how severe, tend to dissipate by the end of the second postpartum week; *postpartum depression,* which affects as many as 20 percent of new mothers even if they don't have a bipolar diagnosis; and *postpartum psychosis,* which includes not only the severe depression, feelings of guilt, and thoughts of suicide that are common in postpartum depression, but also confusion, hallucinations, and delusions. It is this latter form of the disorder that is the scariest, because of the risk of harm to the baby or to you.

But if you've already been diagnosed with bipolar disorder and you're pregnant, you're going to be watched after the baby is born. Heck, you're going to be scrutinized. You and your doctor will talk well before the baby's birth about what you and your family will do if you start to show signs of either depression or psychosis, and you'll have a detailed plan in place. That doesn't mean you should underestimate the risk, of course. It's there, and it's real, and it can happen to you. But if you prepare for it, you have a better chance of beating it back than you would if you were to ignore it altogether.

## In the Thick of Things

When you're stable and well, you have the ability to be as good a parent as anyone else—as good a parent as you can be. But because bipolar disorder isn't curable, and because it almost inevitably does reoccur over time, there might very well be times when your symptoms creep into your parenting—when you're irritable for no reason and you lash out at your daughter, or when your extreme euphoria or impulsiveness becomes unsettling or even scary to your son. You probably can't protect them from this, but you can prepare them. How and when you talk to your children about bipolar disorder is your decision, but you should realize that ignorance is not bliss when it comes to bipolar disorder.

There are things to be on your guard for, however. One of the main ones is making sure not to allow your child to become your caregiver. Watching your moods, reminding you to take your medication, keeping up with your doctor's appointments—these are not his job. They're yours, or your spouse's, or those of whatever adult is helping support you through rough times. Don't let it fall on your child.

Your child is going to have to learn to deal with a lot of different feelings in his life, ranging from anger at you or your illness to guilt and confusion as to his role in it—and you can't protect him from this. But you can help him sort out these things. Or you can find someone else who can help.

You also need to recognize that no matter how much you shelter your child at home, your love alone isn't going to be able to protect him from the social stigmas that are still attached to bipolar disorder. You can't protect him from the reactions of his friends if you have to be hospitalized for depression, for instance, or if you're having hallucinations in the midst of a manic episode. But you can arm him with the information he needs to be able to educate those people who are

### GET PSYCHED

"We all have to play the hand we've been dealt. I was dealt bipolar disorder. My child was dealt a bipolar parent. It's the coping tools we develop to deal with our cards that are invaluable." –Mara McWilliams, artist, parent, living with bipolar

responding out of ignorance. Giving him information gives him a sense of control over a situation that probably feels scary and out of control. And at the same time, you can use the opportunity to drive home to him that your moods are neither his fault nor his responsibility.

Finally, in addition to watching your own moods, you need to be on the lookout for signs of bipolar disorder in your child (see Chapter 15). You're not likely to miss them, knowing them as intimately as you do. And if by chance your child does pull the genetic short straw, try not to spend too much time and energy kicking yourself. If there's anyone who's going to be able to help him through it, it's you.

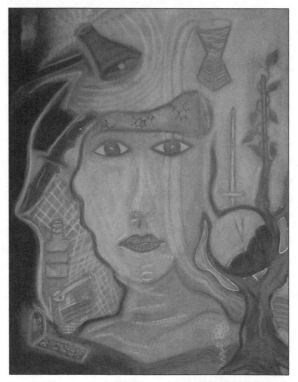

Manic Mind, *charcoal drawing by Mara McWilliams.*
*For more information, or to purchase this or other works,*
*go to www.MaraMcWilliams.com.*

**you're not alone**

# Bipolar Parenting

"As a mother who is also bipolar, I have searched the Internet for websites geared toward helping parents diagnosed with bipolar disorder. I have yet to find one. I believe it would make a big difference if one existed. We all have found, over the years, that sharing our experiences with those who are or have experienced the same thing is healing and therapeutic for all parties involved. The first 12-step program was founded on that basic principle. In this situation, it would be one bipolar parent helping another, and so on.

"I know that as a person raised in a codependent, oppressive environment, I don't want to raise my child in a similar atmosphere. It is important that I raise an independent, responsible, brave young woman who is aware of her boundaries. I am aware that my daughter might be prone to assume the role of caretaker or codependent. It is my responsibility, regardless of my diagnosis, to make sure that doesn't happen. My child is not the parent, I am.

"According to current statistics, my daughter has between a 15 to 30 percent chance of inheriting bipolar disorder. Unfortunately, I cannot protect her from developing this illness, but I can properly prepare her to deal with life and the curve balls it will throw at her. I can teach her to live honestly, to live with compassion in her heart, and to act in kind to all inhabitants on this planet. I can teach her to claim responsibility for her actions and accept the consequences of her decisions gracefully. I can teach her that love comes in all different shapes and sizes and isn't limited to traditional concepts of marriage, tradition, and commitment.

"I am not naive. I know my illness has an effect on my child. What kind of effect, I'm not sure; time will tell. I am honest with my daughter. We have discussed my illness many times: how it is called a brain disorder because there is a chemical imbalance in my brain. She knows that my illness is called bipolar disorder and that I take medication to treat it. She has experienced my moods changing from happy to sad within hours of each other, and she knows that my moods are not a result of something she did. She knows this because we have an open line of communication that is based on honesty and trust. My child knows that it is not her responsibility to change my feelings or make me feel better. I have explained to her that my feelings and moods are my responsibility. Occasionally, when I am feeling blue, she will come up to me, give me a hug, and say, "It's going to be okay Mommy, I love you." And then she will run off and play with her friends, like any other 8-year-old kid. Because of my illness, my child has learned how to be empathetic without becoming codependent. In today's world, that is a very valuable lesson.

"I believe that because of my bipolar disorder and recovery process, my child will grow up in a house that is focused on mental wellness." —*Mara McWilliams, artist and author who lives in Northern California. You can see her artwork in this chapter and on her website, www.MaraMcWilliams.com.*

## What You Can Do

This is where it counts. The effort you put into nurturing your relationships at home is effort that will be paid back thousand-fold. Sure, sometimes that effort is hard to muster. And sometimes it's hard to sustain. But people who watch your back and protect your flanks are worth their weight in gold. So give them your all. Bond with your brother, pamper your parents, give love to get love. Remember, these are the people who are going to be there for you—who have always been there for you—when you have nothing left to give. And if some of your relationships fall a little short of the rosy ideal? Make what you can of them; give as good as you get. Forgive. Forget. Move on. Go home.

- ☐ Work on your communication skills—preferably along with your family or spouse. Learning how to listen actively, to problem-solve, and to make positive rather than negative statements can make a huge difference in your relation-ships.

- ☐ Set limits with your family that will enable you to get the help you need but still retain or regain a sense of indepen-dence and control.

- ☐ Reassess your friendships. Decide which, if any, are doing you more harm than good, and drop them. Use the extra time and energy to nurture those friendships that are worth saving.

- ☐ If you're single, get out there and date once your moods are stable. You deserve to be happy and to be loved; let yourself be.

- ☐ Physical and emotional intimacy in a relationship tends to fall by the wayside when you're in the middle of an episode. Once you've recovered, you and your partner need to make re-establishing that intimacy a priority. If you need the help of a sex or couples therapist, get it. It just might save your relationship.

☐ Talk to your doctor about your treatment choices for pregnancy well before you even begin trying to become pregnant. The hardest pregnancy to manage when you have bipolar disorder is an unplanned one.

☐ Include care of your child in your emergency planning, especially if you are a single or divorced parent. You can't ultimately control whether or not you have a relapse, but you can be sure your child is well taken care of if you have to be hospitalized.

☐ How, when, and what to tell your child about bipolar disorder is up to you. If you choose to explain it to him, be sure to use language that fits his stage of development. "Mania" won't mean anything to an 8-year-old, but "excited" will. Likewise, "depressed" might not really help your 6-year-old understand what you're going through, but "sad" should do the trick.

# The Bipolar Child

I t seems almost cruel to inflict bipolar disorder, with its vagaries of mood and attitude, on a child. It becomes even crueler when you realize that it was only within the past few years—the past decade, at best—that the concept of bipolar disorder in children was even considered, much less explored.

This means that almost any question you might have about bipolar disorder in children—and if you are the parent of a bipolar child, you'll have many—is likely to be answered with a shrug and a "We still don't know for sure."

But we're learning. We're moving farther away from the old Freudian-based views of mental illness, with their focus on conflicts within the psyche, to a more biological view, with its focus on the brain and the internal and external conditions that affect it. It used to seem unlikely that a child could have had the traumas and experiences that would lead to the development of a mental illness, but it now seems clear that brain chemicals and genes can go awry at almost any age.

And so, today, several national organizations and literally dozens of clinical research studies are underway that are attempting to bring the understanding of bipolar disorder in children and adolescents at least to the place where the understanding of the adult version of the disorder is. It's an ambitious undertaking, considering that the very first federally funded grant to study childhood bipolar disorder was awarded just over a decade ago. But it's a critical undertaking, and one that is already starting to pay off.

## Facts and Figures

With so little history, so little study, and so little consensus in the study of bipolar disorder in children and adolescents, there are no good hard-and-fast figures. Perhaps that's not surprising, considering that the numbers and percentages in adult bipolar disorder are still under considerable debate. Still, with adult bipolar disorder, there's at least some consensus—a range of numbers. With childhood bipolar disorder, there's almost nothing. There are, at best, estimates. Some say there are 750,000 kids and adolescents under the age of 18 battling mania and depression. Others say it might be as high as—if not higher than—a million. But privately, almost everyone admits that there's no way to be sure—for all we know, that number could be several times higher.

Part of the problem could be that getting people to even buy into the idea of childhood bipolar disorder has been difficult. In 2003, the Child and Adolescent Bipolar Foundation (CABF) teamed up with AstraZeneca Pharmaceuticals and the research firm StrategyOne to get a glimpse into the public's perceptions of bipolar disorder. StrategyOne interviewed 1,000 people in the United States and found that although almost 79 percent of them knew what bipolar disorder was, only 11 percent believed it could occur at any age. A full 58 percent, in fact, was sure bipolar disorder could only strike adults.

**WEB TALK:** The Child and Adolescent Bipolar Foundation has the results of its survey and more at:

**www.bpkids.org**

"The major discrepancies between what people believe and what research data shows about bipolar disorder can have serious consequences, such as adults failing to recognize symptoms in their children, which could lead to delaying appropriate treatment," noted Martha Hellander, CABF's executive director, in response to the survey. "The survey results indicate there is a great need to educate parents and doctors about treatment and convey the benefit it provides."

## How Bipolar Is Different in Children

The short answer is that bipolar in children is faster and meaner. Children go through essentially the same cycles as do adults, but they do it with such rapidity—several, if not dozens of times each day—that to call it rapid cycling is an understatement. In fact, in children, this sort of constant mood flip-flopping is instead called ultra-ultra rapid or *ultradian* cycling.

Actually, children tend to cycle so rapidly from one pole to the next that you can't really call their manic and depressive moments "episodes." This, according to psychiatrist Barbara Geller, M.D., one of the true pioneers in the study of bipolar disorder in children, makes childhood bipolar disorder particularly dangerous. Children with bipolar disorder aren't exempt from suicidal thoughts and plans, she notes. Add to this the rapidity with which they cycle, and "serious suicidality can appear without warning in a split second."

> **PsychSpeak**
>
> **Ultradian** is a biological rhythm that occurs in less-than-24-hour cycles.

Mania in children also tends toward irritability and anger—with frequent, out-of-control temper tantrums and violent outbursts being not uncommon—more often than it does in adults.

Childhood mania does have symptoms in common with the adult version, but they might not look quite the same. A grandiose adult might think he's God, but a grandiose child is more likely to think he's Spider-Man. A euphoric child tends to act silly, giggly, and out of control.

One of the more disturbing symptoms shared by childhood and adult mania is a tendency toward sexual preoccupation. Children who are manic and hypersexual might touch themselves publicly or even attempt to engage in sexual contact with young friends, siblings, even their parents. In fact, as a recent report about childhood bipolar disorder on National Public Radio pointed out, this sort of behavior often sets off concerns that the child has been sexually abused, when actually it is simply her equivalent of the multiple affairs and rampant sexual experimentation seen in bipolar adults.

In addition to the mania, children with bipolar disorder experience depression just as frequently and just as severely as adults with bipolar disorder do. But recognizing and diagnosing depression in children is a challenge, even when it's unipolar. Boredom, low energy levels, and withdrawing from friends and family are all indicators of depression in kids, and these symptoms are often accompanied by intense feelings of self-hatred and thoughts of suicide. But because of the way bipolar children cycle, they tend to bounce back from these "moods" so quickly that you might not even think to become concerned about them, especially if you're comparing it to the way depression tends to take root and linger for months at a time in adults.

## If You Suspect Your Child Is Bipolar ...

It's hard for most physicians to diagnose bipolar disorder, especially in children. So it's not a real surprise that it can be difficult as well for parents to figure out what's going on with their angry, excitable, energetic children.

Still, as more and more information about bipolar disorder in childhood makes its way into the public consciousness, more and more parents are going to start wondering about their children and their symptoms.

**Q&A**

*What are the symptoms of bipolar disorder in childhood, and how early can they begin?*

"We have interviewed many parents who report that their children seemed different from birth, or that they noticed that something was wrong as early as 18 months. Their babies were often extremely difficult to settle, rarely slept, experienced separation anxiety, and seemed overly responsive to sensory stimulation. In early childhood, the youngster may appear hyperactive, inattentive, fidgety, easily frustrated, and prone to terrible temper tantrums (especially if the word 'no' appears in the parental vocabulary)." *—Demitri Papolos, M.D., and Janice Papolos, Juvenile Bipolar Research Foundation*

Trust your instincts, says Dr. Geller. "What we always recommend to families who have a concern is, if you have a suspicion, get a consultation," she says.

You can look to online mania checklists such as the parents' version of the Young Mania Rating Scale to get an idea of whether or not your child should be seen by a professional. Still, keep in mind that once a diagnosis becomes "popular," it can start to be overused. Geller points to irritability as an example. "A comparison to sore throat may be useful to put irritability in proper perspective," she notes in a paper describing mania in youngsters. "Sore throat is the most common symptom of strep throat, but only 5% or fewer of children who present with a sore throat actually have strep throat. By analogy, only a very small percentage of children with irritability will have mania. Irritability is also a very frequent symptom and a very common reason for clinical referral in children with numerous other child psychiatric disorders."

> **WEB TALK:** You can find the parent's version of the Young Mania Rating Scale at:
> www.bpkids.org/learning/reference/articles/08-20-03.htm

## Diagnosing Children and Adolescents

If diagnosing bipolar in adults is complex, diagnosing it in children can be downright Byzantine.

For one thing, there's so little research on childhood bipolar disorder that it's going to take years for its knowledge base to even begin to catch up with that of adult bipolar disorder—which is particularly ironic when you consider how far behind research into adult bipolar disorder lags behind that of other adult mental illnesses.

Then there's that ultra-rapid cycling to deal with. Pinning down bipolar disorder's symptoms is difficult enough when they're moving at the relative snail's pace of the adult disorder. But when they're zipping back and forth like a hyperkinetic minnow, it becomes nearly impossible to grab them and study them.

Yet despite knowing just how quickly children swing from pole to pole, many clinicians still rely on the *DSM*'s criteria for diagnosing bipolar disorder, which requires a single mood episode to last for days or even weeks. "The *DSM* needs to be updated to reflect what the illness looks like in childhood," notes the Juvenile Bipolar Research Foundation in one of its FAQs.

WEB TALK: Find the Juvenile Bipolar Research Foundation comprehensive FAQ at: www.bpchildresearch.org/ juv_bipolar/faq.html

In addition to the time issues, there are differences in symptomology as well. The hallmark of adult bipolar disorder—mania—can look quite different in children than it does in adults. "It's not intuitive that kids can be too elative or too expansive or grandiose," Geller admits. "Children aren't going to max out credit cards or get married four times. Because of these differences in child versus adult manifestations of the disorder, doctors need to be specifically trained on how to recognize elation and grandiosity in their patients."

You, too, can learn how to tell the difference between the normal child and the bipolar child, Geller says. Oftentimes the mania manifests itself as inappropriately silly, giddy, rowdy behavior that leads to the child being sent to the principal's office or being asked to leave a movie theater. "When these kids are grandiose, you'll realize they're not just playing—they really believe they are Super-Man," Geller says. "Instead of pretending to fly, they'll actually jump out a window."

Children who are bipolar also seem to have a decreased need for sleep, says Geller. "They can be up all night. Sometimes the parents don't even know it, because they don't seem tired the next day."

These symptoms often lead directly down the path of misdiagnosis, spawning labels such as ADHD (attention deficit/ hyperactivity disorder), ODD (oppositional defiant disorder), or conduct disorder (see "Hand in Hand: Disorders Linked to Bipolar in Children"). And as I mentioned in Chapter 2, oftentimes those labels aren't entirely wrong; in fact, with estimates of comorbidity between bipolar disorder and ADHD near the 90 percent mark, they're usually quite right. They're just missing a key component: bipolar disorder.

Finding the right doctor for your child—a specialist, rather than a general pediatrician—is equally difficult. The 2003 Consensus Statement on the Unmet Needs in Diagnosis and Treatment of Mood Disorders in Children and Adolescents—presided over by the Depression and Bipolar Support Alliance (DBSA)—noted that "Patients experience limited exposure to clinicians adequately trained to address their problems and little information to guide care decisions, particularly concerning bipolar disorder." And until that changes, the rest of the issues with getting a quick and accurate diagnosis for your child will likely continue to follow you as well.

There are options, however. You can try calling the nearest children's hospital and asking for a psychiatric referral. If there is no children's hospital nearby, try the nearest academic medical center. They're likely to have experts who can help you find the right specialist—or, if you get lucky, they might have the specialist right there for you.

Another possible tack to take is to contact one of the groups that focuses on bipolar disorder in children: the Juvenile Bipolar Research Foundation (JBRF) and the Child and Adolescent Bipolar Foundation (CABF) are two of the best-known groups. JBRF has discussion groups where you could ask parents who've been where you are for recommendations. And the CABF even has a physician database that lists professional members of the organization.

## Hand in Hand: Disorders Linked to Bipolar in Children

One of the reasons bipolar disorder is so hard to see or to pin down in children is that not only does it often look like any number of other disorders, but quite frequently that other disorder actually does exist in the child. It's just that the bipolar disorder is there, too—and it often gets missed.

In addition to attention deficit disorder (ADD) or ADHD, childhood bipolar disorder often sits side by side with what are called conduct disorders, with an estimated 69 percent of bipolar children fitting the criteria for that diagnosis as well. Similarly, bipolar can willingly share a child's brain with oppositional-defiant disorder, obsessive-compulsive disorder, separation anxiety disorder, and any number of other anxiety disorders.

*My son was diagnosed with bipolar disorder and ADHD. Is there a genetic or biological link between the two, or is he just unusually unlucky?*

"Hyperactivity is relatively common. You'd expect to see it in some kids with mania because the prevalence is so high in the general population. It may be that the genetics of these particular symptoms are linked, but right now we just don't know. I do know, however, that we don't think it's going to be one gene that gives both of these disorders to you—or even one gene that gives bipolar disorder to you." —*Barbara Geller, M.D., professor of psychiatry, Washington University School of Medicine in St. Louis*

There are also certain educational issues—learning disabilities, sensory integration issues, and more—that can come into play with a bipolar child. Some of these may be truly comorbid—in other words, these are separate issues occurring next to, or with, the bipolar disorder itself. But others might be caused by the disorder or its treatments.

## Treating Bipolar Disorder in Children and Adolescents

Finding the best way to treat bipolar disorder in children is the goal of a large, multisite study called TEAM: Treatment of Early-Age Mania. "We're looking to answer two questions," says Geller, who is the study's coordinator and principal investigator. "The first is which of the three classes of drugs should we give a child first: Atypical antipsychotics like Risperdal, lithium, or an anti-convulsant like Depakote. The second question is what's the next best to add on if the first drug doesn't work?"

Studies to date have shown that lithium lasts for a significantly shorter period of time in a child's body than it does in an adult's body—a finding that's not surprising, considering how quickly a child's metabolism runs, and it can cause cognitive impairment in a subgroup of children, even when it's present at relatively low levels in the blood. Nonetheless, studies of adolescents with bipolar disorder have shown that lithium works quite well at stabilizing mood. To reap the benefits of lithium while skirting its most destructive side effects, Geller says that children on lithium need to be closely monitored, especially when treatment is first started. And that, she notes, can be a real problem for parents who may themselves be bipolar or who have other children to take care of.

Studies of Depakote have shown some promising preliminary results, says Geller, but studies of the drug when used in young girls to control epilepsy show an extremely high rate of polycystic ovarian disease as well as obesity. "Obviously, these would be prohibitive side effects for most female children with manic-depressive illness," she notes.

> ## GET PSYCHED
>
> "It is now in the forefront of National Institute of Mental Health interest to find ways to better diagnose and treat children who are presenting with this illness. Great strides have already been made in getting this international attention. This will help because if people pay more attention, more research will be done. I believe that in their children's lifetimes, we're going to know a lot more about this disorder."
> —*Barbara Geller, M.D., professor of psychiatry at the Washington University School of Medicine in St. Louis*

How long a bipolar child should stay on medication is another question that needs to be answered. Geller's gut instinct is that they will need to keep taking a mood stabilizer throughout their childhood and adolescence if they want to keep at least most of the symptoms of their disorder at bay. In the few studies that have been done, mostly of adolescents taking lithium, discontinuing the medication leads to a high rate of relapse.

If this turns out to be the case, however, you'll want to check in regularly with a clinician who can adjust your child's medication dosages. Children can grow at such a rapid rate that a dosage that works like a charm today might start faltering 6 months from now.

Once your child's mood has been stabilized, you'll want to get him into therapy with a psychologist or other clinician who can help him understand what's going on inside him. Bipolar disorder is scary for adults; it must be absolutely terrifying for children. A therapist who can help to calm that terror, and also work with your child to develop a plan for how to deal with his symptoms, will be invaluable.

Unfortunately, there's been even less systematic research into psychosocial treatments for childhood bipolar disorder than there has been into pharmaceutical treatments. So it remains a question as to which form of psychotherapy will best serve your child. But that doesn't mean you shouldn't pursue therapy at all. In fact, it's absolutely essential to the treatment of the child. If you can find someone who practices family-focused therapy (see Chapter 8), that would be ideal. FFT would enable you to get some therapy as well, or at least to gather up the fullest set of tools possible to help your child reach his or her full potential—and prevent yourself from inadvertently aggravating the disorder.

Give the therapy—and the therapist—time to work. But after all is said and done, if you don't think your child is getting what he needs, it's time to start looking for references and referrals again.

You can use a number of behavioral techniques at home to help your child get control over her moods. Ask her clinician for suggestions that are consistent with whatever therapy she's getting, such as the following:

- Relaxation techniques
- Stress-reduction techniques
- Coping techniques
- Implementing structure and routine

- Using music, lighting, water, or touch as coping and relaxation tools
- Channeling creativity and other strengths
- Letting go of little issues; prioritizing larger issues

In addition, mood charting can be as powerful a tool in the prevention or control of bipolar disorder in children as it is in adults. You can find child-oriented mood charts at a number of different websites, including www.bpkids.org.

## Getting an Education for Your Bipolar Child

It doesn't matter what diagnosis your child has or doesn't have: If you're a parent, getting the best possible education for your kids is probably one of your main sources of worry. Add bipolar disorder into the mix, and that worry can turn into terror.

The good news is that the biological havoc bipolar disorder wreaks on your child's brain is usually limited to her moods, emotions, and impulse control. It has nothing to do with her intelligence. She is capable of fulfilling all those dreams you had for her as you watched her drift off to sleep as an infant. It just might be a little harder for her to get there.

In other words, IQ aside, your child is going to face hurdles in getting an appropriate and full education. Concentrating on long division can seem overwhelming to a child whose mind is racing so fast he can't even keep up with it. Completing a science experiment is extremely difficult for a child who's distracted by every sound around her and can't sit still. And studying for a test is nearly impossible for a child who is on medications that make him sleepy and lethargic.

**Your Child's Options** It's entirely possible that your public school system will be able to provide precisely what your child needs. In fact, it's legally required of them. Still, on the chance that there might be places that provide a better educational fit for your child, you might want to consider some of the alternatives:

- **Private or parochial schools.** Private or parochial schools often have smaller class sizes where teachers might be better able to give your child the attention she needs. On the other hand, they might not have special education classes or be able to afford all of the accommodations your child might need. And because they are not funded with public money, they are not required to meet the same legal standards as are public schools (see "Your Child's Legal Protections"). If you do choose to go the private school route, however, be aware that you're still eligible for public school services, such as speech therapy or occupational therapy, should your child require them.

- **Charter or other alternative schools.** These schools are often publicly funded and will be in a better position to provide the services your child might need. Oftentimes, however, these schools are in such high demand that getting in is a matter of random chance.

- **Homeschooling.** Homeschooling can be a wonderful choice for both parents and children with special needs. Certainly, you'd know that your child's educational needs are being met. And as in the case of private school, you're still eligible for services from the public school system. Of course, if you work outside the home or you simply know you wouldn't have the patience necessary to school your high-needs kid, then homeschooling probably isn't a good choice for you.

- **Inpatient/residential treatment programs.** Most often, these are short-term programs where your child will get intensive therapy and learn a variety of techniques to help stabilize his moods. But there are a number of residential treatment centers (RTCs) that can

**GET PSYCHED**

"One of the things they taught Keegan at the Acute Treatment Center was that his actions come with consequences. We still have some of the same behaviors, but we're learning new ways to deal with them. So, all in all, even though it was such a difficult decision for us, it was a good thing to have him go there." —Bobbi Jo, mother of 6-year-old Keegan

provide both medical care and an education consistent with your child's needs. These schools can be prohibitively expensive, but in some cases, you might be able to get the school district to pay some part of the fee.

**Your Child's Legal Protections** There are really two main protections on the books that give you and your child the tools you'll need to get the best education possible.

The first is referred to as Section 504. It's part of the 1973 Rehabilitation Act and the Americans with Disabilities Act, and it protects all people with disabilities from discrimination based on that disability. In part, Section 504 reads:

> No otherwise qualified individual with a disability in the United States ... shall, solely by reason of her or his disability, be excluded from the participation in, be denied the benefits of, or be subjected to discrimination under any program or activity receiving Federal financial assistance or under any program or activity conducted by any Executive agency or by the United States Postal Service ...

What does Section 504 mean? Not as much as you might think. It's somewhat limited in its scope in that it simply requires that schools provide your child with access to the same "free appropriate public education" (FAPE, in special education lingo) that any other child gets. It makes sure that a public school can't refuse to accept your child because of his disorder. And in the case of physical disability, it requires that the school be accessible—it needs to have handicapped ramps, for instance. When it comes to kids with psychiatric issues, it can help you to get some minor accommodations in the classroom—maybe scheduling tests for afternoons, if your child has a hard time getting started in the morning the way so many bipolar children do. And that's undeniably a good thing. But it's perhaps not as sweeping a law as you might want.

Under Section 504, your child gets the exact same access to education as other children—but not access that's specially tailored to him. For that, you need to turn to IDEA, the Individuals with Disabilities Education Act, which was amended in 1997.

The IDEA is all about accommodations. This law gives schools the responsibility for identifying and evaluating any child who needs special education services. Those services can be as significant as a special education class or as minor as a schedule change. It can include a request for a one-on-one aide or regular meetings with a school counselor. It can include almost any service your child might need.

To get these services, however, your child has to qualify for them. For a bipolar child, simply having a diagnosis does *not* qualify him for services. His diagnosis—his disorder—has to be having a demonstrable effect on his ability to learn or participate in the classroom. The impact of his disability on his academic potential is one of the things that will be considered when your child is evaluated.

If the school doesn't suggest an evaluation—or if you know going in that your child will likely need services—you are well within your rights to request an evaluation. Most states have a strict timetable that determines how long the school district has to respond to your request, initiate an evaluation, and give you a report once you've made a request.

The evaluation will include any number of tests, including an IQ test, a psychological assessment, and an academic achievement test to which the IQ test can be compared to determine whether your child is achieving to her potential.

The school district pays for all this testing, although you are welcome to have your child evaluated separately and provide the results of that evaluation as well. If that seems like overkill to you, remember that the school district's testers might not provide the depth or insight you would want to come up with the best plan for your child.

If, after an evaluation, your child qualifies for services under IDEA, only then will the next step be taken: drawing up an Individualized Education Plan, also known as an IEP.

**Navigating an Individualized Education Plan** You are an integral member of the team that will prepare your child's IEP document. And one of the most critical decisions you'll make during this time is about your child's placement: Should she be put in a regular classroom, or would she do better in a special education class or a class for children who are emotionally disturbed? If you have a strong feeling about placement, while the IEP is being drawn up is the time to make those feelings known.

Other members of the IEP team will include at least one representative from the school's administration (a principal or vice principal, school psychologist, or guidance counselor), your child's current teacher, and—if he's interested and old enough to participate in the process—your child himself. You or the school might also wish to include a speech, physical, or occupational therapist; your child's therapist or psychiatrist; the specialist who did any additional testing on your behalf; a legal or mental health advocate; as well as other teachers with whom your child might have contact.

Realize that you are your child's only true advocate in an IEP meeting. The rest of the people there have competing interests— budgets to worry about, scarce resources to divide, limited time and staff. You have only one child to worry about—your own. That doesn't mean you need to be adversarial, but it does mean you need to be prepared. You need to know your rights.

You have the right to ...

- Be a part of the IEP committee. If they come at you with an already-completed IEP, you have the right to refuse to sign off on it. If they schedule a meeting for a time when you're unavailable, request that it be rescheduled.

311

- Bring along people you think might have something important to add to the conversation. As noted earlier, this could be anyone from your independent tester to your child's therapist to a legal adviser or mental health advocate.
- Insist that your child be given all services promised within the timeframe set up in the IEP.
- Ask for the committee to meet again if you don't think things are working well for your child.

All IEPs will have a similar structure. Your child's IEP will include an assessment of where he is, performance-wise, in academics, social interaction, behavior, communication, and other areas of potential concern. You'll put together a list of goals that take into account what your child should be able to accomplish in a single school year, as well as some short-term objectives the team can use to be sure he's on target to meet his overall goals. You'll discuss and document the best placement for your child in the school, specifying to what extent he'll participate in regular education. And you'll list any and all special education services he might need to meet his goals, spelling out the location, frequency, and duration of those services. Finally, the team will put together a list of criteria to determine whether the goals are being met and a timetable for updating goals or reevaluating your child.

**WEB TALK:** You can take a look at a model IEP prepared for a bipolar child at: www.bipolarchild.com/iep.html

In addition, if your child is in high school or over the age of 16, a portion of her IEP will need to address how you and the school plan to prepare her for either college or a job. There are vocational rehabilitation programs that provide not only job training, but often will also provide a job coach to help your child learn how to deal with workplace stresses and pick up on the necessary skills (see Chapter 13).

But if your child doesn't have any significant learning disabilities, chances are that you'll be considering the transition into college. What you might not know is that IDEA provides for publicly funded education and special education services for your child until she reaches age 22, if those services are still necessary. That assistance can range from a tuition break to mentoring and counseling on campus to special education accommodations at the college level. Just as it's illegal to keep a child out of the primary school system because of a disability, it's also illegal for any college—public or private—to do that as well.

This doesn't mean your child is guaranteed a place in the college of her choosing. She still has to show that she is capable of doing college-level work before she can be admitted. But if she is capable of doing the work, no college can keep her out because of her mental illness. In fact, in public universities and community colleges, if she needs special accommodations to reach the level of work she's capable of doing, the schools are mandated to provide those accommodations to her.

## The Challenge of College

College is an unsettling time under the best of circumstances. Stress, sleepless nights, the allure of drugs and alcohol—for many young adults, it's their first taste of true freedom.

That's why it's not so surprising that college—and especially the freshman year—is such a dangerous time for adolescents with bipolar disorder. In fact, for many, it's the time when their first symptoms will start to show. And for others, it's a time when previously stable moods start to swing wildly.

The good news, according to Terence Ketter, M.D., chief of the bipolar disorders clinic at Stanford University Medical Center, is that college also appears to be a time when intervention can have a really positive effect on the course of this illness. In a recent study he and his colleagues conducted, they found that college students who are diagnosed early—and particularly those who are diagnosed before being given antidepressants without a mood stabilizer—have a much better long-term outcome than those students whose diagnosis is delayed or who take unopposed antidepressants.

313

Still, for many young people with bipolar disorder, that diagnosis doesn't come in time to keep the disorder from wreaking major havoc in their lives. Now a lawyer and treatment advocate, Jonathan Stanley remembers when he was asked to leave college during his senior year, after several severe cycles of mania and depression. "That fall, I was so manic, I had the old typical 'I don't have to study a whit, or go to class, because my insight is going to be so incredible in this subject that not only am I going to get an A, but this professor is going to want me to write a book on the subject with him." Jonathan laughs. "When the grades came back, it turned out that it didn't quite work out that way. And so, not because of my bipolar behavior, but because of my grades, they asked me to take a year off."

**Don't Ask, Don't Tell?** College will probably be the first brush with a question you (or your child) are going to deal with for the rest of your life: Whom should you tell about your bipolar disorder, and at what point should you tell them?

You'll need to talk to the school administration if you're going to require any special accommodations because of your disorder, and you'll probably want to get in touch with the people at the student counseling center so there's someone "in the know" in the event that you have a crisis and need immediate treatment or hospitalization. But your professors don't need to know your medical history unless there are specific requests that they can help you with, such as scheduling conflicts or accommodations you need to get through their class.

The real question comes when you consider telling your newfound friends. Despite the increase in numbers of college students battling bipolar disorder, the stigma of mental illness still exists. And many of the people you encounter will have never met anyone with bipolar disorder—or at least, not anyone they know about.

"There were people on campus who knew about my bipolar who would spread rumors," says Alexis Maislen, whose bipolar disorder was diagnosed at the age 19, during her freshman year of college.

"I really felt it the first time after I came out of the hospital. I felt like they were all talking about me. One girl said she'd never known anybody who had a nervous breakdown in college. I just sort of shut down. I started thinking about everyone, 'I'm not going to tell you about what goes on with me, because I don't really trust you.'"

Of course, that's not necessarily a reason to keep your disorder a secret. But it is a consideration; you need to be aware that once you tell someone about your bipolar disorder, they might treat you differently, or look at you differently, or simply fade out of your life.

**Finding Support**  Because the average age of onset of bipolar disorder has dropped from 40 to 19 in the past couple decades, you're going to find larger numbers of people with bipolar disorder on university campuses than there have ever been before. Some of you might have been battling bipolar disorder since childhood; others will be blindsided by its sudden appearance. Both of you will have challenges to face—chief among them being finding stability amidst the chaos and change of college.

The good thing about these skyrocketing numbers and plunging ages is that if you're bipolar and you're on a college campus, you're not alone. Your student counseling center probably has services to help you adjust to campus life and counselors who are undoubtedly no longer strangers to bipolar disorder and crisis intervention. There might even be on-campus support groups you can attend; if not, it's likely that organizations such as the Depression and Bipolar Support Alliance have support groups in your area.

The fact that many others are blazing this trail alongside you also means that you can share war stories, as it were. People who've been there and done that can tell you what they wish they knew when they started college. For instance, a graduate who struggled through her 4 years of college because she insisted on taking a full course load despite being unable to stabilize her moods might suggest you consider being a bit more realistic in your approach to your academic load. Other bipolar college students say they swear by structure in getting through: writing lists of tasks, setting up study schedules, and keeping their sleep cycle as stable as possible.

## Super-Freshwoman

Looking back, Alexis Maislen knows she began her college career in a full-blown mania. "They called me super-freshwoman," she recalls with a laugh. "I joined every organization on campus, and I was on the dean's list. But I would also get into fights with my roommates. I would cut myself. I would have periods where I didn't know what I did. And I got heavily into drinking, which then became part of my symptoms."

Almost a decade later, she still remembers those days with a sort of bewilderment. "I was very linguistically adept when I was manic," she says. "I would be very creative. But then it would get to be too much. People couldn't keep up with me, or I would say something that was totally off. I would hurt people's feelings unintentionally, because I was totally wired and I couldn't pull back."

By the time the end of her sophomore year rolled around, Alexis had been hospitalized and diagnosed and was dating a boy from another school who was also bipolar—and verbally abusive. "He was an artist and would draw me things," she says. "And I would write him pocket poems. It was wonderfully creative. But then he would go into this thing about Jesus Christ and how he was becoming Jesus Christ."

Despite watching her boyfriend degenerate, Alexis wasn't ready to get serious about her medication. "I was still very active on campus, on the newspaper, even with a senator's re-election campaign. I was manic, but I didn't want the meds to stabilize me. I thought now was the time to ride out the high."

That ride eventually dropped her off outside the college gates, with a "medical leave of absence" after she sent some manic emails to a girl who had a college-administered restraining order against Alexis. After another hospitalization and a number of different medication trials, Alexis continued and completed her education at another school.

Still, she says, she regrets the way her college education went. "I got really nothing out of it, because I was so scattered," she says. "I may have ridden the highs, but I was very scattered about it, so I ended up getting a piecemeal education."

That's why she's now taking classes in science writing and working on a book that she hopes will someday help today's bipolar college students avoid her mistakes. "It's going to be a survival guide, based on my experiences," she says. "I want them to hear my story, and I want to tell theirs. I want them to know that we may have an illness, but we can do the work to stay healthy and lead productive lives."

# What You Can Do

The differences between bipolar disorder in children and bipolar disorder in adults are many—and they're significant. If you're the parent of a bipolar child, you need to educate yourself on the options available for your child so you can be her greatest advocate. All that changes in late adolescence, when the time comes for you to let go and for your child to step up to the plate and learn to deal with her disorder on her own.

☐ No one is better equipped to advocate for your child than you. And he's going to need all the advocating he can get. Collect the facts, collect your thoughts, and don't give up until your child has gotten whatever it is you think he needs.

☐ Talk to your doctor about your child's treatment options, particularly about which pharmaceuticals will be able to best control her symptoms without saddling her with too many significant side effects.

☐ Be aware that as a child grows and gains weight, the dosages of his medications will likely need to be modified or the medications themselves changed entirely. Talk to a clinician about how frequently your child should be monitored during and after medication changes are made.

☐ Be sure your child—and your family as a whole—is getting therapy to learn coping mechanisms for the times when the disorder is raging out of control.

☐ If your child is having any persistent difficulty whatsoever in school, ask for an assessment and an IEP meeting. Accommodations can—and, legally, must—be made to ensure her the best possible education.

☐ Keep in mind the differences between childhood and adult bipolar disorder when you're looking for signs and symptoms. If you don't, you might miss some obvious clues to your child's diagnosis.

- ☐ If you think your child has signs of both bipolar disorder and some other psychiatric condition—ADHD, conduct disorder, anxiety disorder—pursue your hunch with her physicians. Considering the frequency with which other conditions tag along with bipolar disorder, you may very well be right.

- ☐ Before going off to college, find a clinician in the area whom you can go to for medication checkups and in case of emergency. You should also find a therapist in the area. You can probably get recommendations, and possibly even therapy, at your campus's student counseling center.

- ☐ Take it easy on yourself at college. Don't overload yourself with course work or stay up all night partying, or you'll find yourself in the midst of a manic episode before the semester is out.

- ☐ If you're away from home, it's a good idea to have at least one person who sees you on a daily basis who knows about your disorder and its symptoms and can warn you of signs that a manic episode is approaching.

# A Survival Guide for Friends and Family

To most of the world, bipolar disorder is something scary, alien, and off-putting. It's something that happens to "them," to those other people, those crazy people. But to you, it's personal. The face of bipolar disorder is that of your daughter, your husband, your sister, your father, or your best friend. It might still be scary, but it's part of your life. It's not them. It's us.

What most people don't think about is that a bipolar disorder diagnosis rocks more than one world. Caregiving for someone with bipolar disorder can be exquisitely stressful at times; as a result, caregivers are plagued with stress-related illnesses and depressions. The ups and downs of mood, the stigma of mental illness, the financial and legal ramifications, the social isolation as people on the periphery drift away—if you're part of a bipolar person's life, you share in all this. And although there's an increasingly large and supportive community ready to help the person you love through this difficult transition, there's not nearly as much for you. You are the forgotten one.

Well, not here. This chapter is for you—to help you think about some of the issues that come with your loved one's diagnosis and to give you the impetus to start brainstorming some solutions. It's here to encourage you to think about yourself now and again, to get help for yourself so you can better help your loved one. And if nothing else, it's to let you know that you're not alone. As the adult child of a bipolar parent, I know how good it feels simply to know you're among people who can not only sympathize, but also truly empathize.

## What to Do If You Think Someone You Love Is Bipolar

Your husband ran up an enormous credit card debt, and now you've found out that he's been picking up women in bars when he tells you he's working. Your daughter lost her job after refusing to leave her apartment for an entire week. Your brother is convinced that the rest of your family is plotting against him and is refusing to come to any more family functions.

You know your loved one needs help, and you know you can't do it on your own. What are your rights? What are his? What are hers? What can you do?

Assuming that your loved one is an adult, there are definite limits to the steps you yourself can take. You cannot force anyone to go into treatment unless he or she meets specific criteria set out by the laws of your state. Few if any doctors will take on a patient who isn't coming to them of his own free will, especially in an outpatient setting. Whether they should or not is a topic of much discussion and debate, but that debate has not yet been settled. And until it is, it's unlikely that you'll be able to force someone in your life to get treatment unless she's an imminent danger to herself or others.

In fact, says Jacqueline Castine, who is not only living with bipolar disorder herself but has three adult children, two of whom are also living with the disorder, you really do have to let the person you love come to the conclusion that she needs help on her own. "There are things that families can do," she says, "but somehow they have more to do with finding ways to support the person, even in their delusions."

There are, however, some things you can do with or without your loved one's permission. The first and most important is to educate yourself. "There's not enough that you can learn," says Kay, whose daughter, son-in-law, and ex-husband all have bipolar disorder. The more you know about this disorder, the more you'll understand what your loved one is going through.

And once you've educated yourself, Kay says, you need to educate the people who are close to the person you think is ill. That way, you can send an unequivocal message to your loved one: you have an illness, and you're not alone. We're here to help. Let us.

## What Your Loved One Needs from You

From a practical point of view, the sicker your family member or friend is at first, the more he'll need your help. When someone hasn't slept in days—or hasn't gotten out of bed in weeks—it's awfully hard for him to get focused enough to find the right kind of help. That's where you, as someone who cares and wants to do what you can, come in. You need to encourage him to get treatment, and maybe even offer to help him find a therapist. If he's willing, help him draw up a list of questions or symptoms for the doctor, or even offer to go with him. If you think he needs a second opinion, say so. And then, when a treatment regimen has been settled upon, offer to do whatever you can to help him stick with it.

The key words here are *offer* and *help*. Bipolar is not your disorder; it's his. You cannot cure him. You cannot take his medication for him. You cannot go to therapy for him. He has to do these things. You can offer your help, and that's all you can do. If it's accepted, great. If it's not, then clearly you need to back down—even if you don't think that's really the best thing for him.

Of course, if you think your loved one is in danger—real, physical danger of harming herself or others—all bets are off. You intervene. You don't ask permission. You call 911 or take her to an emergency room or enlist the help of other friends or family members. If you think your loved one is "only" planning or considering suicide, or seems at risk of becoming violent, you can be a little less intrusive and a little more respectful of her autonomy, but you still need to be sure her therapist or physician knows what's going on. You need to encourage her to call a suicide hotline, or just to talk to you. You need to let her know how important she is to you. And you need to be sure she doesn't have access to knives or guns or piles of pills until you're sure the danger period has passed.

WEB TALK: A great resource for information and links for friends and family of bipolar persons is:

noetic.oathill.com/bipolar/supp.html

Kay, a mother who has dealt with bipolar disorder for almost 15 years now, says she usually just thinks about what she would do for her bipolar daughter if she was dealing with cancer, not mental illness. "If somebody had cancer, you would take them to the doctor, you would take them to treatments, you would take them to chemotherapy. You would help them emotionally; you would help them financially," Kay notes. "Bipolar disorder is the same thing—it's a chronic, devastating disease, and people with it can't do it all on their own, at least not until they're medicated and stabilized."

Neither can you, of course, although in these days of decreasing insurance benefits and increasing mental illness, it often seems to fall on the friends and family of the person with bipolar disorder to provide much of their care and even much of their treatment. Oftentimes, that's simply not possible. There's only so much you can do. But there are some simple, internal gifts you can offer to the person you care about. Here are a few, some of which I'll discuss in more detail later on in the chapter:

- **Acceptance.** There's so much stigma out in the world; your loved one needs to know you're not judging her for having a mental illness.

- **Positivity.** There's no name you can call or fault you can find that your loved one hasn't already labeled himself with. Nagging and lecturing—and most especially, condescending— will almost guarantee that your words will fall on deaf ears. Give your message a positive spin, however, and you're more likely to be heard ... and actually listened to.

- **Respect.** Treat your loved one as your equal, because she is. Having a mental illness makes her no less worthy of respect than you are.

- **Support.** This is your loved one's disorder, but how you handle it can make a big difference. Let him make his own choices about treatment and then back him up with what- ever he decides. It might not be what you want for him, but it's not your decision to make.

- **Space.** Be very, very wary of becoming overly involved in your loved one's illness or, worse yet, becoming a martyr. You can help him manage his disease and then you have to let him do some things for himself. You can point out to him when his moods are changing, for instance, but you can't make him talk to his therapist or take his medication. Those things are up to him. On the other hand, how you respond to them is up to you. Don't trap yourself in a posi- tion where his actions and moods determine how you feel, and what you do with your life.

- **Time.** Healing takes time. Medications don't work immedi- ately. Moods don't usually change overnight. Give your loved one a chance to get into treatment, then give her a chance to let the treatment work. And be aware that this is a disorder fraught with mishaps and relapses. Be patient when those, too, occur. They are not her fault; they are her disease. They, too, will pass.

Much of this, of course, is easier said than done. It's one thing to say that someone has a disease and is not directly responsible for her behaviors when that disease is in control. It's another entirely to smile and completely forgive your wife when she returns home after some manic sexual escapade or a spending spree that wipes out your life's savings. It's another entirely to ignore your son's hateful words and proclamations that you don't love him enough when his depression makes him suicidal.

"It's very difficult," says Kay, who has dealt with bipolar disorder in her daughter and in her ex-husband. "How can you be a normal human being, and not take a lot of this stuff personally?"

You can't. Not completely, at least. But you can try. And that's what your loved one needs—he needs for you to try, to hold on to the good, and to remember who he is when he's not sick. And he needs for you to be open to forgiving him, especially if he's doing all he can to get better. He needs for you, also, to recognize how hard it can be for him, an independent person with a devastating diagnosis, to accept help and to be dependent.

In the end, however, the only person who knows exactly what your loved one needs from you is your loved one. Ask her. Then listen to what she has to say. You might just be surprised by what you hear.

## Support: How Much Is Too Much? How Little Is Too Little?

You'll hear it again and again: what your loved one needs from you is unconditional support. But what does that mean? And more important, what *doesn't* that mean?

If you ask other people who've been in the role of caregiver for someone with bipolar disorder, they'll likely tell you that unconditional support means being sure your friend or family member knows that you are there for him, that you do not think less of him because he is ill, that you love him for who he is, that you are not judging him.

Hopefully, they will also tell you what unconditional support *does not* mean. It does not mean allowing yourself to be manipulated or used. It does not mean patting your loved one on the back and smiling when she decides to stop taking her medication. It does not mean letting her hit you or hurt you emotionally. It does not mean getting drunk or stoned with her when you know that's an invitation to disaster.

Kay, who's been continually supportive of her daughter since her daughter's diagnosis almost 15 years ago, admits that it can seem a little contradictory. But she says she often falls back on a saying she learned in a significant others' support group she's been involved in for many years: "Let go, let God, and maintain the golden thread."

The golden thread, she says, is unconditional support. "People with this disease can't always make the right decisions, because this illness doesn't stay level," Kay says. "It may change over the years. They need a thread they can use to connect, to find their way back when they get lost in their own illness."

There's a big difference, however, between support and smothering, between encouragement and encouraging dependence. It is not your job, nor is it your place, to protect your loved one from life's ups and downs in the hopes of keeping him safe from another episode. Don't shield him from bad news; don't keep him away from people who might ask inappropriate questions. He needs to learn how to keep himself stable even when life is doing its best to unbalance him. And you need to learn how to let him do that on his own.

"One time in my mood disorder group, somebody was saying, 'I keep trying to show him that I love him,' and my friend said, 'You can't love him enough, you can't give him enough money, you can't kiss him enough. There's not enough; he has an illness,'" Kay recalls.

One thing you need to do, say those who've been there, is set some ground rules. Make it a formal contract, if you like. Tell the person you love that you'll be there for her, always, as long as she takes her medication. Or tell her that you'll stay by her side as long as she stays clean and sober.

"My daughter and I made a verbal contract," Kay says. "I said I would be her advocate and I would never bring up bipolar or her behavior in relation to that unless I really felt I knew that something was up. She gave me her permission to interfere and say what I was thinking, and she would either act on it or not."

It's been an effective bargain, Kay says. "She's my daughter; I know when she's at her best, and I know when she's not. I'm not always right, but 99 percent of the time I am. And she knows it."

Basically, says Kay, when you're laying down ground rules, you need to decide what's so important that you can't compromise, and then set that in stone. "With my current relationship," she says, "every time I've left him, it was because he wasn't taking his medication."

And the rest? For the rest, she says, you simply need to be there, supporting.

## GET PSYCHED

"My mother was wise to let me know right up front that I could live with her only if I took my medication. That kind of healthy boundary setting was exactly the way I handled my own children's addiction and mental health problems both before and after my own illness was diagnosed. And they, too, have achieved tremendous things in spite of their own difficulties."
—Jacqueline Castine, living with bipolar disorder and alcoholism, and mother to three adult children, two with bipolar disorder

Finding a middle ground is especially hard if your loved one has a drug or alcohol problem, as do more than half the people diagnosed with bipolar I disorder. You'll probably be tempted to take control—hide the bottles of alcohol, flush his stash down the toilet—but really, all that does is set the two of you up for a power struggle. On the other hand, supporting or condoning your loved one's behavior can be equally damaging, keeping him from getting much-needed help and facing his addiction.

Ultimately, you need to remember that if you make a threat, whether it be real or implied, you'd better be able to carry it through. If you don't, your credibility with your loved one will be shot. So if you tell your wife you're going to leave unless she keeps her appointments with her therapist, you'd better be ready to walk out the door if and when it happens. If you don't think you can do that, try a different tack, something you can actually stick to.

## Avoiding the Pitfalls of Caregiving

As a caregiver, you spend most of your time walking a tightrope. Without a safety net. In a high wind. You know it's just a matter of time before you lose your balance. In fact, ironic as it is, the majority of problems you'll face while trying to deal with bipolar disorder are essentially identical to those faced by your loved one: Both of you need to find balance.

Kay calls living with or loving someone who's bipolar being "bipolar by proxy." While the bipolar person in your life needs to balance mania and depression, you need to balance support and independence—for both of you. You cannot just go on with your life as if nothing has happened, as if you have no added responsibility. You do. You have many new responsibilities. But on the other hand, you also have a continuing responsibility to yourself. And although it's clichéd, it's also very true that you won't be much good to the person who needs you if you yourself become sick or completely burnt out.

> **GET PSYCHED**
>
> "Eventually you may see the silver lining in the storm clouds: your own increased awareness, sensitivity, receptivity, compassion, and maturity. You may become less judgmental and self-centered, a better person." —From "Coping Tips for Siblings and Adult Children of persons with Mental Illness" at www.nami.org

That's why it's important to know some of the pitfalls of being with, loving, or caring for somebody with bipolar disorder. It's only in knowing where those pitfalls lie that you can figure out ways around or out of them.

**Stress** There's almost nothing about bipolar disorder that's not stressful: fighting to get the right diagnosis, working to get insurance coverage, dealing with the financial and legal implications of the disease, and, first and foremost, trying to support and help someone you love as he fights to regain or keep some emotional stability in his life.

In a New Zealand study of caregivers to people with bipolar disorder, 71 percent said they experienced major stress because of their loved one's illness: 44 percent said this was mostly when the person was sick, but 27 percent said it hung around pretty much all the time.

But that's not news to you, is it? Nor is the advice that comes with the admission of stress: take some time to focus on yourself. Do things that make you happy, that reduce your stress levels. Don't allow your loved one to put more stress on you by demanding things you're unable to give her—whether it's money, time, or even support. If you don't have it to give, say so. And then duck. Because even as the stress wanes, the guilt probably isn't far behind.

**Guilt** It used to be that mental illness was all the parent's fault; you were unloving or dysfunctional or abusive and caused these mental breakdowns with your behavior and actions. Today, nearly everyone realizes that assertion to be the rubbish it is. Sure, how you act and react to your child or loved one who is mentally ill can play a role in how the illness develops and how easily it can

# you're not alone

"That night in December 1997 will always remain one of my more painful memories.

"I'd heard from my father earlier in the week, a rather cheerful conversation, considering he was calling from yet another mental hospital. He wanted me to know that, after all those years, someone had finally seen what I'd long

ago seen, and diagnosed him with bipolar disorder.

"Now it was 5 days later, and I'd just put my 4-month-old down for the night. Then the phone rang, and it was Dad. He sounded angry and depressed. He wanted me to sign him out of the hospital in New York, to fly him out to California, to let him 'recover' in my home.

"I'd thought this might be coming, and I'd thought I was ready for it. I told him I was proud of him, and then I told him no. No, I wouldn't sign him out of the hospital. No, I wouldn't take care of him. I wouldn't, and I couldn't.

"I've never heard my father so angry in my life. He ranted and raved at me. He threatened to sign

be treated. But that's only one small part of the equation. You did not cause your loved one's bipolar disorder. In fact, scientific evidence is piling up to show that the opposite is true—that the stress and behavioral results of your loved one's disorder can create mental instability in you and other members of your family.

Still, that doesn't mean you're going to live your life guilt-free. And if you're already caring for someone with bipolar disorder, you're probably well aware of that. For one thing, there's the genetic component. If you're a parent of a bipolar child, you have to deal with the possibility that you passed that genetic predisposition on to her. And although we all know we can't pick and choose our genes, this can be a difficult thing to truly internalize and accept.

But even more likely, you spend time feeling guilty for all the things you could be doing for your loved one, but aren't. You might feel guilty for the times you snap under the pressure. You might feel guilty for the times you take off so you *don't* snap under the pressure. You might feel guilty for feeling angry. You might feel guilty for being scared. You might feel guilty for feeling guilty. It's a vicious cycle.

himself out and live on the streets. He broke down and pleaded with me: 'I can't stay here. It's the holidays. How can you do this?'

"I don't know where the resolve came from. Maybe from being a new mother. Maybe from years of knowing that this was coming some day. Maybe from places it really shouldn't have come—from anger, from resentment Probably from all of that. In any case, I refused. And he stayed at the hospital until they were ready to release him. He got stabilized on his new medications. He found a place to live. He found new love.

"I think I did the right thing that night—for him, for me, for my new family. My dad? He doesn't even remember that call, that anger. He doesn't remember the rejection. It's my most painful memory, and he has no memory of it at all." *—Lori Oliwenstein, author of this book*

329

How can you break that cycle? It's not easy. Education is one way. If you know how bipolar disorder works, you'll know how little a role you played in your loved one's disease. Another help is communication. Let the person you love know what he can and cannot expect from you, so that when you do have to say, "No, I can't do this anymore," or "No, I can't give you what you want," it won't come as a surprise. If you know you've thought through your choices, that you've made them with the best interests of both you *and* your loved one in mind, you should be able to shrug off most of the guilt, or at least know it's a price worth paying for doing what you think is best.

**Anger**  If it weren't for your wife's illness, you'd have pristine credit and money to burn. If it weren't for your son's disorder, you could go back to school or back to work. If it weren't for your sister's depression, you would get some attention from your parents. If it weren't for your father's mania, you would actually feel taken care of, rather than feeling like the eternal caregiver.

**WEB TALK:** Beacon of Hope, a website "for partners of those touched with mental illness," offers coping tips at: www.lightship.org/cope.htm

Anger and its twin, resentment, are extremely common, extremely normal reactions to caring for someone with bipolar disorder. Consider some of these statistics, from the New Zealand survey of caregivers:

- 76 percent of caregivers who worked outside the home had reduced their hours or taken time off from work because of their loved one's illness, with 67 percent saying the disorder made their work a strain or stress for them.

- 27 percent of caregivers said their income had dropped since their loved one's illness had begun, with that number rising significantly when you consider only partners of people with bipolar disorder and ignore other caregivers (parents, siblings, friends).

- Half the caregivers had to take "significant" responsibility for their loved one's finances when they were ill.

How do you let go of the anger? How do you kiss resentment good-bye? You start by letting go of the "could have beens" and "should have beens" and by looking at the reality in which you live. Yeah, it would be great if you'd had a more nurturing father or a "normal" son. But you don't. You do have someone you love, someone who's ill, someone who no more wants to destroy your life than you want to destroy hers.

That sort of intellectual exercise might give you a start in ridding yourself of anger and resentment, but the reality is, you're going to need more help than that. Get some therapy—for yourself, not for your loved one. Or join a support group. Learn how to channel your emotions and how to safely let them out. If you don't, you're going to explode. That's a promise.

**Emotional Overinvolvement** If you're going to be there for your loved one, you have to remember a few things. First, she's not always going to be sick. Most people with bipolar disorder have periods of time—hopefully long periods of time—when they don't need much outside help to manage their disease. These are the times when you have to let go. And that can be harder than you might think.

Second, you need to keep your distance. You need to maintain your own identity. Otherwise, you are at risk of losing your sanity and your self. You cannot be responsible for your loved one's moods; you can't let his moods control yours.

Jacqueline Castine knows all about the dangers of becoming overly involved in another person's disorder. In addition to her own bipolar disorder and alcoholism, she spent several years taking care of her alcoholic ex-husband. She then moved on to "helping" her son, whose aggression, violence, and anger have plagued him since he was a child. Jacqueline says she used to fret about him all the time, trying to get him to accept his bipolar disorder diagnosis, trying to get him into treatment, trying to keep him out of jail. None of it worked.

## GET PSYCHED

"I was the one who had to come to my own bottom in this, and it was the most freeing experience. I just thought, 'He's 42, I'm 63, and I'd better just accept that it's his life and I'd better have the best relationship with him that I can.'"
—Jacqueline Castine, living with bipolar disorder and parent to three adult children, two of whom have bipolar disorder

"I finally came to the conclusion that I have to practice what I preach," says Jacqueline, who has written a book, *Recovery from Rescuing*. "It's been so hard to do that I haven't been able to love him just the way he is." Jacqueline's second book, *I Wish I Could Fix It, But …* (Phoenix Publishers), was published in the fall of 2004.

Just remember, helping someone you love is a good thing. But there's a fine line between helping and controlling. If you think you've crossed it, get help for yourself. Both you and your loved one will benefit from it.

## Maintaining Your Own Life

You're tired, you're angry, and you're resentful. You need a break. No, really. *You need a break.*

One of the biggest downfalls for caregivers is martyrdom. It's true your friend or family member needs you. And it's true he is ill. And it's true it's not his fault. And it's true he deserves love and respect. But you know what? It's also not your fault. And you, too, deserve love and respect—from yourself. You need to take care of yourself.

You can start by getting therapy. Many of the psychosocial treatments out there for bipolar disorder—such as family-focused therapy, or FFT—help families to draw boundaries between themselves and the person with the disorder. By going to therapy, not only would you be helping your loved one in her recovery, but you'd be helping yourself to find solutions to your most difficult issues.

But that's not all. Taking care of yourself goes deeper than going to therapy, deeper even than making sure you maintain friendships and outside interests—although you should definitely devote time to all that. It comes down to the basics. When you're knee-deep in drama and disorder, you can forget to eat, or you don't eat well. You stop exercising. You no longer get a good night's sleep. I don't have to tell you how counterproductive that is and how your loved one is really going to be in trouble if you work or worry yourself into the hospital. You know that. You now have to internalize it. You have to *do* it.

That's not to say that in the midst of your loved one's psychotic break or a major depressive relapse you should go off for a weekend at a spa. But someone else in the family can come in and cook dinner one night so you can go to your book club or even just take a half-hour walk. And when the crisis is over, yes, go for the spa weekend. And take a friend. You deserve it.

**Q & A**

*I know it sounds clichéd, but what about me? What about my needs?*

"It is important to take care of yourself, and it is normal for you to have symptoms of stress, anxiety, or depression when someone you care about is ill. It's important for you to build your own support system of people who will listen to you and be concerned about your well-being, including friends, relatives, and possibly a doctor or therapist. There is no shame in looking for help for yourself. You might think your problems are minor in comparison to what your loved one is coping with, but that doesn't mean you are any less deserving of help and comfort. Admit your own feelings, and let yourself experience them.

"Take time out for yourself, and make time to do things that relax you and things you enjoy. You will be best able to support the person you care about when you are healthy, rested, and relaxed. Be honest about your own feelings to your loved one. Speak openly about your needs before you start to feel resentful. For example, if you need some time alone or some time to rest, you have a right to ask about it." —*From the Depression and Bipolar Support Alliance pamphlet, "Helping a Friend or Family Member with a Mood Disorder"*

## Support Groups for Friends and Family

You are no less worthy of love and support than your loved one. And although there's less of it out there for you than there should be, there are places you can go and people who understand:

- **The Depression and Bipolar Support Alliance (www. dbsalliance.org)** has more than 1,000 peer-run support groups throughout the United States, including groups that focus on family members and friends.

- **The National Alliance for the Mentally Ill (www.nami. org)** has chapters and support groups nationwide as well, and also offers a Family-to-Family Education Program, a 12-week course provided for free in hundreds of U.S. communities, as well as in Canada, Puerto Rico, and Mexico.

- **The National Mental Health Association (www.nmha.org)** offers local support groups for both people with mental illness and their families.

You might also find support groups affiliated with major medical centers, especially if they have a bipolar or mood disorders clinic.

In addition, there are online communities galore, where you can find people from around the country or even around the globe who've been where you are and are willing to lend a hand:

- **BPSO (Bipolar Significant Others; www.bpso.org/subscrib. shtml)** maintains a high-volume mailing list, meaning you'll get dozens of messages each day. It's also a closed list, meaning you'll need to subscribe and be approved to join in.

- **Mental Health Sanctuary's Bipolar Disorder Sanctuary (www.mhsanctuary.com/bipolar/board2.htm)** offers a Family Message Board for friends and family of people with bipolar disorder.

- **NAMI (www.nami.org)** has four online discussion groups for families of people with mental illness: "Mental Illness in My Family," "My Parent Is a Consumer," "Parents of Child/ Teen Consumers," and "Siblings of Consumers."

- "Manic Moments: A Bipolar's World" (www. manicmoment.org/support/notsomanicsub.php) maintains an e-mail list called the Not So Manic Support List for spouses and loved ones of people with bipolar disorder.

- SupportPath.com (www.supportpath.com/sl_b/ bipolar_disorder.htm), houses a list of real-time chats hosted by the folks at About.com's Bipolar Disorder page. These include chats about bipolar disorder and the family and bipolar disorder and relationships that might be of interest to you.

- The Guides Community (bang.dhs.org/guides/index.html) is "an online community for people who are living with, friends with, in love with, parent/child/brother/sister/third cousin of someone afflicted with a depressive illness, including bipolar disorder." It has a couple mailing lists, chat information, and a list of "real-world" support groups if e-mail lists aren't filling all your support needs.

And finally, you shouldn't pooh-pooh the idea of getting some therapy for yourself, to have someone who's looking out for you and you alone. "I think when a family member has had a lot of distress or trauma as a result of this disorder it can be very helpful to get some psychotherapy," says Ellen Frank, Ph.D., director of the Depression and Manic Depression Prevention Program at Western Psychiatric Institute and Clinic in Pittsburgh. "I think just supportive psychotherapy that helps someone try to cope with living with someone who has this disorder can be hugely important."

# Into Her Own Hands

The pain—the emotional anguish—was more than Kay could stand. She didn't know how to ask for the help she so clearly needed—and there was nobody offering help, not even when she carved the letters H-E-L-P into the skin on the inside of her arm. "I just wanted somebody to see the pain," she recalls. She was so desperate to get away from bipolar disorder and what it had done to her life that she looked into taking an adult-education course on changing your identity. She just wanted to run.

The thing is, Kay doesn't have bipolar disorder. It was the pain of dealing with her now-ex-husband and her adult daughter—both of whom have since been diagnosed bipolar—that pushed her so close to the edge.

"I kept getting on the phone with my sister, saying 'Help me, help me.' I wanted them to just come. They said, 'How can we help you?' but they would never come," Kay recalls. "I remember thinking they're just not there for me. Nobody's coming; there's no white horse when you look up the street."

What brought her back from the edge, she says, was a support group for friends and family at a New York hospital she had read about in a magazine.

"You need to be with people who understand the pain you're going through," Kay says. "In general, people just don't get it. They say, 'You can do it. Just push.' They have no idea."

When she first walked into her support group, Kay says, "I just totally fell apart. I was so happy to be with people who understood. It just helped me so much."

It wasn't long before the group's leaders came to her and asked her to be a facilitator—to lead other groups like the one that had helped her so much. "I got my training, and since then, I've facilitated groups for bipolars, groups for the depressed—I've done everything," she says. "But most of all I've worked with groups for friends and families. Those are the ones I get the most out of. After all, I still need all the help I can get."

Having support doesn't take all the pain away, Kay admits, but it does give you a safe place and a safe way to express it. And it taught her the value of a sense of humor. "There is a way out," she says. "There is someone coming to help. This is a treatable illness and we can all live normally."

# What You Can Do

You have enough on your plate. I'm not going to tell you what you should or should not do for the person you love or are caring for. But I am going to tell you what you can do for yourself—what you *should* do for yourself. Because in the same way that you've come to understand that your loved one is no less worthy of love and respect because she's ill, you need to recognize that you're no less worthy of love and respect because you're not ill.

- ☐ Try not to take your loved one's disease personally, and try not to blame yourself. His bipolar disorder is not his fault, but it's not yours, either.

- ☐ Cry, yell, kick, scream—but be sure someone hears you and is watching your back.

- ☐ Find and join a support group, whether it be online or in person. Or better yet, do both. There's no such thing as too much support.

- ☐ Educate yourself. If you haven't already, go back and read the first few chapters of this book. Check out some of the websites listed in Appendix C. Read some of the books recommended in Appendix B.

- ☐ Get involved. Advocate on behalf of the mentally ill, facilitate a support group for significant others, or simply be there for another person who's in the same spot you're in.

- ☐ Get therapy for yourself. This disorder can have just as much impact on your life as on your loved one's, and you need to know how to deal with that.

- ☐ Be realistic in terms of what you expect from your loved one. Treatment takes time; he will not get better overnight.

- ☐ Recognize that support is one thing; trying to fix everything by yourself is another. You can encourage your loved one to see a therapist or take her medication, but you can't do those things for her.

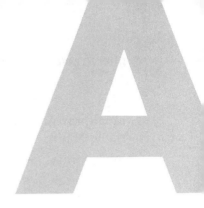

# Glossary

**Abilify**   *See* aripriprazole.

**acute mania**   Mania that comes on very suddenly, gets worse quickly, and lasts over a fairly short, defined period of time. In bipolar disorder, it usually refers to a single episode of mania.

**advocate**   Someone who pushes forward an idea, pleads for a cause, or argues in favor of a particular point.

**affective disorder**   A disturbance of emotions, such as bipolar disorder or depression, in which the disturbance is not caused by an unrelated medical problem.

**agranulocytosis**   A reduction in the number of certain white blood cells in the circulation.

**amino acids**   The fundamental building blocks of proteins; there are 20 primary amino acids that are generally used in the synthesis of a protein strand.

**amygdala**   The brain's almond-shape "seat of emotion"; the place from which your feelings and impulses arise.

**anosognosia**   An inability to recognize, acknowledge, or act upon a set of symptoms such as those of mania. Literally, it means "to not know a disease," and comes from the Greek words for "diseases" (*nosos*) and "knowledge" (*gnosis*).

**anticonvulsant**   A medication that prevents or relieves seizures.

**antidepressant**   A medication that prevents or relieves depression and stimulates positive mood.

**antipsychotic**   A medication that is effective in the treatment of psychosis.

**aripriprazole**   An atypical antipsychotic that goes by the brand name Abilify.

**arrhythmia**   Any kind of variation from a normal heart rhythm.

**attention deficit disorder (ADD)**   A pattern of behaviors—difficulty paying attention, restlessness or constant motion, and lack of impulse control—that are out of synch with a child's level of development.

**attention deficit/hyperactivity disorder (ADHD)**   *See* attention deficit disorder (ADD).

**atypical antipsychotic**   Novel drugs that differ chemically from the older antipsychotics and that are able to quell psychosis at doses that don't bring on the severe movement disorders common with the older drugs.

**autoimmune disease**   Any of a number of medical conditions in which the body's immune system responds to and attacks the body's own tissues.

**axon**   A long, hairlike projection from the body of a neuron, down which nerve impulses travel.

**bipolar disorder**   A mental disorder characterized by alternating periods of mania and depression, usually with periods of normal mood in between. Also known as manic-depression.

**bipolar I disorder**   A version of bipolar disorder in which the person in question has experienced at least one full-blown manic episode.

**bipolar II disorder**   A version of bipolar disorder in which the person in question has never experienced a full-blown manic episode but experiences hypomania.

**bipolar III disorder**   A version of bipolar disorder in which mania is triggered by treatment with antidepressant medications.

**bipolar spectrum**   The entire range of ways in which bipolar disorder can manifest itself.

**borderline personality disorder**   A mental illness marked by impulsivity (often involving risk-taking), unstable moods, and chaotic relationships.

**calcium channel blockers**   Medications that slow, or block, the movement of calcium into cells. In the brain, this blocks the flow of electrical impulses.

**carbamazepine**   An anticonvulsant medication that goes by the brand name Tegretol.

**catatonia**   A behavior disturbance during which you spend long periods of time in a virtual stupor. Physical symptoms characterizing catatonia include very stiff, rigid muscles, especially in the arms and legs.

**chromosome**   Structures that contain a cell's genetic information. There are generally 46 chromosomes in humans, and they are found in the nucleus of all cells.

**circadian rhythm**   From the Latin *circa,* meaning "about," and *dies,* meaning "day," *circadian* literally means "about a day." A circadian rhythm is a biological cycle that lasts for approximately 24 hours.

**clinical social worker**   A therapist who has been trained to make diagnoses and provide a full range of psychotherapeutic services.

**clinical trial**   A scientific study involving human subjects, which is designed to evaluate the safety and efficacy of a new treatment under strictly controlled conditions.

**clozapine**   An antipsychotic medication that goes by the brand name Clozaril.

**Clozaril**   *See* clozapine.

**comorbidity**   A state in which two or more medical conditions exist simultaneously and usually independently of one another.

**conduct disorder**   A pattern of behavior in which a child repeatedly or persistently acts with aggression toward other people or animals, destroys property, lies or steals, and deliberately violates parental and societal rules and norms.

**cortex**   The outer layer of brain tissue (or of any organ's tissue); the gray matter of the brain.

**cyclothymia**   A mild form of bipolar disorder in which a person goes through periods of both hypomania and depression that are shorter in duration and less severe than in bipolar I or II.

**delusion** A false belief that is maintained despite strong evidence to the contrary.

**dementia praecox** An obsolete term for schizophrenia.

**dendrite** Short, branching arms that extend from the body of a neuron and receive signals from the axons of adjacent neurons.

**Depakote** *See* divalproex.

**differential diagnosis** A systematic compare-and-contrast method physicians use to determine which condition a patient is suffering from when there are two or more possibilities that share a number of similar symptoms or signs.

**disability** A physical or mental impairment that substantially limits one or more major life activities.

**disclosure** The deliberate informing of one or several people in your workplace or life about your psychiatric disability.

**divalproex (valproate or valproic acid)** An anticonvulsant and mood stabilizer sold under the brand name Depakote.

**dominant gene** A gene that is fully expressed even when there is only one copy in the cell.

**dopamine** A neurotransmitter in the central nervous system that plays a role in such processes as movement and balance.

**double-blind study** A clinical trial in which neither the patient nor the physician knows what treatment, if any, the patient is actually receiving.

**durable power of attorney** A document that gives another person the right to make legal and financial decisions on your behalf when, if, and for as long as you are either physically or mentally incapable of making them yourself.

**dysphoria** An unpleasant mood, often characterized by depression and restlessness.

**dysphoric mania** Mania jumbled with the symptoms of depression.

**electroconvulsive therapy (ECT)** A treatment for mood disorders in which a mild convulsion is produced by passing an electrical current through the brain. It is also called electroshock therapy.

**electrode**   A conductor that allows electricity to enter a nonmetallic part of a circuit.

**employee assistance program (EAP)**   A program that offers support and education to employees who are trying to cope with emotional or behavioral problems that might have an effect on job performance. Oftentimes, an EAP will allow you a certain number of visits, then provide you with a referral to an outside therapist covered by your insurance.

**epilepsy**   A disorder in which brain activity is briefly disturbed, resulting in seizures, loss of consciousness, abnormal movements, and more.

**episode**   A significant event in a disease process; a bipolar episode is a pathological disturbance of mood, either manifesting as mania, hypomania, major depression, or a mixture thereof.

**essential fatty acid (EFA)**   A type of fat your body cannot synthesize and, therefore, has to be included in your diet.

**euphoria**   An exaggerated, over-the-top feeling of well-being, particularly when there is no external reason for feeling that way.

**euthymia**   A normal, tranquil mood. Euthymia is how you feel between episodes of mania and depression; it's the goal of treatment for bipolar disorder.

**expressed emotion**   Negative attitudes (criticism, anger, emotional overinvolvement) that relatives might hold toward someone in the family who is psychiatrically ill.

**facilitator**   The DBSA's term for a peer or a consumer who keeps an eye on the meetings to be sure they stay within the organization's set of rules.

**fatty acids**   Any compound derived from breaking down fats; they generally include long chains of hydrogen and carbon atoms.

**fluoxetine**   An antidepressant medication that goes by the brand name Prozac.

**folie circulaire**   Literally, "circular madness"; a nineteenth-century term for bipolar disorder.

**formulary**   A list of prescription drugs covered by a specific health plan. If a drug is not on a company's formulary, they generally won't cover its costs.

**frontal lobe**   The part of the brain's cerebrum found directly behind the forehead. It's responsible for voluntary movement, thought, and feelings.

**gamma-aminobutyric acid (GABA)**   A neurotransmitter that works to inhibit the excitation or activation of brain cells.

**Geodon**   *See* ziprasidone.

**gene**   A segment of DNA that allows for the production of a product such as an enzyme or other protein.

**gene chip**   A sliver of silicon that can grab and hold on to a very large number of DNA samples in a tiny grid pattern. Gene chips have enabled scientists to make genetic discoveries at a previously unimaginable pace because they can now analyze the activity or function of hundreds of genes in the time it used to take to look at just one.

**glutamate**   A form of the amino acid glutamic acid. Amino acids are the building blocks of proteins. Glutamate is the most commonly found neurotransmitter in the brain and spinal cord.

**grandiosity**   An exaggerated belief in your own importance or intelligence or power. It is usually linked with delusions of fame and wealth.

**hallucinations**   Perceptions of an object that does not exist. Hallucinations are often either visual (seen) or auditory (heard).

**hallucinogen**   A chemical that distorts perception to create delusions or hallucinations.

**hypersexuality**   Excessive sexual activity, desire, or interest.

**hyperthyroidism**   An overly active thyroid gland, resulting in an overabundance of thyroid hormone in the circulation and a speeded-up metabolism.

**hypomania**   A mood state that is much like mania, but is less intense and does not have any associated psychotic symptoms.

**hypothalamus**   An area of the brain that includes the suprachiasmatic nucleus, which plays a role in setting circadian rhythms.

**hypothyroidism**   An underactive thyroid gland, resulting in a lowered metabolic rate.

**impaired insight**   *See* anosognosia.

**Individualized Education Plan (IEP)**   A document that lays out a complete educational plan for a child with a disability.

**intrusiveness**   Aggressively advancing yourself and your ideas without invitation or regard for the appropriateness of your meddling.

**kindling**   A concept originally associated with epilepsy, in which a first seizure, caused by an outside influence, sets up conditions that allow future seizures to occur without provocation. The same idea is being considered for episodes of mania and depression in bipolar disorder, with the idea being that each episode that occurs makes future episodes more likely.

**Lamictal**   *See* lamotrigine.

**lamotrigine**   One of the newest anticonvulsant medications approved for the treatment of bipolar disorder. It is sold under the brand name Lamictal.

**libido**   Sexual energy or sexual drive.

**linoleic fatty acids**   *See* omega-3 fatty acids.

**linolenic fatty acids**   *See* omega-6 fatty acids.

**lithium**   An elemental metal used as a mood stabilizer in the treatment of bipolar disorder and particularly mania.

**lumen**   A measure of the energy of light in all directions.

**lux**   A measure of illumination over a specified surface area. One lux is the uniform lighting of one square meter by one lumen of light.

**major depressive disorder**   A several-week-long abnormal mood characterized by sadness and emptiness, markedly decreased pleasure or interest in normal activities, or significant irritability.

**mania**   A pathological mood state characterized by grandiosity, euphoria, sleep disturbances, and sometimes delusions and hallucinations.

**manic-depression**   A synonym for bipolar disorder that is only now starting to fall out of common usage.

**MAO inhibitors**   Drugs used to treat depression that work by blocking the action of the enzyme MAO, or monoamine oxidase, which otherwise works to break down certain key neurotransmitters. It has the effect of prolonging the action of such neurotransmitters.

**melatonin**   A hormone made and secreted by the brain's pineal gland in response to light exposure. Melatonin acts as a kind of natural sleep aid.

**mental health insurance parity**   Mental health insurance that is equal in function to physical health insurance.

**methionine**   An amino acid that is the body's principal supplier of sulfur.

**mixed state**   A blend of manic and depressive symptoms that appear at the same time.

**monotherapy**   A form of treatment that employs only one drug rather than a combination of pharmaceuticals.

**mood stabilizer**   A drug that evens out mood by calming mania without causing depression, and lightening depression without causing mania. The U.S. Food and Drug Administration (FDA), however, doesn't recognize any such class of drug, and scientists have thus far been unable to come to a consensus definition themselves.

**mutation**   A permanent change at the DNA level that is transmitted genetically.

**myelin**   A layer, or sheath, of proteins and lipids, or fats, that covers and protects a neuron's axon.

**neuroleptic**   An antipsychotic drug that has a tranquilizing effect. Haldol and Thorazine are two well-known neuroleptics.

**neuroleptic malignant syndrome**   A severe and sometimes life-threatening side effect of neuroleptic drugs in which the patient experiences muscle stiffness, high fever, sweating, unstable blood pressure, stupor, tremor, confusion, and sometimes even coma.

**neuron**   The brain's signal-conducting cell. Neurons have a "body" surrounded by short branching arms called dendrites, which pick up signals from nearby neurons. Those signals are then passed down the neuron's long, hairlike axon to get to the next neuron in the circuit.

**neuropsychopharmacology**   The use of drugs to treat psychiatric diseases by manipulating the rate of transmission of messages between neurons. *See also* psychopharmaceutical.

**neurotransmitter**   A class of chemicals that travel from the end of one nerve cell to the beginning of another, giving that second cell the signal to fire—that is, to send its electrical message on down the line to the next nerve cell.

**nonessential amino acids**   Protein building blocks the body itself can synthesize or create. In contrast, the essential amino acids cannot be synthesized by the body and can only be acquired through ingesting foods that contain them.

**norepinephrine**   A hormone produced by the body's adrenal glands that, in the brain, acts as a neurotransmitter, affecting such basic processes as heart rate and blood pressure.

**obsessive-compulsive disorder (OCD)**   An anxiety disorder characterized by uncontrollable thoughts (obsessions) or behaviors (compulsions) that tend to focus on orderliness, perfection, or control to ward off distress or a feared event. These obsessions and compulsions become a disorder when they affect normal functioning.

**olanzapine**   An atypical antipsychotic medication approved for the treatment of bipolar mania. It is sold under the brand name Zyprexa.

**omega-3 fatty acids**   Fatty acids found in the leaves and seeds of plants, in egg yolks, and in cold-water fish.

**omega-6 fatty acids**   The most common polyunsaturated fatty acids in foods.

**opiate**   A type of pain-killing drug that's related to morphine and binds to the morphine receptors in the brain, and includes such drugs as heroin, oxycodone, and methadone.

**optic chiasm**   The spot where the two optic nerves cross at the base of the brain, in the hypothalamus.

**optic nerves**   The nerves that carry visual signals from the eye's retina to the brain.

**oxcarbazepine**   An anticonvulsant medication sometimes used in the treatment of bipolar disorder. Its brand name is Trileptal.

**peer-run services**   Services developed and led by people who have a mental illness for other people with that same mental illness. The peers participate fully in the group and are not treatment professionals.

**phase delay**   A sleep pattern in which a person consistently lags behind a "normal" circadian rhythm, going to sleep later and waking later than light cues would suggest.

**phototherapy**   A form of treatment for a disease or condition using light in carefully controlled doses.

**pineal gland**   A tiny hormone-secreting organ in the cerebrum of the brain; it produces melatonin, which is a critical hormone in the sleep-wake cycle.

**placebo**   A completely inactive substance that is administered or taken in a clinical trial so researchers will have something to compare with the effects of the active substance being studied.

**placebo-controlled study**   A clinical trial in which neither the researchers nor the patient knows who is getting the drug being investigated and who is getting a placebo.

**postpartum depression**   A mood disorder that begins after childbirth and usually lasts for at least six weeks.

**postpartum psychosis**   An extreme mental disorder that begins after childbirth and involves confusion, hallucinations, delusions, and sometimes suicidal or homicidal thought processes.

**priapism**   A painful condition in which the penis becomes and remains erect for hours, generally without any sexual arousal.

**prodromal symptoms**   The signs of illness that appear during the prodrome. Prodromal symptoms indicate that a disease is developing or a relapse is about to occur.

**prodrome**   The period of time between the first recognition of a disease's symptoms and when it reaches its more severe form.

**Prozac**   *See* fluoxetine.

**psychiatric rehabilitation**   Services designed to provide skills and support to people whose ability to function on one or more levels is affected by a mental illness.

**psychiatrist**   A physician concerned with diagnosing, treating, and preventing mental illness. Psychiatrists are M.D.s and are able to prescribe medications.

**psychoeducation**   An intervention that teaches people with mental illness about their condition, what its effects and consequences might be, and concrete strategies that can be used to deal with those effects and consequences.

**psychologist**   A professional trained to provide counseling and therapy. Psychologists have Ph.D.s; they are not M.D.s and cannot prescribe medications.

**psychopharmaceutical**   A chemical compound that has an effect on your mental state; a drug that acts on your mind.

**psychosis**   A mental disorder in which the ability to perceive or recognize reality and control impulses becomes impaired. Psychosis is often characterized by hallucinations and delusions.

**psychosocial treatment**   Any therapy that focuses on how psychological and social conditions interact and how they affect mental health.

**psychotropic drug**   *See* psychopharmaceutical.

**quetiapine**   An atypical antipsychotic medication approved in 2004 for use in the treatment of bipolar mania. It is sold under the brand name Seroquel.

**rapid-cycling bipolar disorder**   Four or more major mood episodes (either mania or depression or both) within a 12-month period.

**reasonable accommodations**   On-the-job changes in things such as scheduling or job requirements and expectations that help provide a level playing field on which you have as much chance to succeed as do your co-workers.

**recessive gene**   A gene that is fully expressed only when two copies of it are in a cell.

**recurring**   An event or condition that occurs repeatedly.

**relapse**   The return of the signs or symptoms of a disease after it has gone through a period of improvement or remission.

**remission**   The disappearance or complete regression of the signs and symptoms of a disease.

**rescue medication**   A drug that brings quick relief from an acute episode or attack of an illness.

**Risperdal**   *See* risperidone.

**risperidone**  An atypical antipsychotic approved in December 2003 for the treatment of acute bipolar mania. It is sold under the brand name Risperdal.

**schizoaffective disorder**  A mental disorder that has signs and symptoms of both schizophrenia and bipolar disorder, with those symptoms being so intertwined that neither diagnosis can be made on its own.

**schizophrenia**  A mental disorder that causes a break between thought and emotion. It is characterized by delusions and hallucinations; disorganized speech; flattened or blunted emotions; and unusual, often bizarre, behavior or inactivity.

**seasonal affective disorder (SAD)**  A mood disorder connected to seasonal changes in light duration. Generally, it is characterized by depression that begins in fall or winter and dissipates in spring or summer.

**sedative**  A chemical that reduces mental activity or excitement.

**seizure**  A sudden burst of abnormal electrical signals that temporarily interrupts normal brain activity and often results in an altered state of consciousness.

**selective serotonin reuptake inhibitor (SSRI)**  A type of antidepressant medication that blocks the reuptake of the neurotransmitter serotonin by neurons, leaving it available to continue to act on other receptors in the brain.

**Seroquel**  *See* quetiapine.

**serotonin**  A neurotransmitter involved in sleep, memory, aggression, sex drive, and appetite. Serotonin causes blood vessel constriction and stimulates smooth muscle action in the body.

**social rhythms**  Daily routines that, when disrupted, might trigger the onset of a mood episode.

**spectrum**  The entire landscape of a disease, with all the combinations and permutations of its symptoms. A spectrum is the full range of ways a disorder can make itself known or felt.

**stigma**  A symbol of disgrace or shame, or a negative label that often results in someone being rejected or shunned by others.

**stimulant**   A chemical that increases activity in the brain and central nervous system.

**suprachiasmatic nucleus (SCN)**   An area of the brain that sits just above the optic chiasm. The SCN feeds off the light signals sent by the optic nerves and passes the information on to the pineal gland. It is also known as the brain's biological clock.

**Symbyax**   A combination of the atypical antipsychotic olanzapine and the antidepressant fluoxetine. In December 2003, it became the first-ever FDA-approved medication specifically aimed at bipolar depression.

**tardive dyskinesia**   A neurological syndrome that results from the use of antipsychotic medications. It is characterized by abnormal, involuntary body movements, especially in the lower face and tongue.

**taurine**   An amino acid that stabilizes excitability in cell membranes, including those of the neurons in the brain.

**Tegretol**   *See* carbamazepine.

**thyroid**   A large gland near the base of the neck that produces thyroid hormones.

**thyroid hormones**   Any of a number of compounds secreted by the thyroid gland that work to regulate metabolism.

**Topamax**   *See* topiramate.

**topiramate**   An anticonvulsant medication with some utility in treating bipolar mania. Its brand name is Topamax.

**total sleep deprivation**   An antidepressant therapy in which a person is deliberately kept awake for 36 or more hours before being allowed a recovery sleep. This cycle is often repeated several times in a row to get the best results.

**Tourette's syndrome**   A neurological disorder characterized by uncontrolled and recurrent vocalizations and movements called tics.

**tricyclic antidepressant**   A mood-elevating drug that works by inhibiting reuptake of the neurotransmitters serotonin and norepinephrine and by interfering with the metabolism of nervous-system compounds called amines.

**Trileptal**   *See* oxcarbazepine.

**tryptophan**   An amino acid that plays a role in the creation of serotonin.

**tyrosine**   An amino acid that's a precursor to the neurotransmitters norepinephrine and dopamine.

**ultra-rapid cycling**   Cycling between depression and mania at such a quick pace that it's impossible to even tell one from the other. Ultra-rapid cycling includes mood switching that typically occurs more than once a day.

**ultradian**   A biological rhythm that occurs in less-than-24-hour cycles.

**undue hardship**   In legal terms, an action that carries with it significant difficulty or expense to the extent that it would do more harm than good.

**unipolar depression**   A mood disorder in which a person experiences one or more episodes of persistent sadness and apathy without any intervening episodes of mania or hypomania.

**unspecified episode**   An episode in which your current symptoms of bipolar disorder do not meet the criteria (in terms of either time or severity) to be considered mania, hypomania, or depression, although one or most past episodes have met the criteria.

**valproate**   *See* divalproex.

**valproic acid**   *See* divalproex.

**ventricle**   A sac or cavity; one of the fluid-filled spaces in the center of the brain.

**zeitgeber**   German for "time-giver," zeitgebers are external influences or cues that work to regulate circadian rhythm.

**ziprasidone**   An atypical antipsychotic being considered for FDA approval for the treatment of bipolar mania. It is marketed under the brand name Geodon.

**Zyprexa**   *See* olanzapine.

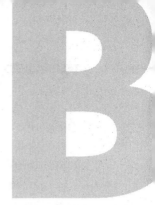

# Further Reading

From technical tomes to highly personal prose, the literature on bipolar disorder offers views of this mental illness from just about every vantage point imaginable. Are you living on the outside of the disorder, trying to understand what it's like on the inside? Patty Duke's story will inspire you; Andy Behrman's story will shock you. Are you someone who's looking for a better understanding of what's going on inside your body? Frederick Goodwin and Kay Redfield Jamison's much-cited volume covers every topic you can think of.

And those provide only a taste of the informational feast that's awaiting you at your local library or at your favorite bookstore. Here are some other offerings you might want to consider:

Barondes, Samuel H. *Mood Genes: Hunting for Origins of Mania and Depression*. W.H. Freeman and Company, 1998.

Behrman, Andy. *Electroboy: A Memoir of Mania*. Random House, 2002.

Castine, Jacqueline. *Recovery from Rescuing*. Health Communications, 1989.

Castle, Lana. *Bipolar Disorder Demystified: Mastering the Tightrope of Manic Depression*. Marlowe and Company, 2003.

Conner, Avery Z. *Fevers of the Mind: Tales of a Roaming, Wounded Critter*. PublishAmerica, Inc., 2002.

Cronkite, Kathy. *On the Edge of Darkness: America's Most Celebrated Actors, Journalists and Politicians Chronicle Their Most Arduous Journey*. Delta, 1995.

*Diagnostic and Statistical Manual of Mental Disorders, Fourth Edition.*
American Psychiatric Association, 1994.

Duke, Patty. *Call Me Anna: The Autobiography of Patty Duke.* Bantam, 1988.

Duke, Patty, and Gloria Hochman. *Brilliant Madness: Living with Manic Depressive Illness.* Bantam, 1997.

Fast, Julie A., and John D. Preston. *Loving Someone with Bipolar Disorder: Understanding and Helping Your Partner.* New Harbinger Publications, 2004.

Fisher, Carrie. *The Best Awful.* Simon & Schuster, 2004.

Geller, Barbara, and Melissa P. DelBello, eds. *Bipolar Disorder in Childhood and Early Adolescence.* Guilford Press, 2003. (highly technical)

Ghaemi, S. Nassir. *Mood Disorders: A Practical Guide.* Lippincott Williams and Wilkins, 2003.

Goodwin, Frederick K., and Kay Redfield Jamison. *Manic-Depressive Illness.* Oxford University Press, 1990.

Hershman, D. Jablow, and Julian Lieb. *Manic Depression and Creativity.* Prometheus Books, 1998.

Hinshaw, Stephen P. *The Years of Silence Are Past: My Father's Life with Bipolar Disorder.* Cambridge University Press, 2002.

Jamison, Kay Redfield. *An Unquiet Mind: A Memoir of Moods and Madness.* Vintage, 1997.

———. *Night Falls Fast: Understanding Suicide.* Alfred A. Knopf, 1999.

———. *Touched With Fire: Manic Depressive Illness and the Artistic Temperament.* The Free Press, 1993.

Maj, Mario, Hajop S. Akiskal, Juan José Lopez-Ibor, and Norman Sartorius, eds. *Bipolar Disorder.* John Wiley and Sons, 2002.

Miklowitz, David. *The Bipolar Disorder Survival Guide: What You and Your Family Need to Know.* Guilford Press, 2002.

Miklowitz, David J., and Michael J. Goldstein. *Bipolar Disorder: A Family-Focused Treatment Approach.* Guilford Press, 1997.

Mondimore, Francis Mark. *Bipolar Disorder: A Guide for Patients and Families.* Johns Hopkins University Press, 1999.

Nettle, Daniel. *Strong Imagination: Madness, Creativity and Human Nature*. Oxford University Press, 2001.

Papolos, Dimitri, and Janice Papolos. *The Bipolar Child: The Definitive and Reassuring Guide to Childhood's Most Misunderstood Disorder, Revised and Expanded Edition*. Broadway Books, 2002.

Pollard, Marc. *In Small Doses: A Memoir about Accepting and Living with Bipolar Disorder*. Vision Books International, 2004.

Raeburn, Paul. *Acquainted with the Night: A Parent's Quest to Understand Depression and Bipolar Disorder in His Children*. Broadway Books, 2004.

Simon, Lizzie. *Detour: My Bipolar Road Trip in 4-D*. Washington Square Press, 2003.

Styron, William. *Darkness Visible: A Memoir of Madness*, Vintage, 1992.

Torrey, E. Fuller, and Michael B. Knable. *Surviving Manic Depression: A Manual on Bipolar Disorder for Patients, Families, and Providers*. Basic Books, 2002.

Waltz, Mitzi. *Adult Bipolar Disorders: Understanding Your Diagnosis and Getting Help*. O'Reilly and Associates, 2002.

———. *Bipolar Disorders: A Guide to Helping Children and Adolescents*. Patient Centered Guides, 2000.

Whybrow, Peter. *A Mood Apart: The Thinker's Guide to Emotion and Its Disorders*. HarperCollins, 1997.

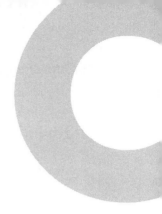

# Resources

It might feel like you're out here on your own. But the truth is, there's help all around you. From mental health organizations to academic medical centers to the far reaches of the World Wide Web, there is information to be uncovered, support to be given, and help to be found.

I've divided this appendix into three sections. The first lists some of the national and international organizations with information and resources you can turn to with almost any request or question.

Second is a short list of clinics and academic centers that have specific and well-regarded programs for research and treatment of bipolar disorder. These are the places where you'll find cutting-edge care and state-of-the-art science, and where you can not only get the best care available, but also give back by helping to advance knowledge of your disease.

Finally, there's a list of websites that can provide you with a range and breadth of resources you simply can't find elsewhere. And it's right there, waiting for you, 24/7.

Of course, none of these lists is complete or comprehensive. And keep in mind that the World Wide Web is a rather fluid universe. Web addresses that work fine today might be nothing but broken links tomorrow—if they exist at all.

# National and International Organizations

**American Psychiatric Association (APA)**
www.psych.org

The APA, "the nation's oldest national medical specialty society," includes on its website information on its treatment guidelines for physicians, abstracts from its annual meetings, and more. To search and read issues of the APA's monthly newspaper, *Psychiatry News*, go to pn.psychiatryonline.org.

**Child and Adolescent Bipolar Foundation (CABF)**
www.bpkids.org/
847-256-8525

CABF is a web-based organization led by parents of children who are either living with or at risk for bipolar disorder. Their mission is to educate families, professionals, and the public; connect families with resources and support; advocate for and empower affected families; and support research on pediatric bipolar disorder.

**Depression and Bipolar Support Alliance (DBSA)**
www.dbsalliance.org/
1-800-826-3632

DBSA is arguably the most extensive resource available for information and support for people with bipolar disorder. Until recently, this organization was known as the National Depressive and Manic Depressive Association.

**International Society for Bipolar Disorders (ISBD)**
www.isbd.org/
412-605-1412

ISBD was created "in response to the need for further awareness, education, and research on this severe mental illness."

**Juvenile Bipolar Research Foundation (JBRF)**
www.bpchildresearch.org

JBRF is "the first charitable foundation devoted solely to support research in childhood-onset bipolar disorder," funding promising research into the disorder's causes, treatments, and prevention.

**National Alliance for the Mentally Ill (NAMI)**
www.nami.org
1-800-950-NAMI (1-800-950-6264)

With more than 1,000 affiliates in the United States, NAMI calls itself "the nation's voice on mental illness." On its site you can search for a local chapter, get legal support, participate in a bipolar disorder discussion group, and more.

**National Alliance for Research on Schizophrenia and Depression (NARSAD)**
www.narsad.org
1-800-829-8289

NARSAD says it is the "largest donor organization in the world devoted exclusively to funding scientific research on psychiatric brain disorders."

**National Foundation for Depressive Illness, Inc. (NAFDI)**
www.depression.org/
1-800-239-1265

NAFDI, which focuses on the full range of affective disorders, was established in 1983 as part of an "ongoing public information campaign addressed to this pervasive, costly, and hidden national emergency.

**National Institute of Mental Health (NIMH)**
www.nimh.nih.gov
866-615-NIMH (866-615-6464)

The NIMH is one of the National Institutes of Health; its stated mission is "to reduce the burden of mental illness and behavioral disorders through research on mind, brain, and behavior." To go directly to a page dedicated to information about bipolar research and resources, go to www.nimh.nih.gov/publicat/bipolarmenu.cfm.

**National Mental Health Association (NMHA)**
www.nmha.org
1-800-969-6642

NMHA proclaims itself "the country's oldest and largest nonprofit organization addressing all aspects of mental health and mental illness." Its 340 affiliates nationwide are charged with improving the mental health of all Americans through advocacy, education, research, and service.

**Organization for Bipolar Affective Disorders Society (OBAD)**
www.obad.ca/main.htm
403-263-7408

OBAD is a provincial organization based out of Calgary, Alberta, Canada, aimed at helping people with bipolar disorder, anxiety, and depression. The site includes a downloadable book on bipolar and other affective disorders, an "ask the experts" column, and information about meetings and resources for people living with affective disorders.

## Clinics and Academic Centers

**Harvard Bipolar Research Program at Massachusetts General Hospital**
www.manicdepressive.org
617-726-6188

This site includes general information about bipolar disorder, as well as a downloadable and printable mood chart, a nationwide referral database to help you find a bipolar specialist in your area, and more.

**Stanford Bipolar Disorders Clinic**
www.stanford.edu/group/bipolar.clinic/about/index.html

Provides information about bipolar disorders, as well as news reports and links to local support groups and county services in the Stanford, California, area.

**Stanley Center for the Innovative Treatment of Bipolar Disorder**
www.wpic.pitt.edu/stanley/

Located at the Western Psychiatric Institute and Clinic, part of the University of Pittsburgh Medical Center, the Stanley Center "is a research center whose goals are to increase our knowledge about and understanding of bipolar disorder (manic depression) and to promote the development of comprehensive and innovative treatments for bipolar disorder."

**Systematic Treatment Enhancement Program for Bipolar Disorder (STEP-BD)**
www.stepbd.org/
866-240-3250

STEP-BD is a 5-year project that will study approximately 5,000 volunteers with bipolar disorder. The website calls it "the largest treatment study ever conducted for bipolar disorder." Its goal is to find out which are the most effective treatments for treating episodes of mania or depression and for preventing future episodes.

## Online Resources

**bipolar.about.com**

This is About.com's comprehensive look at just about everything you need to know about bipolar disorder, from links to lists to forums for discussion with your peers. There's information on medications, your legal rights, substance abuse, and even articles on adopting a child if you have bipolar disorder.

**directory.google.com/Top/Health/Mental_Health/Disorders/ Mood/Bipolar_Disorder**

Google's awesome and sometimes overwhelming list of websites that talk about bipolar disorder.

**dmoz.org/Health/Mental_Health/Disorders/Mood/ Bipolar_Disorder**

The Open Directory Project's bipolar disorder link list.

**medwebplus.com/subject/Bipolar_Disorder**

MedWeb provides free searches of health and sciences information for both layperson and professional alike.

**www.athealth.com**

At Health offers mental health information and services for both providers and patients. The site includes treatment center and mental-health practitioner directories, as well as a comprehensive discussion of bipolar disorder and a bipolar disorder FAQ.

**www.bipolar.com**

This site is full of information about the disorder, as well as a mood questionnaire. The site is put together and run by Glaxo-SmithKline, the pharmaceutical company that makes Lamictal (lamotrigine). Still, the site itself makes absolutely no mention of any specific drug treatments and does have useful information.

**www.bipolarchild.com**

Based on Dimitri Papolos's book, *The Bipolar Child,* this website also includes links, a FAQ, a sample IEP (Individual Education Plan), and information on subscribing to a free newsletter.

**www.bipolarworld.net**

Bipolar World is an online educational resource for people with bipolar disorder and "the friends and families who care for them." There are "ask the psychologist" columns, a bipolar spectrum diagnostic scale, a chat room, and more. As the site proclaims, "We have walked many miles in your moccasins and truly understand the need for understanding."

**www.electroboy.com**

Andy Behrman's personal website provides information on mania and depression, informative links, a FAQ, a mania quiz, and information on Andy's book, *Electroboy: A Memoir of Mania* (Random House, 2003).

**www.healthcyclopedia.com/mental-health/disorders/mood/ bipolar-disorder.html**

Healthcyclopedia calls itself "the complete guide to health care resources on the internet." This is their list of relevant links for people interested in bipolar disorder.

**www.maramcwilliams.com**

Mara is an artist, poet, author, and mother who writes about living with bipolar disorder on this website filled with colorful, energetic, and disturbing pieces of art. She also provides links to a variety of other websites.

**www.medscape.com**

Medscape requires registration before viewing much of its contents, but it's free and worth the effort. Although the range of information on the site is aimed primarily at clinicians, it's incredible and well worth a look. Specifically go to www.medscape.com/pages/ editorial/resourcecenters/public/bipolardisorder/rc-bipolardisorder.ov or click on Psychiatry and Mental Health under the specialty homepage listing.

**www.mentalhealth.com/dis/p20-md02.html**

The Internet Mental Health site's extremely comprehensive list of links are presented in unique and extremely useful tables of information about the disorder.

**www.mental-health-matters.com/articles/print.php?artID=550**

Shay Villere put together this free, online booklet on living with bipolar disorder simply to help others who need it. As he notes on his site's home page: "I'm just a guy that has what bipolar patients need most—answers."

**www.mental-health-matters.com/research/bipolar.php**

Another site that's chock-full of links to information on bipolar disorder. Mental-Health-Matters.com provides "information and resources for consumers, professionals, students and supporters."

**www.mentalhelp.net**

Mental Help Net is a free service that "seeks to advance the state of online health communications." The Mental Help Net has a therapist search engine and an entire topic section devoted to bipolar disorder, including a mania questionnaire, lists of symptoms and treatments, bipolar news updates, and links to other resources on the web.

**www.mhsanctuary.com/bipolar**

The Mental Health Sanctuary offers a therapist locator, dozens upon dozens of links, chat rooms, bulletin boards, even a recently added list of mental-health related blogs. The bipolar section of the Sanctuary also includes articles on self-care and articles written by people living with the disorder.

**www.neurotransmitter.net/bipolar.html**

Links abstracts from medical journals on almost any topic you can think of relating to neurology and bipolar disorder.

**www.nlm.nih.gov/medlineplus/bipolardisorder.html**

A comprehensive listing of links courtesy of the National Institutes of Health and the National Library of Medicine.

**www.patientcenters.com/bipolar**

Although the Patient-Centered Guides' Bipolar Disorders Center is actually aimed at parents of a child or adolescent with bipolar disorder, this site has a huge amount of information applicable throughout the life span. The site is chock full of excerpts from the bipolar disorders guide, as well as links to resources on almost any topic imaginable.

**www.pendulum.org**

Pendulum Resources is the web presence of the Pendulum e-mail list, an online bipolar disorder support group. This site includes links, writings from people with bipolar disorder, and plenty of information on how to get support if and when you need it.

**www.psycom.net/depression.central.bipolar.html**

A list of links regarding bipolar disorder that is maintained by psychiatrist Ivan Goldberg, M.D.

# Index

# E

# F

## Q-R

# T

## U

ultradian cycling, 299-300
unconditional support, 325
unemployment, 268-269
unipolar depression, 4
University of Milan School
of Medicine, connection
between sleep loss and
mania, 142
Unmet Needs in Diagnosis and
Treatment of Mood Disorders
in Children and Adolescents
(Consensus Statement), 303
*An Unquiet Mind: A Memoir of
Moods and Madness,* 228
unspecified bipolar episode, 30
Usenet/News groups, 244

## V

valproate (Depakote), 107,
111-113
valproic acid. *See* valproate
venlafaxine (antidepressant),
124
violence (manic episodes), 226
vitamins, 172

## W

Weiss, Roger, M.D., Alcohol
and Drug Abuse Program, 217
Western Psychiatric Institute
and Clinic, 105
WHO (World Health
Organization), 214
Winds of Change Bipolar
Disorder Support group, 245
Winokur, George, M.D.,
"Alcoholism in Bipolar
Disorder," 204

Wong, Grace, Coping Inventory
for Prodromes of Mania, 186
workplace, 253-269
accommodations, 264-265
dealing with cognitive
demands, 265-267
finding and keeping a job,
262-264
management, 269
revealing illness, 257-262
stigma of mental illness,
254-257
World Health Organization.
*See* WHO
Wylie, Mary, 41

## X–Y–Z

Yonkers, Kimberly, M.D., drug
risks in pregnancy, 286
Young Mania Rating Scale, 301
young onset, 38-39

*zeitgebers* (biological pacemakers), 140
ziprasidone, 122-123
Zis, Anthanosios, 144

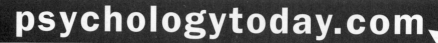
# psychologytoday.com

## You want to talk to someone ...
### but how do you find the right person?

# FIND A THERAPIST
PROFILES | SPECIALTIES | PHOTOS | FIND THE THERAPIST WHO SUITS YOU

* **Review profiles, photos and fees**

* **Explore therapists' specialties, in their own words**

* **Thousands of professionals listed**